D1231857

SPORTS MEDICINE
for the PRIMARY
CARE PHYSICIAN

SPORTS MEDICINE
for the PRIMARY
CARE PHYSICIAN

WITHDRAWN

Editor

Richard B. Birrer, M.D., M.P.H., F.A.A.F.P.

Assistant Professor, Family Medicine
Clinical Instructor, Internal Medicine
State University of New York
Downstate Medical Center and
　Kings County Hospital; and
Director of Academic Affairs
Associate Director of the
　Family Practice Residency Program
Department of Family Medicine
Downstate Medical Center
Former Director of Medical Services
East New York Neighborhood Family Care Center
Brooklyn, New York

 APPLETON-CENTURY-CROFTS/Norwalk, Connecticut

0-8385-8651-1

Copyright © 1984 by Appleton-Century-Crofts
A Publishing Division of Prentice-Hall, Inc.

84 85 86 87 88 89 / 10 9 8 7 6 5 4 3 2 1

Prentice-Hall International, Inc., London
Prentice-Hall of Australia, Pty. Ltd., Sydney
Prentice-Hall Canada, Inc.
Prentice-Hall of India Private Limited, New Delhi
Prentice-Hall of Japan, Inc., Tokyo
Prentice-Hall of Southeast Asia (Pte.) Ltd., Singapore
Whitehall Books Ltd., Wellington, New Zealand
Editora Prentice-Hall do Brasil Ltda., Rio de Janeiro

Library of Congress Cataloging in Publication Data

Main entry under title:

Sports medicine for the primary care physician.

  Bibliography: p.
  Includes index.
  1. Sports medicine.   I. Birrer, Richard B.   [DNLM:
1. Sports medicine.   QT 260 S77045]
RC1210.S73   1984   617'.1027   83-11870
ISBN 0-8385-8651-1

Design: Lynn Luchetti

*To our wives, families, and friends,
who supported us during our writing
endeavors*

Contributors

Eleanor H. Bell, R.D.
Chief Nutritionist
Baltimore Multiple Risk Intervention Trial
Baltimore, Maryland

Burton L. Berson, M.D., F.A.C.S.
Associate Clinical Professor of Orthopedics
Mount Sinai School of Medicine; and
Associate Attending in Orthopedics
Chief, Sports Medicine Section
Mount Sinai Hospital
New York, New York

Emidio A. Bianco, M.D., J.D.
Associate Professor of Family Medicine
University of Maryland School of Medicine
Baltimore, Maryland; and
Chief, Division of Medical/Legal Education
Department of Legal Medicine
Armed Forces Institute of Pathology
Washington, D.C.

Richard B. Birrer, M.D., M.P.H., F.A.A.F.P.
Assistant Professor, Family Medicine
Clinical Instructor, Internal Medicine
State University of New York
Downstate Medical Center and
    Kings County Hospital; and
Director of Academic Affairs
Associate Director of the
    Family Practice Residency Program
Department of Family Medicine
Downstate Medical Center
Former Director of Medical Services
East New York Neighborhood
    Family Care Center
Brooklyn, New York

Joel R. Bonamo, M.D.
Attending, Orthopedic Surgery
Staten Island Hospital
Staten Island, New York

J. David Busby, M.D.
Director, Family Practice Program
Area Health Education Center; and
Associate Professor of Family and Community
    Medicine
University of Arkansas for Medical Sciences
Fort Smith, Arkansas

Stuart Cherney, M.D.
Fellow, Cincinatti Sports Medicine & Institute
Cincinatti, Ohio
Former Resident, Orthopaedics
Mount Sinai Hospital, New York, New York

Ruben S. Cooper, M.D., F.A.A.P., F.A.C.C.
Assistant Professor of Pediatrics
Division of Pediatric Cardiology
State University of New York
Downstate Medical Center; and
Physician in Charge, Diagnostic Cardiology
Brookdale Hospital Medical Center
Brooklyn, New York

Daniel Garfinkel, M.D.
Assistant Professor of Family Medicine
University of North Carolina
Chapel Hill, North Carolina; and
Associate Director, Family Practice Program
Moses Cone Memorial Hospital; and
Team Physician
Greensboro Hornets
Greensboro, North Carolina

Peter M. Hartmann, M.D.
Clinical Associate Professor of Family Medicine
Co-Director, Sports Medicine and Fitness Center
University of Maryland School of Medicine
Baltimore, Maryland

Maynard A. Howe, Ph.D.
Assistant Director
Graduate School of Clinical Psychology
United States International University
San Diego, California

I. Martin Levy, M.D.
Assistant Professor of Orthopaedic Surgery
Albert Einstein College of Medicine; and
Assistant Attending Orthopaedic Surgeon
Montefiore Medical Center
Bronx, New York; and
Visiting Scientist (Research Division)
The Hospital for Special Surgery
New York, New York

James T. Marron, M.D.
Assistant Professor of Family Medicine
State University of New York
Upstate Medical Center; and
Attending Physician
St. Joseph's Hospital Family Practice Residency
Syracuse, New York

Bruce C. Ogilvie, Ph.D., F.A.C.S.M.
Professor Emeritus, Department of Psychology
San Jose State University
San Jose, California; and
Director, Graduate Program in Sport Psychology
United States International University
San Diego, California

Franklin E. Payne, Jr., M.D., F.A.A.F.P.
Associate Professor of Family Medicine
Medical College of Georgia
Augusta, Georgia

Douglas W. Pollack, P.T., M.A.
Founder and Director
Marathon Physical Therapy Center
Manhasset, New York

John P. Reilly, M.D.
Resident, Orthopedic Surgery
Lenox Hill Hospital
New York, New York

Andrew B. Rohen
Clinical Instructor, Division of Cardiology
Downstate Medical Center and
   Kings County Hospital
Brooklyn, New York

Mark F. Sherman, M.D.
Director of Sports Medicine
St. Vincent's Hospital
New York, New York; and
Attending, Orthopedic Surgery
Staten Island Hospital
Staten Island, New York

Richard A. Stein, M.D.
Associate Professor of Cardiology
Director of Heart Exercise Laboratory
State University of New York
Downstate Medical Center
Brooklyn, New York

James B. Tucker, M.D.
Associate Professor of Family Medicine
State University of New York
Upstate Medical Center; and
Attending Physician
St. Joseph's Hospital Family Practice Residency
Syracuse, New York

M. William Voss, M.D., F.A.A.F.P., F.C.C.P.
Associate Professor
Department of Family Medicine
University of Maryland School of Medicine
Baltimore, Maryland

Elmer J. Walker, M.Ed., J.D.
Former Vice Principal
Baltimore County High School System
   of Maryland
Baltimore, Maryland

Contents

Preface

And is not bodily habit spoiled by rest and idleness but preserved for a long time by motion and exercise?
(Plato, Theaetetus)

Exercise, in the natural form of work, was a necessary and regular part of life before the Industrial Age. With the advent of work-saving machinery, people turned more and more to the "sedentary studious life."* Despite the clairvoyant exhortations of some of our nation's political leaders (Thomas Jefferson and Benjamin Franklin) and the world's medical giants (George Cheyne and Joseph Addison) the "pamper'd Race of Men" prospered.† Only during the past several decades has the temper of the times pointed to the benefits of regular exercise. Serendipity played a significant role in the observations that physically active individuals did not suffer proportionately from atherosclerosis, strokes, myocardial infarctions, and other chronically debilitating diseases as did their sedentary counterparts. Rudimentary exercise research began to yield the secret successes of regular fitness training. The general socio-cultural swing back to naturalism, homeopathy, holism, and self-help has embraced exercise and sports activities as a necessary component, and has once again brought us full cycle to our ancestors' philosophies.

Science naturally holds hands with cultural evolution. It is not suprising, therefore, that a great need has arisen to elucidate the fitness profile and to care for the active athlete. Because the world of

---
Cheyne G: Letter to Samuel Richardson, April 20, 1740.
†Dryden J: To John Driden of Chesterton, in Fables Ancient and Modern. c1680.

sports encompasses all ages, both genders, as well as the entire health spectrum, it is fitting that the primary care physician should be the front-line sports medicine specialist. It is this physician who first sees the injured athlete at home, on the field, or in the office. Very often it will be he or she who recognizes the family or personal problem affecting an individual's performance. Above all, it is the primary care physician who is best suited to integrate an athlete's work, sport, family, and school environments, so that maximum exercise potential under the safest health conditions can be realized.

This text sprang from these conceptual roots and the unique opportunity that I had as Chief Resident to sit on the Society of Teachers of Family Medicine Sports Medicine Panel in 1980. It was this Panel, its Chairman, Daniel Garfinkel, M.D., and invigorating members who designed the sports medicine curriculum for the family practice programs of this country. It seemed to me at the time that the assembled resources should also direct their energies into passing on their enthusiasm and expertise to the graduates and grandfathers of primary care. Over the past three years we have labored toward this goal. As the youngest of the group, I take credit only for providing the necessary catalyst; my knowledge of sports medicine comes from the teachers and consultants who wrote these chapters. It is to each of them that I give my sincerest thanks and praise for a job well done. It is my hope that the reader will profit as much as I have.

Acknowledgments

Illustrations...R. Jeffrey Alexander and Shelley Eshleman

Suggestions and assistance
in preparation of Chapter 30 .... Sheena D. Benjamin   Department of Legal
Medicine, Armed Forces Institute of Pathol-
ogy, Washington, D.C.

Careful and diligent review of
Chapter 19 ....Teresita A. Laude, M.D.   Assistant Direc-
tor, Children's Receiving Ward; and Assistant
Professor, Pediatrics, State University of New
York, Downstate Medical Center and Kings
County Hospital, Brooklyn, New York

Careful and diligent review of
Chapters 14 to 18 ....Shephard H. Splain, D.O.   Physician in
Charge of Sports Medicine, Brookdale Hos-
pital Medical Center, Brooklyn, New York;
and Assistant Clinical Professor, Department
of Surgery, Orthopedics, New York College
of Osteopathic Medicine, New York, New York

Typing assistance .... Jo Ella Douglas, Roberta Hilbert, Odessa
M. Jones, Dianne Rabon, and Kathleen M.
Tucci

SPORTS MEDICINE
for the PRIMARY
CARE PHYSICIAN

1

The History of Sports Medicine*

HISTORICAL PERSPECTIVES

The history of sports and recreational medicine is nearly as long as the history of medicine itself. Although ancient Babylonian, Egyptian, and Chinese medical texts make no explicit reference to the treatment of sports-related injuries, it is likely that ancient physicians treated injured runners, boxers, chariot drivers, wrestlers, and archers as well as their more sedentary contemporaries. *The Edwin Smith Surgical Papyrus,* an Egyptian surgical treatise dating to the Old Kingdom (ca. 2600 to 2200 BC), prescribes prudent treatment for a variety of sprains, dislocations, and fractures.[1] Many of the injuries described could well have resulted from sports-related trauma.

The earliest recorded Panhellenic Olympic competition was held in 776 BC, but the Games apparently began much earlier. Homer wrote that until the eighth century the Games were merely local fairs held in temple precincts. According to Paul and Moran,[2] after these humble beginnings:

> The Olympic Games became the greatest festival of a mighty nation. Once every four years trading was suspended, the continuously warring states and fighting tribes laid down their arms, and all of Greece went forth in peace to watch the Games, pay tribute to the nation's manhood and honor its gods.[2]

Prepared by the Information Management Department of Franklin Research Center, a division of The Franklin Institute, Philadelphia, Pa. 19103 and The Institute of Sports Medicine and Athletic Trauma at Lenox Hill Hospital, 130 East 77th Street, New York, N.Y. 10021.

Athletes in ancient Greece were required to train under medical supervision for 10 months before participating in the Olympic Games, held every 4 years. The athletes' physicians, called *gymnastes,* not only were responsible for the physical conditioning of their charges, but also took an interest in their dietary regimens and overall health. Apparently, the theoretical consensus among ancient Greek sports medicine practitioners was no better than it is among modern counterparts. For example, Ryan and Allman[3] discuss Philostratus, who, writing in the third century AD, had sharp words for his fellow sport physicians:

> He describes the rigorous training of athletes of a former day who ate a Spartan diet, slept on animal skins spread on the ground and bathed in cold mountain streams. He contrasted this with the practices of his own day, in which a more clear-cut separation had occurred between the physicians and the trainers. He blames the physicians for overstuffing the athletes, for encouraging them to eat fish, for failing to develop the endurance of the athletes, and for not enforcing more rigorous training.[3]

Galen of Pergamon, practicing in Rome in the second century AD, compiled an impressive research record of anatomy, physiology, physical therapy, and biomechanics while treating gladiators in the public circuses. Galen's patients seem to have been more fortunate in his treatment than in his opinion of them, however. Ryan and Allman[3] use the following example from Galen's writings:

1

Athletes live a life quite contrary to the precepts of hygiene, and I regard their mode of living as far more favorable to illness than to health. They lose their eyes and their teeth, and their limbs are strained. Even their vaunted strength is useless. They dig and plow but they cannot fight. . . . It is easy to discover they are always in debt. While athletes are following their profession their body remains in a dangerous condition, but when they give up their profession they fall into a condition more parlous still; as a fact, some die shortly afterwards; others live for some little time but do not arrive at old age.[3]

Galen's insight that exercise is necessary for the maintenance of health was recognized and put into practice by medieval and renaissance successors such as Avicenna, Maimonides, Mercuriale, and Cagnatus. In the fourteenth century, Vittorino da Feltre established the training of physicians as part of the educational curriculum at a school for children of the court founded by the Marquis Gonzaga of Mantua.

Throughout the sixteenth to nineteenth centuries, research in physiology and biomechanics was carried out by such scientists as Hieronymus Fabricius, Aquapedente, and Ulisse Aldrovandi. The importance of exercise in improving and maintaining health was continually reemphasized.

Ryan and Allman[3] discuss the weakening of the centuries-old bond between exercise and sports medicine during the 1880s, when an interest in physical training became more a military than a medical preoccupation:

Modern physical education, apart from therapeutic exercise and no longer under medical direction, was developed by the work of Jahn in Prussia, Ling in Sweden, Nachtegall in Copenhagen, Clias in Berne and Amoros in Paris. Exercise continued to be a mainstay of physical therapy since there were relatively few specifics that were effective in spite of the enormous empiric pharmacopeia.[3]

But the late nineteenth through early twentieth centuries saw the publication of what is perhaps the first English language treatise on sports medicine[4] and the first comprehensive treatment of the subject of sports medicine.[5] In 1913 an international conference on sports and exercise physiology was held,

but the work of this group was interrupted by World War I.

Appropriately, the revival of the Olympic Games in the nineteenth century also revived, and has helped sustain, the interest in sports medicine so integral to the ancient Greek Olympic Games played 2000 years ago. However, Ryan and Allman[3] suggest that medical support for the early Games seems to have been indifferent, if not sometimes dangerous:

At the Games in St. Louis in 1904, the air temperature in the shade was 104 degrees and the humidity very high. Only 14 of the 27 starters finished the race. The winner, T.J. Hicks of Cambridge, Massachusetts, was treated during the race by a physician who followed him in a car and gave him several injections of strychnine as well as eggs and brandy by mouth. Suffering from severe heat exhaustion, probably aggravated by the treatment given him during the race, he required the services of four physicians who treated him in a nearby gymnasium after the race.[3]

In 1928, 33 physicians met at the Second Olympic Winter Games held at St. Moritz to plan for the establishment of the International Congress of Sports Medicine at the August Olympics and to create a permanent International Assembly on Sports Medicine. In 1933, this organization became the Federation International Medico-Sportive (FIMS), meeting every 4 years at the Olympic Games. The International Congress also continued to meet every 2 years. The operation of both organizations was suspended during World War II, but surviving members of the Federation reconvened in Brussels in 1947. The plenary assembly of the Federation currently meets every 4 years; the Board of Representatives meets every 2 years.

RELEVANT ORGANIZATIONS AND THEIR VIEWPOINTS

Important international sports medicine groups in addition to FIMS are the UNESCO International Council of Sport and Physical Education, established in 1960; the International Committee for the Standardization of Physical Fitness Testing, established in 1964; the Conseil International du Sport Militaire, established in 1948; the Groupement Latin de Medicine Physique et Sport, established in 1961; and the South American Congress on Sports Medicine, established in 1953. Other more specialized international organizations include the International Symposia on Problems of Competition at Moderate Altitudes, the International Symposia on Underwater Medicine, the International Seminars on the History of Physical Education and Sport, the International Seminars on the History of Physical Education and Sport, the International Association of Ski Traumatology and Winter Sports Medicine, the International Meetings of the Hygiene of Sports Installations, and the Medical Commission of the Association Internationale Boxe Amateur.

The creation of sports medicine committees on the international level has proceeded simultaneously with the development of sports medicine organizations on the national level in the United States. One of the earliest such organizations established in the United States was the National Athletic Trainers Association (NATA). Ryan and Allman state that NATA was created in 1949 for "the advancement, encouragement, and improvement of the athletic training profession in all of its phases."[3]

In 1954, the American College of Sports Medicine (ACSM) was founded as a multidisciplinary professional and scientific society organized to encourage research on the health aspects, responses, and motivations of those involved in sports. The ACSM established the journal *Medicine and Science in Sport* in 1969 and in 1971 began publication of the *Encyclopedia of Sport Science and Medicine*.

The year 1954 also saw the appointment by the American Medical Association (AMA) of an ad hoc Committee on Injuries in Sports. This group subsequently became the Committee on the Medical Aspects of Sports. In 1964 a Committee on Exercise and Physical Fitness was also appointed by the AMA.

The President's Council on Youth and Fitness was established by President Eisenhower in 1956, reorganized under President Kennedy, and renamed the President's Council on Physical Fitness and Sport under President Johnson. More recently, federal interest in physical fitness and sports medicine has been reflected in the passage of Public Law 95-626,

which establishes the Office of Physical Fitness and Sport Medicine, and Public Law 95-606, The Amateur Sports Act of 1978.

In 1962, the American Academy of Orthopedic Surgeons established the Committee on Sports Medicine. Other important groups in the field of sport medicine and physical fitness are the American Association for Health, Physical Education and Recreation, the American College Health Association, and the Women's Sports Foundation. Many states and cities have established councils on physical fitness as well.

International and national concern with sports medicine and physical fitness, great as it has been, has been surpassed by the interest of the American public in exercise, health, and sports. Steadily accumulating scientific evidence that systematic, prudent exercise programs promote health and wellbeing—and the extensive promulgation of this information by organizations such as the President's Council on Physical Fitness and Sport—have prompted an unprecedented number of Americans to undertake physical exercise programs, despite the lack of readily available guidelines for sensibly pursuing fitness regimens. Responsible advertising suggests that adults consult a physician before beginning an exercise program; however, few primary care physicians are better informed than their patients regarding the benefits and risks of exercise.

In 1962, the Parke-Davis Company conducted a survey of 3753 American physicians. Although 96 percent of respondents agreed that moderate, controlled exercise is beneficial, most physicians were unable to define physical fitness or how best to attain it. According to Burke and Hultgren,[6] more recent research has yielded similar findings:

A study conducted in 1973 by the Opinion Research Corporation and sponsored by the President's Council on Physical Fitness and Sport showed that physicians, when asked, are among the most enthusiastic advocates of proper exercise as a form of preventive medicine and health care. However, many doctors apparently do not feel they know enough about exercise to prescribe it for their patients. The survey indicated that four of every five Americans have been told to exercise. . . . According to survey results, when physicians do prescribe exercise, their instructions tend to be rather mild and general in nature. Due to the growing body of literature concerning the effects of exercise and in particular that which deals with the topic of prescribed medicine, these findings are discouraging.[6]

Burke and Hultgren[6] also suggest one plausible reason for the primary care physician's hesitancy to prescribe exercise programs. These investigators report the following results from a survey designed to assess the importance of understanding exercise physiology in the current medical school curriculum:

A tabulation of the results indicates that in the majority of our medical schools, very little time, an average of about four hours, usually in conjunction with the medical physiology course, is spent studying the effects of exercise.[6]

Despite the lack of publicly available information on a rational approach to exercise programs, public participation in rigorous, unsupervised sports and recreational activities has continued at a high level. The expanding number of recreational athletes has resulted in concomitant increases in sports-related injuries.

REFERENCES

1. Breasted JH: The Edwin Smith Surgical Papyrus, vols 1 and 2. Chicago, University of Chicago Press, 1930.
2. Paul CR Jr, Moran RM: The Olympic Games. United States Olympic Committee, 1979.
3. Ryan AJ, Allman FL: Sports Medicine. New York, Academic Press, 1974.
4. Byles JB, Osborn S: In Peck H, Aflalo PE (eds): The Encyclopedia of Sport. New York, Putnam, 1898.
5. Weissbeing S: Hygiene des Sport. Leipzig, Greuthlein, 1910.
6. Burke EJ, Hultgren PB: Will physicians of the future be able to prescribe exercise? J Med Ed 50(6):624–626, 1975.

2
The Role of the Team Physician

Daniel Garfinkel

Sports medicine for a local grammar school, high school, or college is a natural extension of a primary care physician's practice.[1] More than 20,000 physicians now serve as team physicians or medical consultants for teams or school systems. It is estimated that 80 percent of those physicians serving in this capacity are primary care physicians. Sports is a ubiquitous feature of twentieth-century society and has proliferated in American society during the 1970s. Although many sports are biased toward individual achievement of excellence, most youngsters and adolescents gain formal exposure through scholastic programs and the concept of team or team-based sports. It is in this area of organized team sports that the role of primary care physician as sports team physician is most fully developed.

THE SPORTS-TEAM FAMILY

It is helpful to anyone serving or planning to serve as team physician to view the sports team metaphorically as a family.[2] In this mobile, heterogeneous, and changing industrial society, the sports team represents a valid surrogate family, that is, a family within families. The 1979 Pittsburgh Pirate World Championship Baseball Team proudly announced itself as "The Family." The structure of most athletic organizations generates a strong emotional base; therefore, the prototypical roles of the nuclear family appear time and again. The primary care physician's role is a natural complement to the organization. For example, again in a metaphoric sense, it might be helpful to view the manager or coach as a father or other authority figure. The trainer typically plays the role of a nurturant mother, and the assistant coaches play the role of big brothers or big sisters. Team members represent siblings, and ancillary personnel and cheerleaders can be considered the extended family. Putting the team in this perspective is helpful in two ways: (1) it facilitates an understanding of the emotional and organizational relationships among team members, and (2) it provides a working perspective for the physician. Since the team is viewed as a family, the ideal person to oversee the health needs of the team is the primary care physician. It must be kept in mind that the team physician will play a vitally influential role in the sports community and will be expected to provide not only physical aid, but also philosophical and psychological counseling to young athletes who may be concerned about poor sports performance, schoolwork, and the opposite sex. It is not necessary for a team physician to be an orthopedist, because the comprehensive, continuous care provided by the primary care physician makes him or her uniquely qualified.

One study has estimated that on a high school football team roster of 40 to 50 players, 1 or 2 of the athletes will manifest symptoms of nervous breakdown during the season, and another 12 to 15 could benefit observably from some type of counseling.[3] The etiology of these problems is not completely clear, but probably originates as the outcome of a constellation of factors including type of sports activity involved, insufficient ability to compete successfully, lack of aggressiveness, parental pressures, fear of injury, or inability to tolerate the upheaval of success as well as failure. The pressures attending competitive athletics merely exacerbate personality problems already extant in development. Some definable personality types such as hypochondriasis, obsession–compulsion, perfectionism, hyperaggressiveness, overdependence, or a combination thereof might be overrepresented among athletes with problems.[4] It is entirely possible that some problems emergent among young athletes are characterized as normal variants of adolescence under the stimulus of undefinable success, failure, or intolerable ambiguity.

As the practitioner becomes involved with an athletic program as team physician, a very subtle process takes place. The team physician becomes familiar with the personnel in the program and practice environment. He or she sees the peer group in the locker room, at practice, on the game field, and in the contexts of victory and defeat. Over time, this growing familiarity makes it easy for the team physician to relate to these young men and women, perhaps better than any other nonpeer adult. Usually, the physician will encounter team members in their own environment rather than in the confines of a medical office. At first this situation can be uncomfortable for the physician, but it might be the only way in which, with time, to surmount the professional barrier often misunderstood and resented in this age group. It is important for the physician to realize that when an athlete presents for consultations, there might be other problems behind what appears to be a trivial symptom. Under the right conditions, which for the student athlete include respect and privacy, a short systems-psychological review can elucidate any underlying problems. Counseling sessions can then be held either on a short term or more lengthy basis. In most instances involving high school athletes, short-term counseling is all that has been necessary, with psychiatric consultations being warranted only rarely. It is most important to be a good listener in these encounters and to be concerned about the athlete as a total person.

Illnesses are a major concern of the team physician. Usually the primary care physician is attuned to adolescent illnesses, since he or she is involved with the medical care of this age group. Few illnesses will be beyond the scope of the primary care physician, and consultation will rarely have to be sought. The team physician should have a good knowledge of those illnesses that are contagious and should quickly remove an athlete with such an illness from the surroundings, to prevent the entire team from becoming infected. Ensuring that simple hygienic measures are taken to prevent contamination is a major responsibility of the team physician. Herpes gladiatorium is a simple example of how one infected wrestler can contaminate the rest of the team.

Caring for a person's health from infancy to adulthood makes it much easier to relate to the ill teenager. Adolescents have infrequent need of a physician, but when they do make a rare visit, they like it to be on a very close one-to-one basis. Generally, parents should not be present in the examining room, thus making for easier dialogue between the adolescent and the physician. Confidentiality is also important; permission from each athlete should be obtained via signature by the team physician. The athlete should be questioned to determine whether other problems are present when minor symptoms are the major complaint. Teenagers readily respond to a team physician with whom they are familiar, and such areas as sexuality, parent problems, and venereal disease can easily be discussed.

Because of the status enjoyed by the team physician in the community and in the school, there is usually a standing invitation to become involved with the coaching staff and school officials. Such situations present an opportunity to offer helpful advice in many areas of concern, beyond the immediate treatment of injuries. The primary care physician can intervene to make sure that sports activities and examinations do not conflict, help in the care of those athletes who are chronically anxious and depressed, and allay the anxiety of athletes who are acutely stressed before a game or meet. For those athletes who are unusually depressed after a loss or similar disappointment, the familiar presence of the team physician can go a long way toward alleviating the symptoms by simple reassurance and a warm "pat on the back." The team physician is also the first to be called when team members have behavioral or disciplinary problems and is in an ideal position to deliver the appropriate family counseling.

Other useful functions that the primary care physician as team physician can serve are in the areas of preventive health and guidance. The team physician should assess the degree of physical activity of team members. The choice of safe playing conditions, advice concerning specific dangers in certain sports, and aid in establishing adaptive physical education programs fall within the jurisdiction of the team physician. As a school physician, he or she will be asked to consult with a poorly performing athlete who has chosen the wrong sport. The physician should write out a complete exercise prescription, based on the clinical exam, clearly detailing the range of sports suitable for the young athlete, as well as the degree of participation allowable.

The sports team physician should be a qualified, licensed person who has good standing in the community. He or she must have time to devote to a grammar school, high school, or college program, and should be interested in its development. The sports team physician should have a thorough knowledge of sports medicine and should be interested in sports and young people. In addition, the final authority to determine the physical and mental illness of the athlete should rest with the team physician. This unique ability must be understood by the school officials. The team physician should have a complete medical history of all the athletes. Before the season (opening of practice sessions) the team physician should evaluate the health of all athletes and review the history and physical examinations completed by other physicians. The team physician should personally check any positive findings that might be related to athletic performance.[5]

The sports team physician is responsible for the health and safety of the persons participating in sports activities during the game and on the practice field. Although traditionally attending only the local seasonal games, the physician should try to attend practice sessions and "away" events as much as possible. Contact sports such as rugby, lacrosse, and soccer would benefit from a physician in attendance or on call. Considerable data have been accumulated to indicate that most injuries occur during practice, and support the importance of a good communication system that would allow the physician to render care during practice sessions. The team physician should assess the first-aid knowledge of coaches and trainers of the team and should see that they are supplementing current training or correcting any deficits in their knowledge. They should be certified in cardiopulmonary resuscitation (CPR), and their renewals should be up to date.[6]

THE DAY-TO-DAY CONCERNS OF THE TEAM PHYSICIAN

The team physician assumes the responsibility for the complete history, physical examination, and, when indicated, laboratory examination for each player.[7] This role varies in different communities. In some communities group examinations are done. These are mentioned only in passing and should be deplored. Another method is by station, whereby a team concept is employed, and a doctor along with nurses, coaches, trainers, and student managers accept "stations" and perform the necessary parts of the examination. The most efficient and humane way is for each athlete to have his or her own primary care physician do a *sports-specific examination*. This involves the completion of the necessary form by the physician, who should conduct a thorough examination with particular emphasis on the part of the body that will be involved in that particular sport, such as the entire muscular skeletal system in football, basketball, and lacrosse, and feet and knees in runners. Yearly examinations are not only unnecessary, they are not cost effective; millions of man-hours and dollars are wasted yearly on this outmoded form of physical examination.[8] However, a thorough history and physical examination should be done upon entrance to school and should be repeated if a student becomes ill or if performance declines without obvious cause. Coaches should be taught to do yearly performance tests of speed, endurance, flexibility, strength, and agility.[9]

Rehabilitation is an area in which the primary care physician must be extremely well versed (Chapter 22). As is well known, returning a player to activity before complete healing of an injury is unjustified and can lead to complications and unfortunate circumstances. The team physician, as well as the coach and trainer, must understand all aspects of stretching and flexibility.[10] The sports team physician must know about the many forms of progressive resistance training that are used, including Nautilus, Hydragym, Universal, concentric and eccentric methods, and free weights. The physician must know how to improvise rehabilitation techniques for schools that cannot afford the more expensive equipment. The team physician must involve the trainers, student trainers, and coaches in learning and improving their rehabilitation techniques. Such interest on the part of the team physician is an invaluable investment, since coach, trainer, and athletes will listen carefully to the physician's recommendations.[11] When rehabilitation or a training method is outside the team physician's realm, he or she should know when and how to make proper referrals, should work closely and cooperatively with orthopedists, physiatrists, and other specialists, and should keep abreast of new trends.[12]

During the hot summer months the team physician should make frequent trips to the practice sessions and consult with the coaches and trainers regarding fluids, electrolytes, and heat and humidity problems. Preventive medicine can be practiced at this time. Although most coaches are now well aware of frequent water replacement and the hazards of salt tablets, reminders might be necessary. In addition, the team physician should oversee equipment fitting, particularly headgear and shoulder pads. Athletes with previous head injuries must be carefully monitored for recurrent neurologic symptoms or signs during helmet fittings.[13]

Adolescents are motivated to improve their performance by all possible means and will appreciate discussing rest and nutrition with their team physician (Chapter 11). The team physician may help prevent faddism and superstitions about food by stressing the absence of scientific justification for food supplements, megadoses of vitamins, or high-protein diets. Balanced diets sometimes up to 5000 to 6000 calories should be drawn from the four main food groups of protein, cereals, fruits, and vegetables. "Junk foods" are a favorite of young adolescents, and a word from the team physician about proper diet might discourage their ingestion. When consulted about the pregame meal, the team physician should stress that energy is derived from glycogen, which is usually stored in the liver and muscles in advance of a contest or lengthy practice. Thus, the present thinking is that food consumed 48 hours before a contest should be high in carbohydrates, such as bread, cereals, pancakes, potatoes, rice, and spaghetti. Nevertheless, the physician should bear in mind that most young athletes eat what they want and when they want.[14]

As one who has gained the athlete's trust, the team physician must continually give advice about drug use. Studies have shown that drug use among young athletes is lower as compared with use among nonathletes. The team physician must explain to the young athlete that vitamins and mineral supplements are both expensive and unnecessary, with the exception of iron supplements for menstruating females. The youngster should be assured that a well-balanced diet will provide essential nutrients. Much study has been done on the effects of anabolic steroids. It has been shown that anabolic agents increase muscle mass when accompanied by a vigorous conditioning program and a high-caloric diet; however, no agreement has been reached as to whether strength, endurance, or athletic performance is improved, and the side effects make routine use of the drug contraindicated. Such effects include acne, voice deepening, hirsutism, breast enlargement, premature arrest of growth, decrease in testicular size, and oligospermia. Several cases of hepatocellular neoplasms have also been reported in connection with the use of anabolic steroids.

Psychomotor stimulants such as amphetamines and other diet pills are sympathomimetics and produce effects resembling stimulation of the sympathetic nervous system. Users experience increased alertness, elation, euphoria, excitement, or instability, as well as delayed onset of fatigue associated with anorexia. These effects are usually followed by depression. Tolerance may be reached, requiring more frequent use and larger amounts of the drug. Amphetamines can produce serious and life-threatening conditions by masking fatigue or causing cardiovascular collapse secondary to impaired temperature regulation. Other effects are hypertension, cardiac arrhythmias, and necrotizing angiitis. The presence of amphetamines in the bloodstream can also complicate the use of surgical anesthesia given in emergency cases, which is a possibility in contact sports.[15]

Some athletes have also resorted to faradic electromuscular stimulation and intravenous antifatigue medication, such as calcium gluconate, caffeine, or vitamin B_{15} in order to improve their athletic performance. These practices have proved not only valueless, but often harmful. At times athletes have used cocaine, marijuana, barbiturates, and local anesthetics. None of these agents has a place in sports, although it has been conservatively estimated that 70 percent of amateur athletes take some drug before competition. It is essential that the team physician be cognizant of the extent of drug misuse and abuse in this particular population.

Weight loss is another area in which the team physician will become involved, usually with wrestlers or gymnasts. Stern advice is usually necessary to keep young high school wrestlers from losing weight rapidly or excessively. Young wrestlers always feel that they will perform better in a low-weight class but in most cases cannot afford to lose the weight. One way to convince young wrestlers that they are not fat is to familiarize them with the skinfold calipers and the estimation of body fat. The critical measurement is 6 millimeters at the mid-triceps area: a rough indication of the 6 percent body fat that is a safe lower limit. If these skin folds are thicker, young athletes can safely lose weight, but not more than 9 kilograms (2 pounds) per week. Crash diets are not recommended because the weight is usually lost from muscle rather than from fat. Weight loss should be from reduced caloric intake and exercise and should be under the careful supervision of coach, trainer, and team physician.

The primary care physician as team physician should work closely with the athletic trainer. It is best for all concerned that the athletic trainer be certified by the National Athletic Trainers Association (NATA), having completed an approved curriculum or apprenticeship program. Usually, the trainer, who is also serving as a teacher in a school, should be available to all the athletic teams throughout the school year. Under the supervision of the physician, the trainer designs, coordinates, and implements the athletic training program, obtaining pertinent medical history and maintaining current injury records. The team trainer should know how to apply the necessary taping, wrapping, padding, braces, and so on, and should be able to recognize and evaluate injuries and render first aid if the physician is not present. The team trainer should make decisions regarding further participation by the ath-

TABLE 2-1. CHECKLIST FOR CONTENTS OF FIRST AID KIT

_____ Acetaminophen, antacid tablets, ammonia capsules, aspirin
_____ Adhesive tape—3.75 cm (1.5 inch) (ample supply)
_____ Elastic tape—7.5 cm (3 inch)
_____ Tape adherent
_____ Underwrap
_____ Tape remover
_____ Cotton-tipped applicators
_____ Tongue depressors
_____ Scissors—bandages and surgical
_____ Sterile gauze pads—3 × 3, 4 × 4
_____ Adhesive bandages
_____ Petroleum jelly
_____ Alcohol or equivalent
_____ Liquid soap
_____ Safety pins
_____ Thermometer
_____ Flashlight
_____ Nail clippers
_____ Tweezers
_____ Cotton
_____ Tourniquet
_____ Hemostat or tongue forceps
_____ Coins for pay telephone
_____ Saline in plastic squeeze bottle

[From Shaffer TE: So you've been asked to be a team physician. Pediatr Basics (copyright Gerber Products Company) 15(4):4–7, 1976, with permission.]

letes, making sure that athletes with significant injuries receive appropriate care. The trainer supervises the transportation of the injured athletes and at all times stays in close contact with the team physician. The trainer, under the direction of the team physician, performs treatment and rehabilitation programs. In addition, most schools have student trainers who work in conjunction with the head trainer and the team physician in all duties relating to prevention, rehabilitation, and follow-up management of athletic injuries. The student trainer is directly responsible to the head trainer; when the head trainer is absent, the student trainer contacts the team physician to see whether there are any outstanding problems. At all times, both the student trainer and the trainer should make sure that hygienic conditions in the training room are of the highest caliber.

The training room must have a separate area with controlled access that can be used for taping, injury evaluation, and treatment. Equipment (Tables 2-1 and 2-2) should be an integral part of every athletic training setup in the schools under the direction of the team physician.[16]

TABLE 2-2. MINIMUM EQUIPMENT FOR TRAINING ROOM OR LOCKER ROOM

_____ Scales
_____ Chart for recording athletes' weights
_____ Tables for examination, taping, treatments
_____ Refrigerator
_____ Whirlpool bath(s)
_____ Telephone (coins available if pay phone)
_____ Bulletin board for emergency phone numbers
_____ List of phone numbers of each athlete's parents or guardian
_____ Locked cabinet for medication
_____ Sphygmomanometer
_____ Stethoscope

[From Shaffer TE: So you've been asked to be a team physician. Pediatr Basics (copyright Gerber Products Company) 15(4):4–7, 1976, with permission.]

THE HANDLING OF TEAM INJURIES

It is of utmost importance that the team physician have an ambulance present or available for emergency situations, with arrangements made before the game time with the help of the trainer, coaches, or the opposing team's physician. In some communities the ambulance is visible; in some it is hidden from the fans in order to reduce parental apprehension; and in others, the paramedics and emergency medical technicians (EMTs) are on short call and respond readily if they are needed. Finally, the telephone numbers of ambulances, hospitals, and parents should be readily available, either in the training kit or training room. Team physicians should, at all times, let the trainer know where they are or who is covering for them. These master plans should be set up in advance.

If the team physician has difficulty remembering the players and their health history, it is advisable to have the medical records secured safely and taken along with the team so the team physician can refer to them if the need arises. In this way quicker diagnosis and treatment can be instituted.

The physician is always in charge unless absent, in which case the trainer oversees athletic supervision. While at an athletic contest, the team physician should stay in the background and not lose perspective of his or her functions. The team physician must be alert to the action on the field, since injuries can be more easily assessed if the mechanism of injury is known (Fig. 2-1). However, the physician must avoid becoming so wrapped up in the competition that he or she forgets to be available and ready to take care of the injured. The first 20 minutes after an injury constitutes the so-called "golden period," during which swelling has not yet occurred, permitting a more accurate diagnosis. Team protocol requires that only the trainer go out onto the field to assess an injury. This will help cut down on parental apprehension, especially with many transitory, minor injuries. If the physician is needed, the trainer should use a prepared signal to call the physician onto the field. Once the team physician moves out onto the playing field, the athlete becomes the physician's patient. The physician's initial responsibility involves assessing the extent of injury and deciding if, when, and how to move the player. If an injury is judged not to be critical or life threatening (Chapters 12 and 13), the player should be removed to the sidelines for further evaluation. It is unwise to determine the disposition of an athlete who is fully clothed. Usually the player will be able to walk off the field by his or her own power. However, if it appears that the player has refused needed assistance in order to impress the spectators, the physician must be forceful and insist that assistance be given to prevent a progression of injury.

Once on the sidelines, the team doctor must assess the injury rapidly. Diagnostic acumen is extremely important, and it is easier to examine the patient at the time of injury rather than after swelling has occurred. Diagnostic acumen begins with a thorough understanding of sports medicine and sports injuries and easily grows with the confidence gained through experience. Many times it will not be possible to make a complete diagnosis at the time of injury. However, the physician must attempt to keep the injury from worsening. Splints and ice are a necessity on the sideline; an easy and inexpensive means of applying ice is to keep ice cubes or shaved ice in sealed plastic bags. Team physicians should carry their own equipment unless they have easy access to the trainer's equipment.

One of the most important and often very difficult decisions a team physician must make on the sidelines is whether or not to allow an injured player to return to the game. It is not unusual for a team physician to take the helmet away from an injured or overly anxious player in order to prevent the player from returning to the game. On the other hand, it is important to allow the player to return

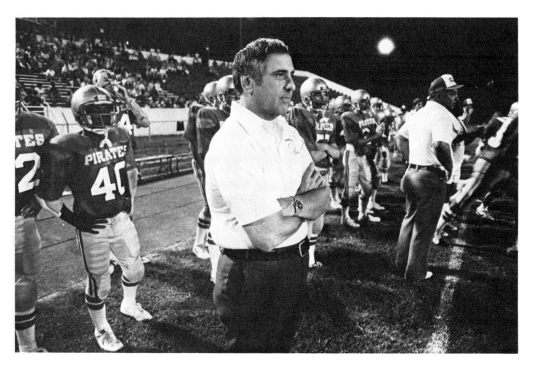

FIGURE 2-1. The alert physician is better able to assess injuries. *(Courtesy of Jim Stratford.)*

to the game as soon as possible if the injury is minor. Most coaches will accept the physician's word as final and will not pressure the physician to return their injured stars to the game. However, the team physician must be prepared to handle the rare situation quickly when the coach questions the physician's judgment. The coach must understand that the physician's word is final insofar as injuries and playability are concerned. The physician who makes an early contract with the coach and trainer will usually avoid this problem.

The team physician should always follow up on the injured athlete at halftime and after the game in the dressing room, or later in the private office, depending on the seriousness of the injury and whether the player wishes to be consulted. The day after a game, the team physician should be available to see the injured athletes. At times a phone call to the anxious athlete and the parents might be all that is necessary to allay any fears. If a serious injury occurs, the team physician should try to accompany the injured athlete to the hospital. The location of the nearest hospital and an emergency protocol (alternate coverage) must be established before the athletic event. The physician for the opposing team, if available, will then be called upon to serve both teams during the game. All concerned—parents, coaches, and players—should be advised of the location of the hospital to which an injured athlete is to be taken in order to expedite the situation and reduce anxiety. A follow-up hospital visit is appropriate.[17]

As a team physician, one must always bear in mind that one's demeanor is being witnessed by an anxious crowd of parents and spectators. The ability to act immediately and with authority helps dispel the fear that often permeates the stands after an injury.

Coaches, trainers, and athletes appreciate the continued interest by the team physician in the life of the team. This includes supportive locker room visits by the physician at pregame and halftime talks, even if an injury has not taken place. When a loss occurs, a friendly ear or a pat on the back are often reassuring to the players when the physician is doing the postgame physical check-up.[18] In addition, the team physician should check on the team as often

as is deemed necessary; this helps develop continued rapport with the young athletes. It is essential that the team doctor drop by the locker room and clubhouse to talk to players and coaches at least once a week when practice sessions are in progress.

Injuries often occur away from actual practice. Athletes might sustain injuries at home, on the way to or from school, or after hours. The team physician must understand and alert the coaches to the possible influence of these injuries on the performance of the athlete as well as on other team members. Nothing is more disturbing to the coach than to find out that a star quarterback was injured while fooling around with other teammates in the locker room and will not be able to play in the big game.

MAINTAINING BALANCE

Every effort must be made to preserve and nurture the coach/trainer–physician–athlete triad:

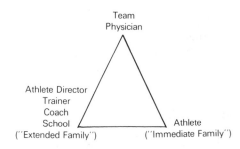

Balance is achieved by the free flow of information between each member of this triad. The team physician, within the athlete's confidence, informs the coach and trainer of any pertinent medical information. At the same time the coach/trainer informs the physician of performance problems and other sport-related difficulties. Even academic problems often need to be discussed within this triad. Equilibrium is best achieved by regular weekly meetings. Midweek is a good time for the meetings since light practice sessions prevail. In such a manner warmth and trust will pervade the team and allow for better-integrated performance of all members.

The team physician should endeavor to be available to the "team family." It is the responsibility of the team physician to make an effort to know every player on the team, and players appreciate the support. When the players sense that their physician is interested in them they become more loyal in their response, and patient compliance and treatment effectiveness are considerably enhanced. Many of these young athletes will become lifetime friends, and after graduation become loyal and responsive patients. As the team physician's relationship with the athletes grows, the breadth of problems encountered and discussed may extend far beyond the playing field and become extremely confidential. It is imperative that the team physician always bear in mind the concept of the team as "extended family," for in so doing, a unique balance will be struck between athlete and community that will provide optimal athletic performance as well as a memorable experience for the team physician.

Sports activities during the formative years help build character in young athletes, and proper input by the primary care physician can favorably enhance their appreciation of the possibilities and limitations of athletics in this and later life cycles.[19] Team physicians wield a good deal of influence and should use all their strengths for the enrichment of the athlete as well as the good of the sport.

REFERENCES

1. Garfinkel D: The family doctor as sports team physician. Fam Med Rev 1(1):91–98, 1980.
2. Garfinkel D: The family doctor as sports team physician. Part II. Fam Med Rev 1(2):37–53, 1981.
3. Cratty B: Psychological health in sport. In Straube W (ed): Psychology. New York, Movement Press Ethica, 1976, pp 209–215.
4. Missildine D: Caring for the emotions of the high school athlete. The Association 56:885, 1961.
5. Zlotsky N: The Team Physician—A Brochure for Team Physicians, Coaches and Trainers. New Haven, Conn, Medical Aspects of Sports Committee of the Connecticut State Medical Society, 1974.
6. Noble B, Bachman J: Organization and administration of a high school program. Northwestern University Center for Sports Medicine, Maui, Hawaii, March 8–15, 1981, pp 1–3.
7. Shaffer TE: The health examination for participation in sports. Pediatr Ann 7:10, 1978.
8. Ryan A: Qualifying exam: A continuing dilemma. Physician Sportsmed 8(8):3–10, 1980.
9. Shaffer TE: The adolescent athlete. Pediatr Clin North Am 20:837, 1979.
10. Anderson B: Stretching. Bolinas, Calif, Random House, Shelter Publications, 1980, p 11.
11. Shaffer TE: The young athlete—new guidlines in sports medicine. Pediatr Consult 1(5):1–8, 1980.
12. Sperryn P: Sports medicine and the student. Br Med J 1:502–507, 1977.
13. Arnold JA, Cohen T, Nelson C: Characteristics of the sports medicine practitioner. J Arkansas Med Soc 74(2):105–107, 1971.
14. Smith N: Food for Sport. Palo Alto, Calif, Bull Publishing, 1976, pp 35–38.
15. Munch L: Drugs and the athlete. In Haylock C (ed): Sports Medicine for the Athletic Female. Oradell, NJ, Elonies, 1980, pp 351–361.
16. Shaffer TE: So you've been asked to be a team physician. Pediatr Basics 15(4):4–7, 1976.
17. Hartmann D, Voss W, Welliver D: The family physician and sports medicine. J Fam Pract 8(2):383–385, 1979.
18. Goldbert G: Varying role in sports medicine. Sports Medicine for Children and Youths, Tenth Ross Round Table, San Antonio, Tex, Jan 29, 1979.
19. Damel WA Jr: Psychogenic Problems in Adolescents in Health and Disease. St Louis, CV Mosby, 1977, pp 221–233.

3
Landmarks and Surface Anatomy

I. Martin Levy

Stepping onto a playing field to evaluate an injured athlete presents a new challenge to the diagnostic skills of the physician. The arsenal of diagnostic aids that one learns to rely on are not readily available. Therefore, physical examination becomes the means by which the nature and extent of an injury are determined. Return to play or even ultimate treatment can be predicated on the impressions made during the initial examination. Often the first examination will be the most revealing, as it is accomplished without the influences of swelling, pain, and muscle spasm; it is essential that this examination be accurate and complete, lest an injured element be overlooked.

Physical examination is intimately related to structural anatomy. Nowhere is this more apparent than in the evaluation of the extremities, where most structures are available to the palpating hand, with significant insight to be gained as to their structural integrity. This section reviews topographic anatomy with special interest directed toward the anatomic basis of physical examination. The objective is to review surface landmarks so that structures can be found easily and their functional competence and structural integrity rapidly determined.

THE SHOULDER

The anterior contour of the shoulder is determined by the S-shaped clavicle and anterior border of the acromion process of the scapula (Fig. 3-1). The clavicle is subcutaneous (or more precisely subplatysmal) throughout its length, as are its medial and lateral articulations with the sternum and acromion, respectively. Because these two articulations are available to the palpating hand, disruptions are easily appreciated. After shoulder separation, the dislocation of the acromioclavicular joint, the lateral limb of the clavicle can be palpated (and seen) as it pushes up the skin overlaying the shoulder. More medially, disruptions of the sternoclavicular joint are less common and can occur in an anterior or posterior direction. Clearly, posterior displacement of the clavicle on the manubrium puts the medial end of the clavicle in a precarious position in regard to the underlying great vessels and trachea. Fractures of the clavicle are not uncommon and are easily appreciated because of alterations in clavicular contour as well as palpable discontinuity.

The smooth lateral contour of the shoulder results from the deltoid muscle mass as it originates from the distal clavicle, acromion process, and scapular spine. Lying deep to the acromion are the tendons of insertion of the short rotators of the shoulder, the supraspinatus, infraspinatus, and teres minor. Separating the rotator tendons from the overlying acromion arch is the subacromial bursa.

The spine of the scapula and the posterior third of the deltoid and trapezius muscles combine to form the posterior contour of the shoulder. The spine extends from the medial border of the scapula to within one fingerbreadth of the glenoid fossa laterally. The scapula has three angles (superior,

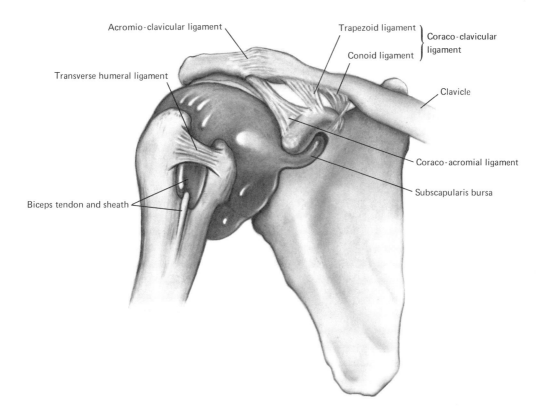

FIGURE 3-1. Bony and ligamentous landmarks of the shoulder. *(Adapted from Anderson JE: Grant's Atlas of Anatomy, ed 7. Baltimore, Williams & Wilkins, 1978, fig 6-43.)*

lateral, and inferior) and three borders (superior, medial, and lateral). The vertebral edge is readily palpated just to the side of the spinal gutter. The lateral border becomes more apparent with the elbow flexed and the arm internally rotated.

The coracoid process is a beak of bone emanating from the anterior scapula and lies below the clavicle inferomedial to the acromion under the cover of the anterior fibers of the deltoid. The coracoid is readily palpated in the relaxed patient and serves as a superficial landmark to the glenohumeral joint, which lies inferior and lateral to its base.

The humeral head sits in the shallow glenoid fossa and is surrounded by the musculotendinous insertions of the rotator cuff—subscapularis anteriorly, supraspinatus superiorly, and infraspinatus

and teres minor posteriorly. The anterior aspect of the humeral head can be palpated, albeit indistinctly, underneath the anterior fibers of the deltoid. With the arm abducted, the inferior glenoid cavity as well as the humeral head can be felt in the axilla. With the arm at the side, internal rotation will permit one to feel the greater tuberosity as it moves from under the acromion. The anterior and posterior surfaces of the humeral head can be grasped in the relaxed patient, and its position in regard to the glenoid cavity as well as its stability within the joint can be evaluated by gentle anterior and posterior displacement of the head with the arm in varying degrees of flexion, abduction, and rotation.

The anterior axillary fold is formed primarily by the pectoralis major and to a lesser extent by the pectoralis minor muscles. Subscapularis, teres major, and latisimus dorsi collectively make up the posterior wall.

The axillary artery is the extension of the subclavian artery as the latter courses over the first rib. Its pulsations can be felt just proximal to the middle third of the clavicle. The vein lies medial to the artery but does not enter the neck. The brachial plexus surrounds the artery as both travel to the arm. The axillary artery is palpable high in the axilla. The cords of the brachial plexus can again be felt surrounding the artery.

THE ELBOW

The elbow articulation permits flexion–extension and pronation–supination of the forearm on the arm. To accomplish these motions and maintain stability of the upper extremity as well as allow significant motion necessitates significant structural demands. The distal humerus widens and flattens distally into medial and lateral supracondylar ridges, which continue more distally into medial and lateral epicondyles (Fig. 3-2). The medial and lateral epicondyles are important landmarks and serve as the origin of the wrist extensor muscle group laterally and wrist flexor group of muscles medially. The ulnar nerve courses posterior, and inferior to the medial epicondyle on its way to the forearm. The tip of the olecranon and the medial and lateral epicondyles form a straight line in the normal, extended elbow. In the flexed elbow, the three points form an isosceles triangle with the apex of the triangle at the olecranon. The humerus articulates with the head of the radius and proximal ulna at the capitellum and trochlea of the humerus, respectively.

Anteriorly, the cubital fossa is a triangular space lying distal to the elbow crease, bounded by the extensor muscles laterally and the flexor muscles medially. The inferior boundary is created by the intersection of the brachioradialis (laterally) and the pronator teres (medially). The median nerve travels medially to the brachial artery as both pass through the fossa.

The radial head is easily palpated at the hu-

meroradial articulation; its movement is appreciated as one pronates and supinates the forearm. In the flexed arm the radial head lies inferior and anterior to the lateral epicondyle. The olecranon lies medial to the radial head. Posteriorly it is largely subcutaneous. The triceps tendon can be palpated as it inserts into the olecranon tip.

The common tendon of the extensor muscle group of the forearm originates in the lateral epicondyle. Taking origin from the epicondyle are the extensor carpi radialis brevis, extensor digitorium, extensor digiti minimi, extensor carpi ulnaris, and anconeus. From the medial epicondyle another common tendon of origin gives rise to the flexor carpi radialis, the palmaris longus, and part of the flexor carpi ulnaris and pronator teres.

THE WRIST AND HAND

Distally, the radius widens out into a flat, triangular end to form most of the proximal wrist articulation. Dorsally, the radial tubercle of Lister is easily palpated at the center of the distal radius. It serves as a pulley for the extensor pollicis longus tendon, which passes medially, on its way to the thumb. The distal, lateral tip of the radius is the radial styloid into which the brachioradialis inserts. Distal and dorsal to the styloid is the "snuffbox" of the wrist, bounded radially by the abductor pollicis longus and extensor pollicis brevis and ulnarward and dorsally by the extensor pollicis longus.

The tubular ulna narrows to form the ulnar head and styloid. The ulna is separated from the carpus by an articular disc but articulates with the distal radius. The styloid of the ulna is easily palpated medially. A deep groove is palpable on the posteromedial aspect of the ulna head, which serves as a channel for the tendon of the extensor carpi ulnaris.

The volar wrist crease is a constant landmark for the location of the proximal carpal row (Fig. 3-3). One can appreciate the tuberosity of the scaphoid distal and radial to the wrist crease and just proximal to the bulk of the thenar eminence. Medial to the scaphoid, at the ulnar limit of the wrist crease, the

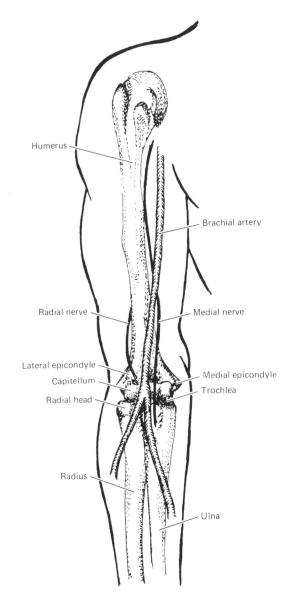

Humerus

Brachial artery

Radial nerve — Medial nerve

Lateral epicondyle
Capitellum — Medial epicondyle
Radial head — Trochlea

Radius

Ulna

FIGURE 3-2. Anterior aspect of the elbow.

pisiform can be palpated. Distal to the pisiform, beneath the hypothenar fat pad, lies the hook of the hamate.

The thenar crease is the medial border of the thenar eminence. The eminence derives its bulk

from the three thenar muscles: the abductor pollicis brevis, the flexor pollicis brevis, and the opponens pollicis.

When present, the palmaris longus tendon is visible volarly in the middle of the wrist as it courses

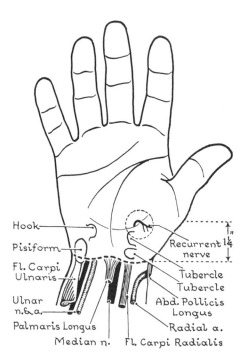

Hook

Pisiform

Fl. Carpi Ulnaris

Ulnar n.&a.

Palmaris Longus

Median n.

Recurrent 1¼ nerve

Tubercle

Tubercle

Abd. Pollicis Longus

Radial a.

Fl. Carpi Radialis

FIGURE 3-3. Suface landmarks of the anterior wrist. *(Reprinted from Basmajian JV: Grant's Method of Anatomy by Regions Descriptive and Deductive, ed 10, p 367. Copyright 1980, The Williams & Wilkins Company. Reproduced by permission)*

to the hand and inserts into the palmar fascia. The tendon is a landmark for the median nerve almost directly underneath, just slightly to the radial side. The radial artery is palpable at the lateral limit of the wrist on its way to the aforementioned "snuffbox."

On the dorsum of the hand, the metacarpal shafts can be palpated for their entire lengths from base to head. The carpometacarpal articulations are smooth and regular, so that disruptions are easily appreciated. Similarly, the metacarpal heads can be evaluated and their camlike contour palpated directly.

The metacarpophalangeal joints are covered only by the extensor retinaculum posteriorly, permitting evaluation of the continuity of the joint as

well as its stability. It is the motion of the metacarpophalangeal joint that results in the distal palmar crease on the volar surface.

The flexor tendons make their way to the fingers through the palm, being well protected by the palmar skin. Two flexor tendons to each finger pass out of the palm into the fibrous digital sheath of each finger. The digital vessels and nerves lie on both sides of each pair of flexor tendons at the base of the digits. More distally, the neurovascular bundles lie between septa stretching from the phalanges to the skin approximately at the dorsal limit of the digital skin creases.

THE HIP

The lower extremity is joined to the pelvis at the hip joint. The round femoral head is well seated into the acetabular socket and held in place by a strong capsule. The confinement of the head restricts range of motion of the hip.

The contour of the buttock results from the gluteus muscle mass and overlying fat (posteriorly). Laterally the hip abductors and vastus lateralis contribute to the shape of the thigh. The landmarks of the hip region are most easily appreciated around the pelvis. The iliac crests are lateral, running from anterior to posterior (Fig. 3-4). Anteriorly they end abruptly at the anterior superior iliac spine and posteriorly at the posterior superior iliac spine. The inguinal ligament courses from the anterior superior iliac spine, terminating at the pubic tubercle. The pulse of the femoral artery can be palpated as it passes under the ligament on its way to the thigh. The vein lies medial and the nerve lateral to the artery.

Laterally, a handsbreadth below the iliac crest, the bony prominence of the greater trochanter can be felt. Internal and external rotation of the hip confirms its position. The buttock has a fold posteriorly, deep to which the ischial tuberosity can be palpated. A bursa separates the tuberosity from the skin. Coursing midway between the greater trochanter laterally and the ischial tuberosity medially is the sciatic nerve.

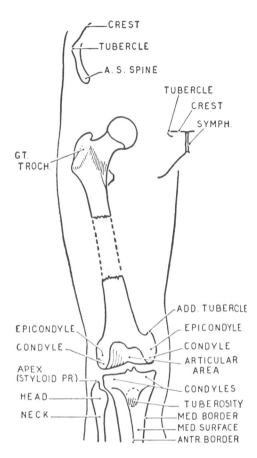

CREST
TUBERCLE
A. S. SPINE
TUBERCLE
CREST
SYMPH.
GT. TROCH.
EPICONDYLE
CONDYLE
APEX (STYLOID PR)
HEAD
NECK
ADD. TUBERCLE
EPICONDYLE
CONDYLE
ARTICULAR AREA
CONDYLES
TUBEROSITY
MED. BORDER
MED. SURFACE
ANTR. BORDER

FIGURE 3-4. Bony landmarks of the thigh. *(Reprinted from Basmajian JV: Grant's Method of Anatomy by Regions Descriptive and Deductive, ed 10, p 246, Copyright 1980, The Williams & Wilkins Company. Reproduced by permission.)*

THE KNEE

Flexion of the leg on the thigh is accomplished by the knee joint. Bony architecture, muscular motors, ligament restraints, and meniscal components act in concert to provide stability for the joint during activity. The thin layer of soft tissue covering the knee permits a very clear insight into the structural integrity of the supporting elements.

Because knee joint contour reflects underlying structure, careful scrutiny can be rewarding. From the front, the patella is seen seated between the medial and lateral femoral condyles, in the femoral groove. It is enveloped by the condensation of the four tendons of the quadriceps muscle mass and is anchored firmly into the tubercle of the tibia by the patellar tendon. The quadriceps group is sensitive to alterations in normal knee function and responds with a rapid loss of muscle girth. Measurement of thigh circumference 10 centimeters (4 inches) above the patella in the relaxed, extended knee can give the examiner a recordable means of evaluating muscle girth.

On both sides of the kneecap are two depressions, one situated inferior to the vastus medialis and one inferior to the vastus lateralis. Absence of the hollows could indicate underlying articular effusion. A ballottable patella might indicate the same. The borders of the hollows are the tibial plateau inferiorly, the patella and its tendon centrally, and the femoral condyles medially and laterally. Just superior to the tibial plateau are the meniscal cartilages. Although the cartilages cannot be palpated directly, inferences of meniscal irritation can be gained when the palpating finger elicits pain.

The medial collateral ligament is a well-defined condensation of collagen, but its limits are not easily palpated (Fig. 3-5). Therefore, in order to evaluate the integrity of this structure, knowledge of its anatomic position as well as its stabilizing function is essential. It has a broad origin on the medial femoral condyle inferior to the adductor tubercle. Its fibers extend distally, inserting broadly well below the level of the tibial plateau into the medial shaft. Palpation of the course of the ligament can provoke pain indicating the site of injury or disruption. Structural competence is evaluated by stress-testing the ligament in 30 degrees of knee flexion. Abduction of a joint that causes widening of the joint line in excess of the normal side can indicate sprain or total disruption. The postero-medial aspect of the knee joint is strengthened by the complex insertion of the semimembranosus. Passing over the insertion of the semimembranosus are the tendons of the pes anserinus: the sartorius,

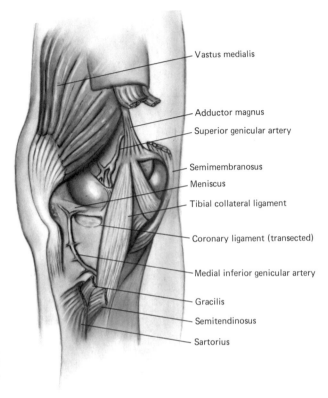

Vastus medialis

Adductor magnus

Superior genicular artery

Semimembranosus

Meniscus

Tibial collateral ligament

Coronary ligament (transected)

Medial inferior genicular artery

Gracilis

Semitendinosus

Sartorius

FIGURE 3-5. Medial aspect of the knee. *(Adapted from Anderson JE: Grant's Atlas of Anatomy, ed 7. Baltimore, Williams & Wilkins, 1978, fig 4–65.)*

gracilis, and semitendinosus. These tendons create a ridge from the medial aspect of the thigh that extends to their insertion on the proximal tibia.

Lateral stability of the knee joint is aided by the well-delineated lateral collateral ligament (Fig. 3-6). It extends from the lateral femoral condyle to the fibula head and is easily located when the leg is placed in the figure 4 position. The fascia lata of the thigh thickens into the iliotibial band, extending across the lateral joint line and inserting in the lateral tibia at the tubercle of Gerdy. The tendon of the biceps femoris forms a ridge along the posterolateral aspect of the knee as it makes its way to the fibular head. The peroneal nerve courses around the fibular head laterally, where it can be palpated as it emerges from underneath.

Posteriorly the medial and lateral hamstrings

form a quadrangular space with the two heads of the gastrocnemius. Through this space pass the tibial and peroneal nerves, the popliteal artery, and the popliteal vein, on their way to the lower leg. The floor of the fossa is formed by the capsule of the knee joint, and the roof by the deep fascia of the leg.

THE ANKLE AND FOOT

Few sports are exempt from injuries to and around the ankle joint. The frequency of injury is great and the implications of early and accurate diagnosis important. Evaluation might necessitate differentiation between fracture and sprain, making familiarity with landmarks imperative.

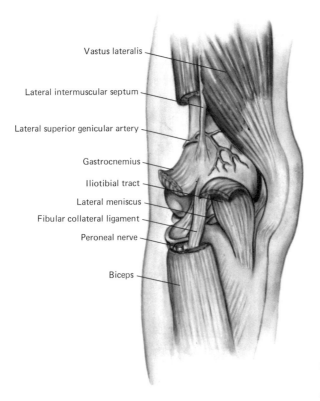

Vastus lateralis

Lateral intermuscular septum

Lateral superior genicular artery

Gastrocnemius

Iliotibial tract

Lateral meniscus

Fibular collateral ligament

Peroneal nerve

Biceps

FIGURE 3-6. Lateral aspect of the knee. *(Adapted from Anderson JE: Grant's Atlas of Anatomy, ed 7. Baltimore, Williams & Wilkins, 1978, fig 4–63.)*

The skin overlying the distal tibia and fibula is closely adherent, separated from bone only by a thin layer of subcutaneous fat. Distally, the tibia flares out medially, to become the medial malleolus. The malleolus extends farther anteriorly than posteriorly and acts as the medial buttress for the talus. Laterally the fibula widens to form the lateral malleolus. It extends farther distally and is set more posteriorly than its medial counterpart, acting as the lateral buttress to the talus. Ankle stability results in a large part, from the bony architecture of the malleoli. Even so, strong ligament supports participate in maintaining the talotibial articulation.

The deltoid ligament is a strong group of collagen bundles extending from the medial malleolus to the talus, calcaneus, and tarsal navicular bone (Fig. 3-7). On the lateral side, three distinct ligament bundles participate in the joint-stabilizing function (Fig. 3-8). The anterior talofibular ligament extends almost horizontally from fibula to talus and is the most commonly injured. Early examination of the injured ankle can permit differentiation between a sprain of the anterior talofibular ligament and fracture of the fibula. The calcaneofibular ligament extends from the fibula to the calcaneus. The posterior talofibular extends from the posterior aspect of the lateral malleolus to the posterior talus.

The tendons controlling foot and ankle orientation hug the underlying bone closely and are held in place by fascial retinacula anteriorly, medially, and laterally. Anteriorly, the tendons of extensor hallucis longus, extensor digitorum longus, and tibialis anterior pass beneath the inferior extensor retinaculum, with the tendon of tibialis an-

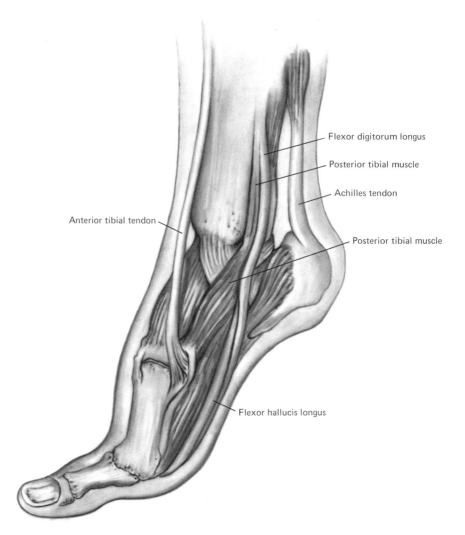

Flexor digitorum longus

Posterior tibial muscle

Achilles tendon

Posterior tibial muscle

Anterior tibial tendon

Flexor hallucis longus

FIGURE 3-7. Landmarks of the medial foot. *(Adapted from Anderson JE: Grant's Atlas of Anatomy, ed 7. Baltimore, Williams & Wilkins, 1978, fig 4–98.)*

terior most medial and that of the extensor digitorum longus most lateral. The dorsalis pedis pulse lies between the extensor digitorum and the extensor hallucis longus.

Behind the medial malleolus pass the tendons

of the tibialis posterior, flexor digitorum longus, and flexor hallucis longus muscles (Fig. 3-7). At the level of the malleolus the tibialis posterior is most anterior and the flexor hallucis longus most posterior. Situated between the flexor digitorum

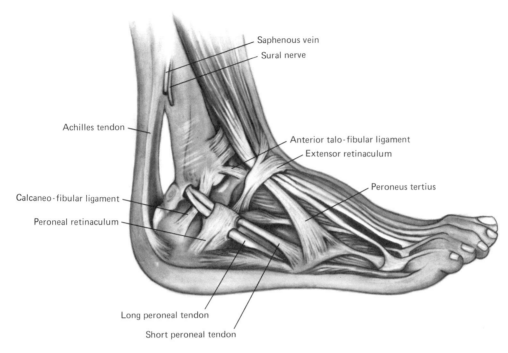

Saphenous vein
Sural nerve
Achilles tendon
Anterior talo-fibular ligament
Extensor retinaculum
Peroneus tertius
Calcaneo-fibular ligament
Peroneal retinaculum
Long peroneal tendon
Short peroneal tendon

FIGURE 3-8. Landmarks of the lateral foot. *(Adapted from Anderson JE: Grant's Atlas of Anatomy, ed 7. Baltimore, Williams & Wilkins, 1978, fig 4–78.)*

longus tendon and the flexor hallucis longus are the posterior tibial artery and the tibial nerve.

Lying just posterior to the lateral malleolus are the tendons of the peroneus longus and brevis: the brevis anterior and longus posterior. Occasionally the superior peroneal retinaculum, which restrains the peroneal tendons behind the lateral malleolus, is disrupted, allowing dislocation of the tendons to a more anterior position.

Posteriorly, the tendon Achilles is formed by the merger of the tendons from the gastrocnemius and soleus muscles. The tendon can be palpated to its insertion in the posterior surface of the calcaneus. If acutely ruptured, a gap is readily palpated in this normally well-defined structure.

Distally, the fibula articulates with the tibia at the inferior tibiofibular syndesmosis. Although the

syndesmosis is covered by soft tissue, widening after diastasis can sometimes be appreciated. Plantar flexion of the foot uncovers the talar dome from the overhanging distal articular surface.

The complexity of the architecture of the foot rivals that of the hand. Multiple joints act in concert to permit adequate foot contact on a variety of geographic contours. The foot is roughly divided into hindfoot, midfoot, and forefoot.

The talus and calcaneus combine to form the hindfoot. The calcaneus transmits the force from the foot to the leg through the talus. It projects posteriorly and inferiorly and forms much of the heel. It is covered by the thick, weight-bearing fat pad of the heel. The plantar aponeurosis is a fascial band that originates in the tubercle of the calcaneus, extends forward as a narrow band broadening distally, and inserts at the bases of the proximal phalanges in the forefoot into the fibrous tendon sheaths and deep transverse metatarsal ligaments. Often osteophytes form at the origin of the plantar aponeurosis. These "heel spurs" are commonly asymptomatic but are sometimes painful, with the site of maximal tenderness just anterior and medial to the tuberosity of the calcaneus.

The bones of the midfoot—the navicular, the three cuneiform, and the cuboid—are readily palpated dorsally. The skin of the plantar surface is thick, and together with the musculature prevents palpation of the deeper neurovasculature structures.

The bases of the metatarsals articulate with the midfoot, and their position is readily evaluated dorsally. The metatarsal heads of the five toes can be palpated on the plantar surface more distally. No one head should be more prominent than another.

THE HEAD AND NECK

Contact and injury are not limited to the extremities. The head and neck are not infrequently burdened by significant stresses that result in injury.

From the front, the most obvious landmarks of the head are the ears, eyes, nose, and mouth. Alterations of the contour and position of those structures are apparent and readily evaluated. The eyeballs are well seated in, and protected by, the bony orbits of the skull. The superior walls of the orbits are formed by the inferior aspect of the frontal bone. The lateral walls of the orbits are formed by the zygomatic bones, which continue laterally as the zygomatic processes of the temporal bones that create the zygomatic arches. The shape and integrity of the zygomatic bone determine the contour of the overlying subcutaneous tissue and the skin of the cheek. The maxilla makes up the inferomedial margin of the orbit and continues inferiorly to form the upper jaw and part of the hard palate. Inferior to the zygomatic arch, the articular surface of the condyle of the mandible articulates with the temporal bone at the mandibular fossa. The condyle of the mandible is continuous with the neck of the mandible, which expands into the ramus of the mandible. The ramus of the mandible joins the body at

the angle of the mandible. The auricle and external auditory meatus lie posterior to the temporomandibular joint. Anterior to the external auditory meatus and below the zygomatic process of the temporal bone, the middle meningeal artery enters the skull at the foramen spinosum and runs in a groove on the inner aspect of the temporal bone. A fracture of the temporal bone can result in laceration of the middle meningeal artery, followed by hemorrhage and cerebral compression.

The contour of the nose is determined by a framework of bone and cartilage. The tip is called the apex, and its inferior aspect is occupied by the two nostrils. The septal cartilage separates the nostrils. The lateral cartilages and major and minor alar cartilages form the flexible distal lateral elements of the nose. The hard proximal contour is determined by the nasal bones centrally and by the frontal process of the maxilla laterally.

The posterior contour of the skull is formed by the union of the two parietal bones and the occipital bone at the lambdoid suture. The trapezius takes its origin from the superior nuchal line of the occipital bone, the external occipital protuberance, and the ligamentum nuchae, as well as the seventh cervical and first thoracic vertebra. It inserts into the posterior surface of the distal third of the clavicle, the medial aspect of the acromion process of the scapula, and the spine of the scapula. Anterior to the lateral borders of the trapezius, lymph nodes can be felt if they are enlarged.

More laterally and anteriorly, on both sides of the neck, the sternocleidomastoid muscles extend from the mastoid process of the temporal bone to the manubrium sterni and upper surface of the clavicle. The carotid artery enters the neck behind the sternoclavicular joint and travels in the neck under the cover of the anterior border of the sternocleidomastoid muscle. Pulsations of the bifurcating carotid artery can be palpated as it emerges from underneath the sternocleidomastoid muscle at the level of the thyroid cartilage. The thyroid cartilage is midline and lies anterior to the fourth and fifth cervical vertebrae. The thyroid gland overlies the cartilages, with the masses of the gland on either side of the midline. The first cricoid cartilage is just inferior to the thyroid cartilage and lies in front of the body of the sixth cervical vertebra. The hyoid is superior to the thyroid cartilage and lies in front of the body of the third cervical vertebra.

THE CHEST, ABDOMEN, AND BACK

Both clavicles converge toward the midline and articulate with the manubrium. The upper border of the manubrium, the suprasternal notch, is concave and thickened. The junction between the manubrium and sternum is at the level of the disc between the fourth and fifth thoracic vertebrae (Fig. 3-9). The angle formed by the junction also marks the level at which the second costal cartilage meets the sternum. Since it is difficult to feel the first rib except at its articulation with the manubrium, the

ribs are more readily counted from the second rib, as its position is reliably located. The 7th, 8th, 9th, and 10th costal cartilages join the rib above it, thereby forming the costal margin. In the male, the nipples are located laterally away from the midline, at the level of the fourth intercostal space, but this anatomic relationship is variable.

The diaphragm rises as high as the fifth rib or to the level of the eighth thoracic vertebra. The lungs, for the most part, fill both thoracic cavities, with the cupola of each protected from behind by the posterior aspect of the first rib. The apex of the heart lies behind the fifth intercostal space, approximately 8.75 centimeters (3.5 inches) to the left of the midline. The superior vena cava enters the right atrium at the level of the third costal cartilage. The aortic arch and left common carotid artery are protected in the front by the manubrium.

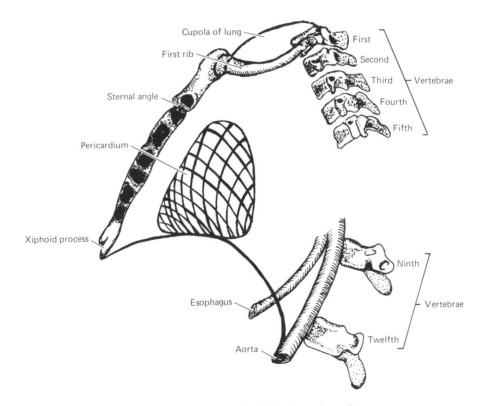

FIGURE 3-9. Landmarks of the thoracic cavity.

The rectus abdominis is attached superiorly to the xiphoid process and bordering costal cartilages, continuing distally to the pubic tubercle and pubic crest. The lateral border of the rectus abdominis extends from the pubis to the costal margin and is quite visible in a muscular person. The medial borders of both straps of the rectus are separated by the linea alba. The linea alba extends from the xiphoid process to the symphysis pubis. The umbilicus is a midline structure located at a level between the third and fourth lumbar vertebrae. Its position is inconsistent, varying with age, sex, abdominal girth, and posture.

In the normal person the spinous processes are midline from the first cervical vertebra to the sacrum. The spinous process of the second cervical vertebra can be felt just below the occiput. The spinous processes of the seventh cervical and first thoracic vertebrae are longer than those above them and are easily appreciated at the base of the neck. The remainder of the thoracic vertebrae have no characteristics that can be readily differentiated by palpation. The fourth lumbar vertebra is at the level of the most superior point of the iliac crest.

BIBLIOGRAPHY

Basmajian JV: Grant's Method of Anatomy by Regions Descriptive and Deductive, ed 10. Baltimore, Williams & Wilkins, 1980.

Hoppenfeld S: Physical Examination of the Spine and Extremities. New York, Appleton-Century-Crofts, 1976.

Snell RS: Clinical Anatomy for Medical Students. Boston, Little, Brown, 1973.

4

The Preparticipation Health Inventory

James T. Marron and James B. Tucker

SCREENING EXAMINATION

The screening physical examination for sports participation is a traditional part of any sports medicine program. Most states require medical clearance before participation at the primary or secondary school level. Likewise, all professional sports teams require some sort of screening examination to help evaluate the health qualifications of prospective athlete employees. Yet, it seems that screening per se has never been shown to reduce the incidence of injuries or prevent sudden death. The number of people who have been spared serious or life-threatening illness or injury cannot be determined from the records of these examinations. Major problems of completing a study on the effectiveness of the screening examination have been variable injury reporting systems and the low incidence of death in the young athlete population. Yet, despite the lack of compelling evidence for its effectiveness, it is very unlikely that the screening examination will be discarded.

There is much to be said for having the athlete's own primary care physician give the screening examination. Diet, nutrition, medical problems, and family and psychosocial history factors may otherwise be omitted. En masse screening examinations emphasize the episodic approach to care, whereas the athlete's physician is specifically concerned with the medical care of the athlete on a longitudinal basis. En masse screening sets minimal standards for participation and precludes a discussion of motivation of the athlete, experiences of success and failure in past athletic endeavors, and goals of the exercise or athletic program. Medical records from en masse screening programs are often unavailable or incomplete. Ideally, sports examinations should be a part of the participants' total medical record.

Despite the drawbacks, en masse screening examinations are common in this country because of their relative low cost and minimal demands on physician time. Some communities have gone to great lengths to create en masse screening programs, and certainly some type of screening is more desirable than none at all. The nature of the screening examination, whether performed in the individual physician's office or in a larger facility en masse, reflects the personal approach of the examiner, as there is considerable controversy over the content of an adequate examination.

The physician should be concerned as much with promoting the participation of athletes with chronic medical conditions as with disqualifying others because of illness or injury. This approach presupposes a working knowledge of the demands of the sports in question and of the limitations set by any illness or disability. An initial thorough preparticipation history and physical examination are strongly recommended by most authorities, particularly for the young athlete competing for the first time. Ongoing medical care for injuries and illness, as well as reexamination (including functional evaluation) before return to activity after an illness or injury that has prevented practice or game participation, are part of a comprehensive program that discourages the annual or frequent "routine" examination.

The timing of the screening examination is an important factor sometimes overlooked because of busy physicians' schedules or summer vacations. The trend is toward physical examinations for fall events performed in the spring, so that the athlete who needs rehabilitation for a fall season can spend the summer obtaining it. Similar lead time should be built into the screening examination for every sport, so that rehabilitation and conditioning programs are promoted rather than left to the last moment when pressure to play might be the most important factor in the young participant's mind.

The screening medical history is the single most important part of the athlete's health appraisal.[1] This document has even more importance when used as part of an en masse screening program, since it can lead the examiner to focus on one particular organ system even though the physician had little or no contact with the athlete before the examination. Ideally, the parents and athlete should fill out the history form, which the primary care physician should review with both parties.

The content of the health history and examination is quite variable. New York State experience indicates that markedly different examination forms are used even in adjacent school systems. These documents should include historical examination information that will screen for the conditions that might disqualify an athlete from competition. A useful tool in this decision is to separate sports into contact, endurance, and leisure classifications according to the demands of different sports. Table 4-1 exemplifies the type of classification currently in use.[1,2] The use of such a classification will help the examiner suggest alternative sports that might be more appropriate given the presence of a restricting condition, an area that requires knowledge of the sport as well as the limitations of the patient's medical condition. Table 4-2 is a guide to medical conditions that may disqualify an athlete from various sports.[3]

TABLE 4-1. SAMPLE CLASSIFICATION OF SPORTS ON THE BASIS OF PHYSICAL DEMANDS

COLLISION/CONTACT SPORTS		
Baseball	Ice hockey	Soccer
Basketball	Lacrosse	Softball
Boxing	Martial arts	Volleyball
Field hockey	Rugby	Wrestling
Football		
ENDURANCE SPORTS		
Badminton	Rowing	Tennis
Cross country	Skiing	Track and field
Fencing	Swimming	Water polo
Gymnastics	Table tennis	
LEISURE SPORTS		
Archery	Golf	Sailing
Bowling	Marksmanship	

In New York State, some school systems use an ongoing health folder as a basic history form; others have no history form and use a physical examination checklist only. The Richmond County, Georgia, en masse screening program uses the history form shown in Figure 4-1.[3] A similar document devised by Dr. Bruce Baker and used at Syracuse University (Fig. 4-2) reflects the differences in approach in two en masse screening programs. The major requirement of such a document is that it offer screening questions that will take into consideration the disqualifying conditions presented in Table 4-2. Physical examination forms should include reference to the following:

1. Snellen test for visual acuity
2. Blood pressure and pulse rate, height, and weight
3. Eyes, ears, nose, and throat examination
4. Cardiopulmonary system examination
5. Abdominal, genitalia, and hernia examination
6. Musculoskeletal system including assessment of flexibility
7. Neurologic examination
8. Assessment of sexual maturity
9. Final review of health history and judgment concerning participation, rehabilitation, and prevention

TABLE 4-2. METHOD FOR DISQUALIFYING ATHLETIC PARTICIPATION BY CONDITION

Condition	Sports Type Disqualified		
	Contact	*Endurance*	*Leisure*
HEENT			
Single eye	X		
Detached retina (even surgically corrected)	X		
Severe myopia (greater than 20/200 in one eye)	X		
Congenital glaucoma	X		
Previous radical mastoid surgery	X		
(Severe) hearing loss	?		
RESPIRATORY SYSTEM			
Active tuberculosis (does not include INH prophylaxis)	X	X	X
Asthma (poor control)	X	X	
Pulmonary insufficiency	O	O	O
Recurrent pneumothorax	X		
CARDIOVASCULAR SYSTEM			
Third-degree heart block	X	X	X
Valvular or cyanotic heart disease	X	X	?
Coarctation of aorta	X		
Recent carditis	X	X	□
Persistent patent ductus arteriosus	X	X	
History cardiac surgery	X	X	
Anomalous A-V node artery	X		
Organic hypertension	X	X	
Uncontrolled hypertension	X	X	?
(Significant) arrhythmia (e.g., atrial fibrilation; paroxysmal atrial tachycardia)	X	X	
Significant coronary artery disease	X	X	
Thromboembolic disease	X	X	
Mitral valve prolapse	O	O	O
ABDOMINAL AREA			
Hepatitis	X	X	
Enlarged liver or spleen	X	X	
Jaundice	X	X	X
GENITOURINARY SYSTEM			
Single kidney or testicle	X		
Undescended or atrophic testicle	X		
Inguinal or femoral hernia/hydrocele	X	X	
Acute nephritis/nephrotic syndrome	X	X	X
Chronic nephritis (uremia)	X	X	
MUSCULOSKELETAL SYSTEM			
Functional inadequacy (physical immaturity)	X		
Inflammatory disease (collagen-vascular)	X	X	O
Spondylolisthesis/spondylosis with pain	X		

(continued)

TABLE 4-2. (Continued)

| | Sports Type Disqualified | | |
Condition	Contact	Endurance	Leisure
NEUROLOGIC SYSTEM			
Seizure disorder (poorly controlled)	X	X	X
Brain–meningeal scarring	X		
[subdural, epidural bleeds; depressed fracture (Fx);			
hydrocephalus; "berry" aneurysm; previous craniotomy]			
OTHER PROBLEMS: HISTORY, LABORATORY FINDINGS,			
ACUTE ILLNESS, CHRONIC DISEASE			
Acute infection			
febrile	X	X	X
severe, afebrile	X	X	X
afebrile	X	X	?
Hemophilia/bleeding tendency	X		
Anemia (severe)—address etiology, gastrointestinal (GI) bleeding,	X	X	
sickle cell trait, thalassemia			
Leukemia/lymphoma	+	+	+
Other malignancy	+	+	+
Diabetes mellitus			
Poor control	X	X	
Good control[a]	O	O	
History repeated concussions	X		
Hyperthyroidism (not controlled)	X	X	
Skin	X	X	X
Boils, impetigo, herpes gladiatorum, pediculosis	X		

X = Disqualify.
? = No concensus.
O = Individualize.
☐ = Disqualify only if condition is acute.
+ = Individualize by diagnosis and phase.
[a]No restriction: Individualize sugar response to strenuous activities. *(Adapted from Lane RM: Maine code of medical qualifications for participants in interscholastic athletics. J Maine Med Assoc 60:247–254, 1969.)*

In the next section we will discuss specific disqualifying conditions.

SPECIFIC DISQUALIFYING CONDITIONS

HEENT (Head, Eyes, Ears, Nose, Throat) System

The presence of monocular vision (i.e., loss of function of one eye means lack of visual correctability to 20/80 or better) is cause for restriction from con-

tact sports. Other eye conditions, including detached retina, presence of a single eye, and congenital glaucoma (Table 4-2) should also restrict participation in contact sports. The use of eyeguards or protectors should be mandatory in certain small ball sports such as tennis, squash, handball, paddle ball, and racquetball (Chapters 14 to 20). Severe hearing loss would probably make contact sports and team sports (where response to officiating is a factor) restricted events. Many schools for the deaf field sports teams with officiating and communications adapted to the special needs of these par-

ATHLETIC HEALTH EXAMINATION RECORD

(1-4)

(Office use only)

School _____ (5-6)

| Last Name | First Name | Middle Initial | | Grade _____ (7-8) |

(9)
Age [ ] _____ Race [ ] Black [ ] White [ ] Other   Male Female
(11)   1   2   3   (12) Sex: [ ] [ ]
Date of Birth   1   2

This application to compete in interscholastic athletics is entirely voluntary on my part and is made with the understanding that I have not violated any of the eligibility rules and regulations of the State Association.

Date _____   Signature of Student _____

Parent's or Guardian's Permission & Release

I hereby give my consent for the above named student to represent his or her school in the athletic activities except those indicated on this form by the examining physician provided that such athletic activities are approved by the State Association. I also give my consent for the student to accompany the school team on any of its local or out-of-town trips. I authorize the school to obtain, through a physician of its own choice, any emergency care that may become reasonably necessary for the student in the course of such athletic activities or such travel. I also agree not to hold the school or anyone acting in its behalf responsible for any injury occurring to the above named student in the course of such athletic activities or such travel."

Typed or Printed Name of Parent or Guardian _____   Signature of Parent or Guardian _____

Address _____   Phone _____   Date _____

HEALTH HISTORY

(13-33)
1   2
(To be completed by student and/or parents)

Yes No

If yes, use the space below to explain

1. [ ][ ] Any chronic or recurrent illnesses? _____
2. [ ][ ] Any illness lasting more than a week? _____
3. [ ][ ] Any hospitalizations? _____
4. [ ][ ] Any surgery other than tonsillectomy? _____
5. [ ][ ] Any injuries requiring treatment by a physician? _____
6. [ ][ ] Presently taking any medications? _____
7. [ ][ ] Any problem with blood pressure or heart? _____
8. [ ][ ] Any dizziness, fainting, convulsions or frequent headaches? _____
9. [ ][ ] Ever been knocked out or had a concussion? _____
10. [ ][ ] Wear eyeglasses or contact lenses? _____
11. [ ][ ] Wear any dental appliance such as braces, bridge or plates? _____
12. [ ][ ] Allergic to ANY medications (aspirin, penicillin, etc.)? _____
13. [ ][ ] Any knee injury? _____
14. [ ][ ] Any knee surgery? _____
15. [ ][ ] Any ankle injury? _____
16. [ ][ ] Any history of neck injury? _____
17. [ ][ ] Any other joint sprains or dislocations (shoulder, wrist, finger, etc.)? _____
18. [ ][ ] Any broken bones (fractures)? _____
19. [ ][ ] Any organ missing other than tonsils (appendix, eye, kidney, testicle)? _____
20. [ ][ ] Any heat exhaustion or heat stroke? _____
21. [ ][ ] Any reasons why this applicant should not participate in sports? _____
Date of last known tetanus (lockjaw) shot _____

Please use this space if needed to further explain any of the above answers or to provide any additional information: _____

Richmond County Medical Society - 1980

FIGURE 4-1. The en masse history form used in Richmond County, Georgia. *(Reprinted from Seklecki RM, Miller M, Strong WB, et al: Richmond County sports medicine preparticipation physical examination program. J Med Assoc Georgia 69:221, 1980, with permission.)*

Nurse _____   Physician _____

PHYSICAL EXAMINATION:

Height _____   Weight _____

Blood Pressure _____   Pulse _____

Facial Scars _____   Teeth _____

Eyes · Lt   20/   Corrected to   20/
       Rt   20/   Corrected to   20/

Are Glasses Required for Sport Participation _____

Ears _____

Nose _____

Mouth _____

Chest _____

Lungs _____

Heart _____

Abdomen _____

Extremities _____

Reflexes _____

Spine _____

Hernia _____

Rectal _____

Urine _____

Wasserman _____

T.B. test or X-ray _____

Polio Immunization _____

Tetanus Toxoid _____

Remarks: _____
_____
_____
_____
_____

FIGURE 4-2. The en masse history form supplied by Dr. Bruce Baker and used at Syracuse University, Syracuse, New York. *(Reprinted by permission of Syracuse University, Syracuse, New York.)*

ticipants. For example, the Amateur Athletic Union (AAU) provides for the participation of deaf boxers in tournaments.

Respiratory System

Respiratory insufficiency, whether from emphysema, bronchiectasis, cystic fibrosis, or severe poorly controlled asthma, constitutes a reason for disqualification from most competitive sports. Such a decision should be individualized. Isoniazid prophylaxis does not necessarily mean that participation should be curtailed for an athlete who is otherwise fit. Recurrent pneumothorax problems probably call for restriction from endurance and contact sports.

Cardiovascular System

The cardiovascular system must be carefully evaluated regardless of the age of the athlete, with particular attention to estimating cardiac size, the adequacy of peripheral pulses, the distinction between functional and organic murmurs, and the persistence of arrhythmias after exercise (see Chapters 6 to 8). Some authorities now recommend routine exercise stress testing in the nonfit athlete starting an exercise program at age 35 or older.[4] Routine use of the cardiac stress test in asymptomatic individuals is controversial because its predictive value depends on the prevalence of coronary artery disease in the population studied.[5] Many authorities recommend its use only in the evaluation of patients with suspected ischemic heart disease.[6] Cyanotic or valvular heart disease, or both, and previous open heart surgery (exclusive of a repaired patent ductus arter-

iosus and repaired septal defect) would disqualify a candidate. In screening for hypertension, the physician should take into account the age-dependent factor affecting its variability. Tables 4-3 and 4-4 show percentiles for blood pressure measurements in the pediatric population.[7] Values above the 95th percentile should be reevaluated, and persistently elevated values should preclude participation until workup is undertaken or treatment begun. Disorders responsible for exercise-related deaths have been categorized in studies by Jokl and McMillan in 1971[8] and Maron et al. in 1980.[9] Congenital defects were the most common cause of autopsy-analyzed deaths in the under-35 age group and were responsible for deaths in many fit people. Hypertrophic cardiomyopathy was the most frequent anomaly, being present in almost one-half of autopsied cases. Anomalies of the right coronary and left main stem coronary arteries, Marfan's syndrome, and hypoplastic coronary arteries accounted for other congenital defects associated with sudden death in Maron's study.[9] Dynamic outflow tract obstruction causes a systolic ejection murmur that increases with the Valsalva maneuver as well as with rising from a squatting position. Marfan's syndrome may be suspected by body habitus, joint findings, or heart murmur. Other anomalies might be associated with the history of syncope yet have no physical examination findings to suggest their presence. Family history can be of primary importance in the evaluation of the athlete with suspected cardiomyopathy, since many with this disorder demonstrate autosomal dominant inheritance with varying degrees of penetrance. As part of the history, the

---

TABLE 4-3. GUIDELINES THAT SHOULD BE EMPLOYED WHEN OBTAINING A CONVENTIONAL OFFICE BLOOD PRESSURE

1. The patient should be supine.
2. The cuff should be at least 20 percent wider than the diameter of the arm and cover approximately two-thirds to three-quarters of the arm, as measured from the elbow to axilla.
3. The examiner should be at eye level with the manometer.
4. The meniscus of the manometer should be checked weekly for zero calibration.
5. While measuring, the rate of fall should be approximately 2 to 3 mm Hg per heartbeat.
6. Readings should be made to the nearest 2 mm Hg.

(From McMillan J, Neiburg P, Oski F. The Whole Pediatrician Catalogue, vol 1, Philadelphia, WB Saunders, 1977, p 260, with permission.)

TABLE 4-4. GUIDELINES FOR THE 95th PERCENTILE OF ACCEPTABLE BLOOD PRESSURE

Age (years)	Systolic (mm Hg)	Diastolic (mm Hg)
0–3	110	65
3–6	120	70
6–11	125	78
11–15	140	80

(From McMillan J, Neiburg P, Oski F: The Whole Pediatrician Catalogue, vol 1, Philadelphia, WB Saunders, 1977, p 260, with permission.)

athlete should be questioned as to a family history of sudden death in a young first-degree relative.

Mitral valve prolapse is now more commonly identified. The risk of sudden death from this benign disorder is remote. For cases involving frequent episodes of palpitation, dyspnea, precordial pain, or fatigue, further evaluation is indicated, since life-threatening arrhythmias occur more commonly in this group.[10] In the great majority of cases no specific treatment or precaution is necessary, with the exception of prophylaxis for endocarditis.

Abdominal Area

Hepatitis or jaundice, or both, from whatever cause, as well as liver or spleen enlargement, should preclude both endurance and contact sports. Hereditary hyperbilirubinemia, such as Gilbert's disease and rotor syndrome, are obvious exceptions.

Genitourinary System

There is little argument that athletes with congenital or surgical absence of one kidney or testicle should refrain from participating in contact sports. Chronic glomerulonephritis, chronic or recurrent nephrosis, chronic pyelonephritis, and any other condition associated with chronic renal insufficiency should preclude all but leisure sports.

Musculoskeletal System

The parameters for examining the musculoskeletal system should be concerned with pain and symptomatology on performing the exercise in question

and functional adequacy as determined by examination. Symptomatic structural abnormalities, whether acquired or congenital, should be individualized to the sport, on the basis of functional adequacy. In a research setting, the use of a Cybex isokinetic dynamometer to analyze muscle strength and detailed goniometric and anthropomorphic measurements to test joint flexibility and strength seem useful in predicting musculoskeletal adequacy for a number of different activities (Chapter 5).[11] The question of large-scale availability and usefulness of such an approach in our secondary schools requires further examination, with equipment and personnel costs a major factor. Matching athletes to the sports for which they are functionally best suited might well help minimize many of the "unavoidable" injuries of our contact sports. Specific testing of ligamentous stability of the knee and ankle joints is a minimal functional evaluation for the screening examination. Previous herniated nucleus pulposus above the L4–5 level or in the cervical area would be cause to prevent a candidate from participating in contact sports, as would spondylolisthesis, previous cervical spine fracture, or symptomatic spondylosis. The Maine Code suggests relegating candidates with joint replacement, intramedullary rods, plates, and screws, to leisure activity only, although this is also somewhat controversial and must be individualized.[3]

Neurologic System

Patients with poorly controlled seizure disorders should be limited to leisure sports. Good control is defined as seizure free for 1 year regardless of the type of seizure disorder. Those athletes with brain or meningeal scarring should not be permitted to participate in contact sports. The question of previous concussion deserves attention because of confusion surrounding its classification. The following is a simplified classification for use by the sports physician[3]: (1) A first-degree concussion is mild and results from a stunning blow and should only be associated with very transitory confusion and/or dizziness; (2) a second-degree concussion is moderate and suggests that unconsciousness has occurred with retrograde amnesia of up to 5 minutes; and (3) a third-degree concussion is severe with unconsciousness for more than 5 minutes and pro-longed retrograde amnesia. Convulsions might be a part of the picture as well. The general consensus is that three or more second- and third-degree con-cussions should exclude the candidate from contact sports, including boxing and the martial arts.

Other Problems: History, Laboratory Findings, Acute Illness, Chronic Disease

In relationship to chronic disease states such as di-abetes, arthritis, and obesity, judgments by the ex-aminer should be individualized. The total picture of the athlete, including motivation, adequacy of support systems, and level of control of the disease process, are important parameters. The athlete must be motivated to gain insight into the disease process in order to monitor the effect of the sports activity on control, particularly in the case of diabetes. This approach demands maturity on the part of the ath-lete, support and cooperation from parents, and a sensitive and flexible physician.

With chronic diseases, the restrictions are gen-erally obvious. For example, there is some concern as to whether candidates with bleeding disorders should be permitted to participate in strenuous en-durance exercises that might cause significant blood pressure elevation and thus cause the athletes to risk intracerebral bleeding. Individualization is the key to restrictions in this area.

PHYSICAL EXAMINATION FORM

The content of each examination is variable but should include sufficient detail to help the physician decide whether any disqualifying conditions are present. Figures 4-3, 4-4, and 4-5 are examples of forms used in en masse screening programs. Ob-viously, there is disagreement as to which condition should be tested for. Differences in content and emphasis are minimal, but obvious, between an examination form devised by Dr. James Garrick (Fig. 4-3)[12] and the one used in Richmond County, Georgia (Fig. 4-4) for example.[2] The form devised by Dr. Bruce Baker and used at Syracuse University includes immunization and VDRL status (Fig. 4-

5). As mentioned above, the more subtle points of the cardiac examination, such as a detailed ques-tioning about sudden death in first-degree relatives and maneuvers to bring out the characteristics of hypertrophic cardiomyopathy are missing in both examination forms. The form used by Daniel Gar-finkel (personal communication, November 30, 1980, Moses Cone Memorial Hospital, Greensboro) in North Carolina tests for stability and flexibility in various joints and includes a routine screening for hemoglobin and hematocrit. We do not know whether these procedures are cost effective. It is not sur-prising that there is neither general agreement on the content of such forms nor a consensus on the type of disqualifying conditions we should be screening for. En masse programs require that a consensus be reached on those conditions that con-stitute an absolute or relative contraindication to play before administration of the examination.

Sports medicine parallels general medicine in that it not only seeks a reliable, effective, cost-effective screening instrument, but continues to em-ploy screening because it has proved beneficial de-spite the lack of proof of its efficacy. Epidemiologic studies, such as the one on sudden death by Maron et al.,[9] should seek to answer questions on various screening efforts. The conscientious sports physi-cian needs to search for new evidence concerning the pathophysiology and epidemiology of sports-related disease.

RESPONSIBILITIES OF THE PHYSICIAN

Disqualification of an athlete from participation in sports is an undesirable task for the sports physician. It is best to focus positively on which sports an athlete is qualified for, rather than concentrating on negative pronouncements. The primary care phy-sician must take into consideration the athlete's mo-tivation within the context of any physical limita-tion. Knowing the potential hazards of participation in contact sports for the athlete who lacks a paired organ, the primary care physician should enforce restriction accordingly. In the extreme situation, the athlete with serious or terminal disease poses an

Conduct of Examination

History:

Undressed athletes are seated and each is given a history/physical form and a black pencil. The physician, nurse, or athletic trainer reads and explains each question on the history form; athletes answer on their sheets. When all the questions have been answered the black pencils should be taken away from the athletes. Athletes with *all* "No" answers on their form line up for the beginning of the examination starting with Station No. 2; athletes with *any* "Yes" answers line up at Station No. 1 to have an individual history taken.*

Station No. 1—Individual History:

All "Yes" items in general history are probed in detail adequate to determine if they constitute a risk when coupled with athletic participation.

Station No. 2—Blood Pressure:

Student trainer or manager. Right arm, sitting. *Diastolic greater than 90.*†

Station No. 3—Snellen vision:

Student trainer or manager. *Vision less than 20/40.*

Station No. 4—Skin, Mouth, Eyes:

Physician, nurse, or athletic trainer. *Pustular acne, herpes, athletes' foot, dental prostheses, severe caries, or pupil inequality.*

Station No. 5—Chest:

Physician. *Murmurs, abnormal rhythm or heart enlargement, incomplete (lung) filling, or wheezes.*

Station No. 6—Lymphatics, Abdomen, Genitalia (Males):

Physician. *Cervical or axillary adenopathy, organomegaly, penile or testicular lesions, undescended testes, or hernia.*

Station No. 7—Orthopedic (Table 1):

Physician or athletic trainer. *Asymmetry, scoliosis, swelling or deformity, decreased range of motion or strength.*

Station No. 8—Urinalysis:

Athlete picks up paper cup, goes to restroom, fills it and gives it to student trainer manager in restroom who tests urine. *Positive test on Lab-Stix.*

Station No. 9—Review:

Physician. One of the following decisions must be made and checked (on the form) for every athlete:

1. No athletic participation.
2. Limited participation (e.g., "no participation in football, hockey, etc."). Specific sports must be listed.
3. Clearance withheld (until additional tests, examination or rehabilitation is completed). Must list precise conditions to be met before clearance can be given.
4. Full, unlimited participation.

Form must then be signed and dated.

---

*One must assume that major historical items will be forgotten or ignored. Part of the purpose of the physical exam is to serve as a "quality control" for the history.

†Items in italics require physician's judgement regarding disqualification.

FIGURE 4-3. The en masse examination form devised by Dr. James G. Garrick. *(Reprinted from Garrick JG: Sports medicine. Pediatr Clin N Am 24(4):741, 1977, with permission.)*

PHYSICAL EXAMINATION

Date _____

Height ☐☐ (34-35)   Vision: Right ☐☐☐ / ☐☐☐   (60) (check one)
Weight ☐☐ (36-38)   (48-50)   (51-53)   Normal 1 ☐ without glasses
Pulse Rate ☐☐☐ (39-41)   Left ☐☐☐ / ☐☐☐   2 ☐ with glasses
                              (54-56)   (57-59)   Abnormal 3 ☐ without glasses
Blood Pressure ☐☐☐ / ☐☐☐   4 ☐ with glasses
                (42-44) (45-47)

(61-80)	Normal	Abnormal	Not Examined	Comments	Examiner	Problem Code (5-44)
1. Eyes						
2. Ears, Nose, Throat						
3. Neck (soft tissue)						
4. Mouth and Teeth						
5. Cardiovascular						
6. Chest and Lungs						
7. Abdomen						
8. Genitalia-Hernia						
9. Sexual Maturity						
10. Skin and Lymphatics						
11. Neck						
12. Spine						
13. Shoulders						
14. Arms and Hands						
15. Hips						
16. Thighs						
17. Knees						
18. Ankles						
19. Feet						
20. Neurological						

Based on this history and physical exam, the following abnormalities were found and may need treatment:

1. _____
2. _____
3. _____

RECOMMENDATIONS

1. ☐ There were no history or physical findings on this exam which would prohibit this student from participating in competitive athletics.
2. ☐ This student should have the following health problems evaluated or treated prior to participating in competitive athletics:
3. ☐ This student has health problems which would **prohibit** him or her from participating in competitive athletics.

FIGURE 4-4. The en masse examination form used in Richmond County, Georgia. *(Reprinted from Seklecki RM, Miller M, Strong WB, et al: Richmond County sports medicine preparticipation physical examination program. J Med Assoc Georgia 69:220, 1980, with permission.)*

Name _____ Date _____

Age _____ Social Security Number _____

School Address _____ Phone _____

Parents or Spouses Name _____

Home Address _____

Home Phone and Area Code _____

Home Insurance Company _____

Sport _____

Year Graduate _____ Fresh._____ Soph._____ Jr._____ Sr. _____

PERSONAL HISTORY:

Allergies _____

Asthma _____

Epilepsy _____

Fainting Spells _____

Frequent Headaches _____

Frequent Nose Bleeds _____

Heart Trouble _____

Hepatitis _____

Mental or Nervous Disorder _____

Mononucleosis _____

Rheumatic Fever _____

Any Serious Illnesses _____

_____

Any Major Operations _____

_____

Any Bone, Joint, or Muscle Problems _____

_____

FIGURE 4-5. The en masse examination form supplied by Dr. Bruce Baker and used at Syracuse University, Syracuse, New York. *(Reprinted by permission of Syracuse University, Syracuse, New York.)*

unusual dilemma. The well-publicized activities of Tim Fox, the Canadian marathoner who underwent an amputation for malignancy and subsequently developed metastasis, provides an excellent example. The motivation and desire of such people to continue to play in the face of serious pathologic processes should underscore the value that athletics have in all young peoples' lives in our society. Supporting the sports activities of terminal patients, despite the higher risks of injury that are present, represents a clear understanding by the primary care physician of these patients' value systems. The determination of whether a particular sport is appropriate for an athlete with a particular medical condition offers both the athlete and the physician an opportunity for problem solving in the finest tradition of the doctor/patient relationship.

REHABILITATION CONDITIONING

Optimal conditioning and the matching of morphologic types to particular sports can be considered the most important factors in prevention of injuries. Timing of physical examinations to facilitate optimal conditioning and rehabilitation before the sports season is an obvious but commonly overlooked factor.

Basic considerations in rehabilitation medicine stress stages of healing and return to maximal flexibility and strength (Chapter 22). The short-term goals of physiotherapy should emphasize control of pain; increase in flexibility; increase in strength, power, and endurance; and various other sports-specific goals. The underlying principle is that movement promotes the health of a joint and increases the nutrition of joint surfaces through increase in synovial fluid production. However, every new movement after the immobilization resulting from injury reactivates the pathologic processes common to injury. The liberal use of ice will help minimize recurrence of the irritation, pain, and edema after active and passive motion of the joint. The collagen in joints and sprained and strained tissue requires a certain amount of movement and stress

to be optimally laid down during the healing process. Lack of movement leads to random deposition of collagen, excessive adhesions, and even revascularization. By contrast, rehabilitation of, and supervised stress to, the injured joint will promote stretching of the capsule and adjacent muscle groups operating across it. An old medical adage is to "take care of the joints and the muscle will take care of itself."

Competitive athletes need rehabilitation for maximum performance, since they make maximum demands on the body. They should be able to run at maximum speed, stop, and reverse direction without pain. Competitive athletes should be able to run in a tight figure-of-eight without pain and then be able to perform each drill for the specific sport without pain. Only when these conditions are met can the primary care physician conscientiously permit an athlete to return to competitive sports. Recently, the use of the isokinetic dynamometer for planning and measuring the progress of joint and muscle rehabilitation has been a useful addition to the armamentarium of the trainer and physician concerned with optimal rehabilitation of the injured athlete (Chapter 22). Unfortunately, the expense and expertise required to use this particular equipment could preclude its wide-spread use, particularly in high school sports.

PREVENTIVE SPORTS MEDICINE

Primary care physicians can provide an important benefit to their patients by being aware of preventive measures in the area of sports medicine.

As many as 100,000 eye injuries occur annually during racquetball play alone in the United States. Tennis, handball, squash, and paddleball are other small ball games in which eye injury can be a significant problem. Estimates show that nearly 40 million people participate in these small ball sports.[13] Industrial safety glasses or plastic eye protectors should be strongly recommended for this group of sports enthusiasts.

Mouthguards to prevent dental injuries should be mandatory in boxing and football. Helmets are an essential protective measure for boxers, football players, and hockey players and are to be encouraged.

Wrestlers need to be cautioned about excessive weight loss, since recent articles have confirmed that performance will be impaired with the food restriction and fluid deprivation that these athletes might inflict on themselves.[14] The effects of such deprivation cannot be corrected in the few hours after weigh-in and should be discouraged. The minimal body weight for wrestlers should consist of at least 5 percent fat, and in some states wrestlers are disqualified if they cannot produce urine with a specific gravity of ≤ 1.015 at weigh-in.[15] The use of such controls will help prevent the hypovolemia and depletion of glycogen stores that characterize the deprived wrestler.

Swimming deaths are the most frequent sports-related deaths in the United States.[16] Clearly, such simple measures as determining individual ability to swim, instituting a buddy system in the water, requiring the use of life preservers while boating, and ensuring adequate knowledge of water depth, currents, and underwater obstructions will reduce the mortality in this sport. The concern of a primary care physician can reinforce the importance of prevention in reducing the high rate of mortality in this sport.

Spotters should be a mandatory part of every gymnastic program. Until the participants have reached a level of expertise that minimizes the likelihood of an accident, the use of hands-on guidance of the young gymnast is to be encouraged. Competitive events involving younger children should not penalize the participant because of the use of a spotter. The use of trampolines and minitrampolines should be prohibited. The difficulty of adequate and effective spotting for their users should preclude their use in high school athletics. This recommendation concurs with that of many national organizations, which likewise deplore the rise in serious cervical spine injuries associated with these devices.[17]

The recent increase in the participation of women in sports events should alert the primary care physician to common concerns from this group. The use of jogging bras can promote comfort and performance, particularly in larger-breasted women. Amenorrhea is becoming more prevalent as women are involved in vigorous training programs in a number of sports events. This phenomenon, common among highly trained ballerinas and noted for years, has only recently been studied in runners. Severe reduction of body fat and nulliparity are factors most highly correlated with the amenorrhea; further study will shed light on this interesting phenomenon.[18] Return of menses upon cessation of vigorous training is the rule. This knowledge will help the primary care physician counsel these women athletes effectively.

REFERENCES

1. Shaffer TE: The health examination for participation in sports. Pediatr Ann 7(10):666–675, 1978.
2. Seklecki RM, Miller M, Strong WB, et al: Richmond County sports medicine preparticipation physical examination program. J Med Assoc Georgia 69:217–221, 1980.
3. Lane RM: Maine Code of medical qualifications for participants in interscholastic athletics. J Maine Med Assoc 60:247–254, 1969.
4. Saleem DN, Isner J: Cardiac screening for athletes. Orthoped Clin North Am 11(4):687–695, 1980.
5. Weiner DA, Ryan TJ, McCable CH, et al: Correlations among history of angina pectoris, S-T segment response, and prevalence of coronary artery disease in the coronary artery surgical study (CASS). N Engl J Med 301(5):230–235, 1979.
6. McNeer IF, Margolis JR, Lee KL, et al: The role of the exercise stress test in the evaluation of the patient with ischemic heart disease. Circulation 57(1):64–70, 1978.
7. McMillan J, Neiburg P, Oski F: The Whole Pediatrician Catalog, vol 1. Philadelphia, WB Saunders, 1977, p 268.
8. Jokl E, McMillan JT: Exercise and cardiac death. J Am Med Assoc 213:1489–1491, 1970.
9. Maron BJ, Roberts WC, McAllister HA, et al: Sudden death in young athletes. Circulation 62(2):218–229, 1980.
10. deLeon AC: Mitral valve prolapse. Postgrad Med 67(1):66–77, 1980.
11. Sapega AA, Minkoff J, Nicholas JA, et al: Sport-specific performance factor profiling: Fencing as a prototype. Am J Sports Med 6(5):232–235, 1978.

12. Garrick JG: Sports medicine. Pediatr Clin North Am 24(4):737–747, 1977.
13. Vinger PF: Excerpt from talk at National Society for Prevention of Blindness, Washington, DC, Nov, 1980.
14. Torranin C, Smith DP, Byrd RJ: The effect of acute thermal dehydration and rapid rehydration on isometric and isotonic endurance. J Sports Med Phys Fitness 19:1–9, 1979.
15. Hursh LM: Food and water restriction in the wrestler. J Am Med Assoc 241:915–916, 1979.
16. Blonstein JL: Sport and medicine. Proc R Soc Med 59(3):649–652, 1966.
17. Kravitz H: Problems with the trampoline. Pediatr Ann 7(10):728–729, 1978.
18. Dale E, Gerlach DH, Willhite A: Menstrual dysfunction in distance runners 54(1):47–53, 1979.

5

The Physiology of Physical Fitness

Franklin E. Payne, Jr.

It is essential that the sports medicine physician have a basic knowledge of the physiologic parameters determining physical fitness. Common office questions such as, How can I improve my athletic performance? What exercises are appropriate for my age? What are my limitations? What exercise will improve my health? can be easily fielded and incorporated into a complete exercise prescription for the patient–athlete. Exercise can be of value on both a preventive and therapeutic basis provided the physiologic foundations are well understood. Obviously, all physicians are not yet convinced that exercise is of merit in either of these two instances. Indeed, the value of exercise is sometimes overemphasized. The explosion of research in many areas of exercise, however, is increasingly providing convincing answers. The goal of this chapter is to provide primary care physicians with a basic understanding of the physiology of exercise, specific examples of exercise programs, and their applicability to specific patients in the form of the exercise prescription.

According to a selected system of classification, several types of exercises develop physical fitness. Basically, these exercises can be divided into two types: aerobic, which require the utilization of oxygen for energy production; and anaerobic, which do not require the presence of oxygen. Synonyms for aerobic exercise include endurance or cardiopulmonary exercise, and it is much more efficient than anaerobic exercise.

The basic characteristic of aerobic exercise is that it produces only small quantities of lactic acid, which can be metabolized as it is produced. Thus, oxygen demand as determined by muscle work does not exceed oxygen supply, as reflected by cardiopulmonary and red cell parameters. Conditioned athletes can continue at high levels of aerobic exercise for hours. Surprisingly, the limiting factor(s) to the duration of such exercise are not known, and probably vary from individual to individual. Maximal aerobic uptake ($M\dot{V}O_2$ or $\dot{V}O_2$ max) is the highest oxygen uptake a person can achieve during exercise. Trained athletes are able to perform aerobically at levels up to 85 percent of this maximum.[1] Examples of aerobic exercise include running, swimming, and cross-country skiing.

Considering health alone, aerobic exercise offers the maximum benefit in terms of investment of time and energy. Western life-styles, which tend to become sedentary even before leaving school, involve less and less activity throughout life. The human body was created for motion and functions best when it is in a regular exercise program. Indeed, the marked incidence of coronary heart disease is partly attributable to the lack of such exercise.[2–4] Furthermore, aerobic exercise can positively modify many cardiovascular risk factors to varying degrees: It can decrease cholesterol and triglyceride levels, increase high-density lipoprotein (HDL), decrease blood pressure in some cases, increase glucose metabolism, improve weight control, decrease stress, improve sleep, and aid in the cessation of cigarette smoking.[5–10] Other physiologic benefits of aerobic exercise are discussed later in this chapter. Aerobic exercise will also increase a person's endurance in any sport, although the type of exercise might be unrelated to the sport. For example, running is a means of increasing endurance in tennis or boxing.

When considering aerobic exercise, one usually thinks of specific sports activities; however, four basic characteristics determine the effective aerobic nature of an exercise. The first factor, intensity, is the degree of effort required and is reflected by the heart rate and respiratory effort. The usual recommendation is 70 to 85 percent of the maximal heart rate, which is age related (Fig. 5-1).[11] If this method is chosen, the pulse must be counted within 10 seconds of the cessation of exercise because of the initial rapid deceleration of the pulse that occurs. A simple method of checking the heart rate is to place the hand over the apex of the heart, which is easily detectable because of its increased impulse during exercise. This method avoids the difficulty of locating the carotid or radial pulses and prevents any arrhythmias that might result from palpation in the vicinity of the carotid body.

Another practical method of measuring inten-

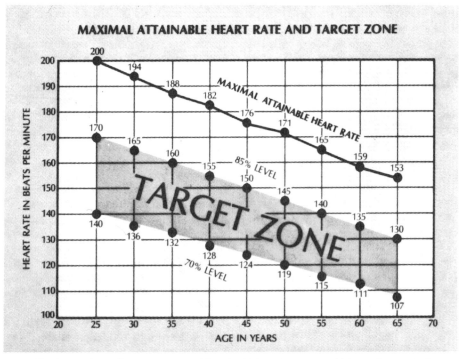

This figure shows that as we grow older, the highest heart rate which can be reached during all-out effort falls. These numerical values are "average" values for age. Note that one-third of the population may differ from these values. It is quite possible that a normal 50-year-old man may have a maximum heart rate of 195 or that a 30-year-old man might have a maximum of only 168. The same limitations apply to the 70 per cent and 85 per cent of maximum lines.

FIGURE 5-1 Maximal heart rate and target zone. *(From Beyond Diet: Exercise Your Way to Fitness and Heart Health, by L Zohman, MD, CPC International, Englewood Cliffs, New Jersey, 1974, p 15. Reprinted with permission.)*

sity can be labeled "conversational pace." This method designates an effort sufficient to produce shortness of breath, but that is limited by the ability of the person to carry on a conversation even though this might be done haltingly. Such a limitation obviously precludes breathing of a gasping nature. Research has shown that this procedure corresponds accurately to the heart rate.[12] This method continues to be effective as the athlete trains, because the intensity must be increased with conditioning.

Duration of activity is the second characteristic of aerobic exercise. Generally, the duration of activity should be at least 20 minutes. The specific activity and the intensity at which the activity is performed can lengthen this period of time. A shorter period of time or less intensity or both, will decrease the aerobic benefit. The heart and musculoskeletal system need warmup time as well as a period of slow cooling. A 5-minute period is suggested for each. Warmup time can consist of light calisthenics or stretching exercises and should not be neglected.

The third characteristic of aerobic exercise is the frequency of workouts. For the most effective results, exercise should be performed three or four times per week. It has been shown that exercising twice weekly will maintain fitness, but this does not necessarily mean that significant fitness will be developed by exercising on such a schedule.[13] An increase beyond three times per week can result in an increased number of injuries, with very little corresponding increase in fitness.[14] In fact, beyond three to four training sessions per week there is an exponential decay in fitness achieved for energy and time expended.

The final characteristic of aerobic exercise is continuity. Running and swimming are relatively constant forms of exercise as long as the person does not exceed aerobic muscle performance. Tennis and the usual approach to weight lifting, however, involve intensive bursts of activity followed by little or no activity. Aerobic development will still occur, but inefficiently, and longer durations of activity will be needed to achieve effective aerobic conditioning. Some sports, such as tennis, can be modified to approach more closely a continuous level of activity and thereby increase aerobic efficiency. With a cooperative partner, a time period

can be designated instead of games and sets. Between points, one player maintains activity by jogging in place while the other person jogs after the ball. In a similar fashion, the partners change sides of the net periodically. Such activity might sound foolish but any athlete's favorite sport could be adapted for improved aerobic fitness, rather than switching to a less enjoyable or even disliked activity. For additional information concerning the cardiovascular effects of exercise, see Chapters 6 to 8.

There are varying opinions about the optimal level of aerobic conditioning desired. Cooper has quantitated many sports activities into a point system.[15] He has also documented physiologic and biochemical changes that result from his recommendation of 30 points of exercise per week for men and 24 points for women. The $\dot{V}O_2$max according to age and sex can be determined from his 12-minute or 1.5-mile run (Tables 5-1 and 5-2). $\dot{V}O_2$max is listed as O_2 uptake (ml/kg/min). The category for the 12-minute distance test is determined by the distance that can be traveled in 12 minutes (i.e., a 0.25-mile track provides a premeasured course). The 1.5-mile test is different in that the outcome is the time required to finish a 1.5-mile course. Two disadvantages are the requirements that the course be completed (this could be difficult for an unfit person), and that the time of administration be indefinite, that is, until the last participant finishes.

Another system is determined by calories burned per week during the periods of exercise. Paffenbarger et al.[16] recommend 1800 calories per week. This level requires a greater expenditure of total energy than does the 30-point system (approximately 700 to 900 calories per week) but is more complex for each person because the program must be adjusted according to age, weight, intensity of exercise, and so forth.

ANAEROBIC EXERCISE

Anaerobic exercise involves short-duration, high-intensity activity and is far less energy efficient than aerobic exercise. At the cellular level, energy for muscle contraction occurs predominantly without

TABLE 5-1. MEN'S AEROBICS FITNESS CLASSIFICATION (PREDICTED)

Category	Measure	Age (years)					
		13–19	20–29	30–39	40–49	50–59	60 +
I. Very poor	O₂ uptake (ml/kg/min)	<35.0	<33.0	<31.5	<30.2	<26.1	<20.5
	T. M. time (min:sec)	<14:30	<12:50	<12:00	<11:00	<9:00	<5:30
	12-min. dist. (mi)	<1.30	<1.22	<1.18	<1.14	<1.03	<.87
	1.5-mile time (min:sec)	>15:31	>16:01	>16:31	>17:31	>19:01	>20:01
II. Poor	O₂ uptake (ml/kg/min)	35.0–38.3	33.0–36.4	31.5–35.4	30.2–33.5	26.1–30.9	20.5–26.0
	T. M. time (min:sec)[a]	14:30–16:44	12:50–15:29	12:00–14:59	11:00–13:29	9:00–11:29	5:30–8:49
	12-min. dist (mi)	1.30–1.37	1.22–1.31	1.18–1.30	1.14–1.24	1.03–1.16	.87–1.02
	1.5-mile time (min:sec)	12:11–15:30	14:01–16:00	14:44–16:30	15:36–17:30	17:01–19:00	19:01–20:00
III. Fair	O₂ uptake (ml/kg/min)	38.4–45.1	36.5–42.4	35.5–40.9	33.6–38.9	31.0–35.7	26.1–32.2
	T. M. time (min:sec)[a]	16:45–21:07	15:30–18:59	15:00–17:59	13:30–16:59	11:30–14:59	8:50–12:29
	12-min. dist. (mi)	1.38–1.56	1.32–1.49	1.31–1.45	1.25–1.39	1.17–1.30	1.03–1.20
	1.5-mile time (min:sec)	10:49–12:10	12:01–14:00	12:31–14:45	13:01–15:35	14:31–17:00	16:16–19:00
IV. Good	O₂ uptake (ml/kg/min)	45.2–50.9	42.5–46.4	41.0–44.9	39.0–43.7	35.8–40.9	32.2–36.4
	T. M. time (min:sec)[a]	21:08–24:44	19:00–21:59	18:00–20:59	17:00–19:59	15:00–17:59	12:30–15:44
	12-min. dist. (mi)	1.57–1.72	1.50–1.64	1.46–1.56	1.40–1.53	1.31–1.44	1.21–1.32
	1.5-mile time (min:sec)	9:41–10:48	10:46–12:00	11:01–12:30	11:31–13:00	12:31–14:30	14:00–16:15
V. Excellent	O₂ uptake (ml/kg/min)	51.0–55.9	46.5–52.4	45.0–49.4	43.8–48.0	41.0–45.3	36.5–44.2
	T. M. time (min:sec)[a]	24:45–27:47	22:00–24:59	21:00–23:59	20:00–22:59	18:00–21:14	15:45–20:37
	12-min. dist. (mi)	1.73–1.86	1.65–1.76	1.57–1.69	1.54–1.65	1.45–1.58	1.33–1.55
	1.5-mile time (min:sec)	8:37–9:40	9:45–10:45	10:00–11:00	10:30–11:30	11:00–12:30	11:15–13:59
VI. Superior	O₂ uptake (ml/kg/min)	>56.0	>52.5	>49.5	>48.1	>45.4	>44.3
	T. M. time (min:sec)[a]	>27:48	>25:00	>24:00	>23:00	>21:15	>20:38
	12-min. dist. (mi)	>1.87	>1.77	>1.70	>1.66	>1.59	>1.56
	1.5-mile time (min:sec)	<8:37	<9:45	<10:00	<10:30	<11:00	<11:15

[a]Treadmill time using Balke-Ware technique. (From THE AEROBICS WAY by Kenneth H. Cooper, M.D., M.Ph. Copyright © 1977 by Kenneth H. Cooper. Reprinted by permission of the publisher, M. Evans and Co., Inc., New York, New York 10017.)

TABLE 5-2. WOMEN'S AEROBICS FITNESS CLASSIFICATION (PREDICTED)

Category	Measure	Age (years)					
		13–19	20–29	30–39	40–49	50–59	60+
I. Very poor	O$_2$ uptake (ml/kg/min)	<25.0	<23.6	<22.8	<21.0	<20.2	<17.5
	T. M. time (min:sec)[a]	<8:30	<7:46	<7:15	<6:00	<5:38	<4:00
	12-min. dist. (mi)	<1.0	<.96	<.94	<.88	<.84	<.78
	1.5-mile time (min:sec)	>18:31	>19:01	>19:31	>20:01	>20:31	>21:01
II. Poor	O$_2$ uptake (ml/kg/min)	25.0–30.9	23.6–28.9	22.8–26.9	21.0–24.4	20.2–22.7	17.5–20.1
	T. M. time (min:sec)[a]	8:30–11:29	7:46–10:09	7:15–9:29	6:00–7:59	5:38–6:59	4:00–5:32
	12-min. dist. (mi)	1.00–1.18	.96–1.11	.95–1.05	.88–.98	.84–.93	.78–.86
	1.5-mile time (min:sec)	18:30–16:55	19:00–18:31	19:30–19:01	20:00–19:31	20:30–20:01	21:00–20:31
III. Fair	O$_2$ uptake (ml/kg/min)	31.0–34.9	29.0–32.9	27.0–31.4	24.5–28.9	22.8–26.9	20.2–24.4
	T. M. time (min:sec)[a]	11:30–13:59	10:10–12:59	9:30–11:59	8:00–10:59	7:00–9:29	5:33–7:59
	12-min. dist (mi)	1.19–1.29	1.12–1.22	1.06–1.18	.99–1.11	.94–1.05	.87–.98
	1.5-mile time (min:sec)	16:54–14:31	18:30–15:55	19:00–16:31	19:30–17:31	20:00–19:01	20:30–19:31
IV. Good	O$_2$ uptake (ml/kg/min)	35.0–38.9	33.0–36.9	31.5–35.6	29.0–32.8	27.0–31.4	24.5–30.2
	T. M. time (min:sec)[a]	14:00–17:29	13:00–15:59	12:00–14:59	11:00–12:59	9:30–11:59	8:00–10:59
	12-min. dist. (mi)	1.30–1.43	1.23–1.34	1.19–1.29	1.12–1.24	1.06–1.18	.99–1.09
	1.5-mile time (min:sec)	14:30–12:30	15:54–13:31	16:30–14:31	17:30–15:56	19:00–16:31	19:30–17:31
V. Excellent	O$_2$ uptake (ml/kg/min)	39.0–41.9	37.0–40.9	35.7–40.0	32.9–36.9	31.5–35.7	30.3–31.4
	T. M. time (min:sec)[a]	17:30–18:59	16:00–17:59	15:00–16:59	13:00–15:59	12:00–14:59	11:00–11:59
	12-min. dist. (mi)	1.44–1.51	1.35–1.45	1.30–1.39	1.25–1.34	1.19–1.30	1.10–1.18
	1.5-mile time (min:sec)	12:29–11:50	13:30–12:30	14:30–13:00	15:55–13:45	16:30–14:30	17:30–16:30
VI. Superior	O$_2$ uptake (ml/kg/min)	>42.0	>41.0	>40.1	>37.0	>35.8	>31.5
	T. M. time (min:sec)[a]	>19:00	>18:00	>17:00	>16:00	>15:00	>12:00
	12-min. dist. (mi)	>1.52	>1.46	>1.40	>1.35	>1.31	>1.19
	1.5-mile time (min:sec)	<11:50	<12:30	<13:00	<13:45	<14:30	<16:30

[a]Treadmill time using Balke-Ware technique. *(From THE AEROBICS WAY by Kenneth H. Cooper, M.D., M.Ph. Copyright © 1977 by Kenneth H. Cooper. Reprinted by permission of the publisher, M. Evans and Co., Inc., New York, New York 10017.)*

oxygen. Without oxygen, cellular metabolism rapidly leads to accumulation of lactate as a result of the biochemical breakdown of glycogen. The increasing accumulation of lactate slows and eventually stops energy production. Symptomatically, muscle fatigue and pain will correspond approximately to the elevation of the lactic acid. The more intense the exercise, the greater the oxygen deficit and the more rapidly the exercise is slowed or halted. In fact, maximal exercise can be maintained for only 1 minute through only the anaerobic pathway.[1] Examples of predominantly anaerobic exercise are weight lifting, tennis, and sprinting.

Strength training, which is predominantly anaerobic, consists of isotonic, isometric, isokinetic, and accommodating resistance varieties of exercise. Isotonic exercise consists of movement against a constant resistance through the full range of motion of a joint. The traditional example is weight lifting with barbells. Isometric exercise is muscle contraction without movement, that is, against a fixed object. An example would be an attempt to lift an object bolted to the floor. Isokinetic exercise involves muscle contraction against a variable resistance at a fixed speed. The emphasis is to complete the exercise as fast as is possible, and for this reason the aerobic/anaerobic ratio is high. Special, costly equipment is necessary, however. Accommodating resistance exercises (Nautilus) provide muscle contraction against a full range of motion, using a machine that rotates on a common axis of the joint. Each of these forms of anaerobic exercise has advantages and disadvantages according to the goals of the athletes in particular sports, but all will develop muscle strength and tone through a regular program.

A basic program for strength training and body building involves 3 days of workout each week. In weight training (isotonic or accommodating resistance), each workout should consist of three sets of five to eight repetitions per muscle group.[17] The first set should be at 85 percent 1 RM (the maximum weight that can be achieved during one repetition after appropriate warmup), followed by the second and third sets at 80 percent and 75 percent 1 RM. Weights are increased when an athlete is able to complete each daily workout at the weights designated for three consecutive (1-week) workouts. One day a month can be used to evaluate increases in the 1 RM accomplished by the training program. An isokinetic program should follow the same three sets, with five to eight repetitions per day, 3 days per week at maximum effort for the best results.

Many athletes combine anaerobic and aerobic exercise. The concept that high resistance with low repetitions will develop strength and low resistance with high repetitions will develop muscular endurance is inaccurate. Either method results primarily in an increase in muscular strength.[18] The increased strength will produce some increase in endurance.[19] However, when combined with weight training, aerobic exercises will markedly prolong general muscular endurance during prolonged exercise. In tennis, for example, strength training will increase the force of the racquet swing, and aerobic training will permit longer and more vigorous activity. Each type of training increases playing ability through its specific effects.

TYPES OF MUSCLE FIBERS

At the cellular level, muscle fiber types can be distinguished on the basis of physiological, biochemical, and histochemical means.[20,21] Muscle fibers are red, slow twitch (ST or type 1) and fast twitch (FT or type 2).

FT fibers can be further divided into types FT_a and FT_b. The significance of these two categories is not fully understood. It is known that with prolonged endurance training, almost all FT fibers are FT_a but will revert to normal ratios of each with deconditioning. It is therefore assumed that these changes represent an adaptive response to endurance training. A third subtype, FT_c has been identified, but such fibers are few in number (1 to 2 percent) except in infants (10 to 50 percent).

ST fibers have a higher capacity for aerobic than anaerobic metabolism and FT fibers have the reverse capacity. As expected, sprinters have mostly FT fibers in their leg muscles and long-distance runners have ST fibers. Throwers, weight lifters, and high jumpers have an even distribution of both types, which is somewhat unexpected, since these events are explosive in nature. Indeed, the sports specificity of the two types of muscle fibers is still questionable. Any predictive counseling made on the basis of muscle fiber typing alone is spurious, considering the lack of scientific evidence. Ironically, one of the top five athletes to finish in the 1972 Olympic marathon was found to have predominantly FT fibers.

AGING AND EXERCISE

The running boom has clearly nullified the myth that older people are only able to play shuffleboard, walk slowly, or sit most of the time. In fact, many people in their 60s and 70s regularly run long distances, and even 26.2-mile marathons. Although quality is not the only consideration, certainly life has an added dimension for those who are active.

In addition, exercise retards the physiologic changes that result from aging. Clinically, the immobilization of a joint results in atrophy of muscles and tendons, muscle shortening, and osteoporosis with loss of strength of all these parts, whereas all musculoskeletal structures are strengthened by active conditioning. With the usual decrease in activity that accompanies the physiology of the aging process, women over 35 years of age lose bone mineral at approximately 1 percent per year.[22] This process can be reversed with physical activity and calcium and vitamin D supplements.[23] In addition to the increased coordination that accompanies physical exercise, this effect presents a real opportunity to reduce many of the musculoskeletal problems of aging: hip and vertebral-compression fractures, reduced joint mobility, low back and neck problems, and osteoporosis.

The risk of strokes, myocardial infarction, and other thromboembolic events may be decreased through physical activity, which reduces platelet stickiness and enhances fibrinolytic activity.[24,25] Although specific causes of death are not well researched, in general, sudden death is reduced if physical fitness is maintained during the later years.[3,4]

A decrease in circulating catecholamines might reduce chronic stress on the cardiovascular system and be synergistic with the other effects presented.[26]

Although maximum aerobic capacity decreases with age, the decline can be minimized. A marked example is a study demonstrating that as few as 3 weeks of bed rest will reduce work capacity by 20 to 25 percent regardless of age.[26] Most older persons are capable of fitness levels exceeding those of sedentary people who are several decades younger. In one instance there was no documented decline in aerobic capacity from age 45 to 55.[27]

JOINT LAXITY AND MUSCLE STRETCHING

The long postulated etiologic relationship between joint laxity and injury was recently tested in a study of professional football players.[28] The initial results showed an increased likelihood of knee ligament rupture with increased looseness. However, subsequent studies performed on high school students[29,30] and college students[31] with the use of a variety of objective measurements[32] have failed to demonstrate such a relationship. As a result, an athlete with an identifiable laxity need not be counseled to withdraw from, or participate in, certain sports as a precautionary measure against secondary injury. That is, injuries cannot be predicted from consideration of laxity alone; recommendations for particular sporting events must be based on more than just the laxity spectrum.

Although studies have also failed to correlate athletic performance with tightness or looseness, a progressive decrease in looseness is observed with increasing age.[33] Laxity varies among individual joints, but it is an inherent physiologic trait, which can be identified and characterized by the summation of the laxity in certain joints. Examples of methods used to determine joint looseness/tightness are ability to (1) flex, extend, or hyperextend the elbow; (2) reach toward or touch the floor with the fingers or palms while the knees are extended; (3) flex the hamstrings by measuring the angle of knee flexion with the palms on the floor; and (4) flex the ankle (maximum degree). Surprisingly, sexual difference has no effect on the final analysis of laxity.

Flexibility refers to the ability of a muscle tendon unit or ligament to lengthen. Unless a person is involved in activities that stretch muscles, they will shorten. A specific example concerns those who sit most of the time either at home or at work. As they get older, such people will discover that they are unable to reach over as far as they once could. This phenomenon is attributable to the shortening of the calf, hamstring, pelvic, and paraspinal muscles. Although solid research is yet to be done, many sports physiologists and physicians are convinced that stretching prevents injuries, promotes healing of certain injuries and prevents many lifestyle-induced musculospinal problems. It is generally agreed that strengthening exercises will decrease the likelihood of injury and that stretching should be recommended for people with tight joints.

Muscle stretching is gaining popularity among most sports enthusiasts, even at the professional level. Many physicians and trainers are convinced that stretching reduces injuries. Certainly, it is easy to demonstrate that flexibility can be increased over a period of only a few weeks, although the medical literature has little documentation that stretching improves performance and decreases injuries. A benefit of stretching that has been documented is its reduction of soreness following exercise.[34]

Disagreement continues as to whether to use ballistic (bouncing or rebounding) or static (slow, gradual pull) stretches. One study has demonstrated that both types possess equal efficacy.[35] Logic suggests a preference for the static stretch because of the possibility of muscle pulls with ballistic movements. It might even be discovered that one type or the other is better for particular individuals. Static stretching involves little risk, and even with the lack of conclusive evidence concerning its efficacy, it can be soundly recommended.

A newer variation of exercise, which involves brief antagonistic muscle contraction before each stretch, has been shown to produce better physiologic lengthening of the muscle group of the joint tested.[36] This study involved the use of a weight–pulley system, but such equipment could be

eliminated by the use of ingenuity, and particularly if a partner were available.

WOMAN AND CHILD ATHLETES

Compared with male athletes, the exercise physiology of women is qualitatively similar; quantitively, however, the aerobic capacity and muscle mass of female athletes is not as great. Even so, it is apparent from modern investigation of various women's sports that women are remarkably capable athletes. In the marathon, for example, women's times have been lowered by more than 30 minutes in the past 10 years. Such developments should stimulate further interest in the need for women to be physically fit. A few distinguishing features of women's physiology are presented.

Menstrual oligomenorrhea and amenorrhea are commonly recognized in highly trained female athletes. This irregularity is cause for concern, especially to women who plan to bear children. Considerable scientific data are available to indicate that an approximate minimum of 22 percent of body fat is necessary for normal menstruation in women beyond the late teens.[37–39] Many coaches and trainers, however, have noted normal menses in women with less than 17 percent body fat.[40] Additional evidence shows that such menstrual problems are not related to exercise alone, since they also occur in patients with anorexia nervosa.[41] When women in training are followed over a period of at least a year, most resume regular menstrual activity.[42] In conclusion, menstrual problems are not necessarily limited to thin athletes or to women with a certain percentage of fat composition. All women have a complex of psychological and physiologic variables that interact differently according to individual makeup. The details of this complex are yet to be unraveled.

The prevailing opinion among sports physiologists is that menstrual regularity and fertility will return with a decrease in the intensity of the training program, as well as with weight gain and possibly the addition of medication.[43] Final conclusions, however, are not available, and women athletes should be made aware of this possibility. If a woman does become pregnant, it is recommended that she continue a fitness program throughout pregnancy. This conditioning will assist in the rigors of labor and in the postpartum period. Exercise has not been shown to be harmful to the unborn child.[44,45]

Women who are athletes or potential athletes will be concerned about the number and frequency of injuries in various sports. Christine Haycock, one of the leading authorities on women's sports injuries, has concluded, in a survey of college teams, athletic trainers, and published studies, that women athletes sustain "the same injuries in relatively the same numbers as their male counterparts, with perhaps only the injuries related to the patella and joints occurring more often in women."[46] Concerning the breasts, Haycock and associates reported that 72 percent of female athletes experience sore or tender breasts after exercise in such sports as running, basketball, and weight lifting.[47] The reason for breast soreness is not known, but current theories locate the etiology in the underlying pectoral muscle: structural damage, spasm, or overstretching of the elastic components (i.e., the connective tissue among the fibers and fibrils). No damage to the breast tissue itself has been recorded, however. These problems can now be prevented with several varieties of sports bras now on the market. The more common brands of sports bras have been studied for linear displacement, velocity, and acceleration of the breast during movement.[48]

The progressive development of aerobic capacity in children is possible. One study noted a 15 percent improvement in the aerobic capacity of 11-year-old boys over a 6-month period of time.[49] Another study demonstrated a 12 to 14 percent increase in aerobic capacity over a slightly shorter period of time.[50] A surprising phenomenon is the lack of change in $\dot{V}O_2$max as expressed per unit of body weight in teenage male middle-distance runners over a period of 2 to 5 years.[51] As expected, absolute $\dot{V}O_2$max, in liters per minute, did continue to increase in direct proportion to body weight.

Children are generally thought of as actively pursuing games and physical activities, but many authorities are concerned that physical exercise is progressively decreasing in children, as well as in adults. Factors contributing to such a decline are (1) inactivity during the school day, (2) television viewing during daylight hours, and (3) the emphasis on competitive athletics, with corresponding neglect of physical activities available to those children who cannot physically "make the team." Since it is commonly held that those adult behaviors that are difficult to change are established in childhood, the most effective, long-range program to increase adult activity would appear to be one directed at school-age children. Programs can be designed that will develop and maintain physical fitness over several years of schooling.[52] Activities that can be carried over into adulthood (e.g., swimming and bicycling) should be emphasized.

FALSE-ABNORMAL FINDINGS

Blood tests can be altered during periods of physical training, as a direct result of the conditioning process or secondary to injury from the specific athletic endeavor. Anemia (low hemoglobin or hematocrit) in runners and other athletes is thought to be an adaptive response to maximize oxygen transport. Other possible explanations include mechanical destruction of red blood cells and an increase in blood volume.[53,54] It might be assumed that such anemia would limit performance because less oxygen would be delivered to the tissues. Studies show conflicting results in this area, but those that indicate limited performance are probably not relevant to athletes. A diagnosis of sports anemia can be made when other etiologies in the athlete have been carefully considered and excluded by appropriate laboratory tests.

Enzymes commonly present in the blood that can be tested in making specific diagnoses of certain diseases might well be abnormally increased in athletes. Three enzymes, serum glutamic oxaloacetic transaminase (SGOT), serum glutamic pyruvic transaminase (SGPT), and lactic acid dehydrogenase (LDH), are commonly elevated during physical exertion in proportion to the intensity of the exercise.[55,56] Although the source of these elevated enzymes is believed to be skeletal muscle, another enzyme, creatine kinase (CK), may be fractionated into isoenzymes in order to distinguish between skeletal and cardiac origins. The myoglobin (MB) isoenzyme is generally thought to be from myocardial muscle but long-distance runners have been found to have elevations of the MB isoenzyme in the absence of myocardial pathology.[57,58] Another enzyme pattern usually diagnostic of heart damage is the "flipped" LDH pattern, which is also seen in extreme physical activity.[59] These findings will present a dilemma to the physician who sees an athlete currently engaged in an extensive program, and yet who has symptoms that suggest myocardial damage. These patients might have to be hospitalized for observation in order for the physician to arrive at an accurate diagnosis, especially if the athlete has collapsed during participation in a sports event. Recently, however, "infarct-avid" scintigraphy has been used to demonstrate the absence of underlying myocardial abnormalities in runners.[60]

The urinalysis is a simple but vital test of kidney function. A common finding in the athlete is the presence of proteinuria and hematuria. It is generally accepted that exercise does not injure the athlete's kidney.[61] The proteinuria is attributed to relative renal ischemia resulting from the shunting of blood to the exercising muscles or direct constriction of the renal vessels. Hematuria can result from repeated mechanical trauma to the bladder or kidneys, such as occurs in contact sports or long-distance running, or from the duration of the sports activity and its intensity.[62] In the Commonwealth Games of 1976, proteinuria occurred more frequently in the endurance events. It should be remembered that proteinuria and, to a lesser extent, hematuria might be normal findings, particularly postural proteinuria. In addition, disease states must be considered concurrent with the athletic participation, for example, glomerulonephritis, which is common in young people.

Myoglobin in the urine (myoglobinuria) secondary to rhabdomyolysis can cause renal failure with accompanying hyperkalemia and hypocalcemia in acute situations.[63] Intense exercise, excessive heat, lack of training, and dehydration are contributing factors. As potassium leaks from muscles and is lost in perspiration and urine, continually exercised muscles will leak myoglobin easily, and often at extremely high rates. Paradoxically, salt

tablets can increase the risk of muscle breakdown. The importance of regular, frequent ingestion of plain, cold water (8 ounces or more, every 20 minutes, depending on the size of the athlete) during exercise, and continued ingestion after exercise until significant urination has occurred, cannot be overemphasized.

DRUGS: FALSE HOPE, DANGER, AND NEW POSSIBILITIES

In the vigorously competitive world of sports, athletes hope and strive for increased performance. Such a drive causes many athletes to seek the supposed benefit of drugs to assist them in attaining this goal. Athletes engaged in power events, for example, weight lifting, shot putting, and wrestling, are frequent users of anabolic steroids, such as methandienone, nandrolonedecanoate, nandrolone phenylproprionate, oxymetholone, or stanozolol. A summary report and position statement has been prepared by the American College of Sports Medicine.[64] The research, based on a double-blind study, found increased strength, lean body mass, and/or body weight in some cases but not in others and recommended that any benefits are likely to be small and not worth the health risks involved. Since these drugs are chemically similar to the androgenic hormones, users could be endangering normal sexual function and future ability to have children.

In men these drugs can cause impotency, decreased testicular size and function, and decreased sperm production, secondary to a variable reduction (30 to 65 percent) of the body's production of testosterone and gonadotropins.[65] Because of their anabolic effects, the growth rate in adolescents can be adversely affected; these steroids can lead to hepatocellular dysfunction, with cases of acute hepatitis, hepatic carcinoma, and leukemia being reported. In women these drugs also produce undesired side effects, such as masculinization, hirsutism, and enlargement of the clitoris.

It is possible to detect traces of these drugs in urine and blood, although the methodologies often are not available. Unfortunately, the conclusion that steroids do not improve performance cannot be stated definitively, but their known potential side effects can be severe.

Stimulants are another common drug group often used by athletes. Examples of these drugs by general classes are psychomotor stimulants (e.g., amphetamine, its derivatives, and cocaine), sympathomimetic amines (e.g., ephedrine, methylephedrine, and methoxphenomine), and miscellaneous stimulants (e.g., amiphenzaole, nikethamide, pentylenetetrazol, and strychnine). A summary article on the use of these drugs among athletes reports that there is no conclusive evidence to support that their use will result in such effects as improved ability to exercise, alertness and wakefulness, decreased sensitivity to pain, and increased ability to concentrate.[66] Increased hostility and aggressiveness are common sequelae to these drugs and can result in brutality in contact sports.

Serious toxic side effects of these drugs include hypertension, dizziness, disturbed perception, life-threatening cardiac arrhythmias, convulsions, hallucinations, paranoid ideation, panic states, and suicidal or homicidal tendencies. Prolonged use of amphetamines has been known to lead to irreversible cardiac hypertrophy, with eventual failure and lethal arrhythmias. These drugs are of no proven benefit, produce serious toxic effects, and are thus contraindicated as an aid to performance in athletic participation. They can be detected in urine and blood by laboratory screens.

Many other agents are commonly used by athletes: dimethyl sulfoxide (DMSO), pituitary snuff, lecithin, ginseng, bee pollen, special diets, and others, which are frequently common to a specific sport. It must be concluded from studies of certain of these agents that none has been proven consistently beneficial. Furthermore, the toxicities of some of these substances have the potential to produce severe or lethal effects, either directly or indirectly. Many of these agents are not easily detectable by laboratory testing. Physicians should take every opportunity, especially during the health history and examination, to educate athletes about drugs and discourage their use in sports. Trainers and coaches are often ignorant of drug problems, making it incumbent on the primary care physician to take the opportunity to continue their initial educational efforts in the locker room and on the field.

Blood doping and caffeine might be exceptions in relationship to performance. An internationally recognized researcher, Dr. David Costill, found improved work production with caffeine usage in cyclists who were exercised for 2 hours.[67] It should be noted, however, that the work involved an endurance event, a specific dosage of drug, and concomitant carbohydrate ingestion. In a review of 18 studies, blood doping was found to increase endurance performance significantly in sports that are dependent on sustained high levels of oxygen, for example, distance running and swimming: "The increase in $\dot{V}o_2$max, due to increased oxygen transport, is the underlying physiological rationale."[68] One reservation to its use would be the possibility that strict protocols developed by the American Red Cross for the handling of all transfused blood would not be followed. Serious injury or death could result from such failure.

In addition, the question of legality must be settled by the various governing bodies of athletic competition, as well as the ethical contention that such aid is a breach of proper sportsmanship. The acceptance and benefit of caffeine and blood doping await future application and experimentation before they become an established fact of modern sports medicine.

REFERENCES

1. Åstrand P, Rodahl K: Textbook of Work Physiology. New York, McGraw-Hill, 1977, pp 289–330.
2. President's Council on Physical Fitness and Sports: Physical activity and coronary heart disease. Phys Fitness Res Dig 2(2):1–13, 1972.
3. President's Council on Physical Fitness and Sports: Update: Physical activity and coronary heart disease. Phys Fitness Res Dig 9(2):1–25, 1979.
4. Paffenbarger RS, Hale WE: Work activity and coronary heart mortality. N Engl J Med 292:545–550, 1975.
5. President's Council on Physical Fitness and Sports: Update: Exercise and some coronary risk factors. Phys Fitness Res Dig 9(3):1–22, 1979.
6. Cooper KH, Pollock MI, Martin RP, et al: Physical fitness levels vs selected coronary risk factors. J Am Med Assoc 264:166–169, 1976.

7. Kentala E: Physical fitness and feasibility of physical rehabilitation after myocardial infarction in men of working age. Ann Clin Res 4(suppl 9):1–84, 1972.

8. White JR, Hunt HF: When doctors test themselves, the prescription is exercise. Phys Sportsmed 3(12):72–77, 1976.

9. Hartung GH, Foreyt JP, Mitchell RE, et al: Relation of diet to high-density-lipoprotein cholesterol in middle aged marathon runners, joggers and inactive men. N Engl J Med 302:357–361, 1980.

10. Folkins CH, Sine WE: Physical fitness training and mental health. Am Psychol 36(4):373–389, 1981.

11. Zohman LR: Beyond Diet: Exercise Your Way to Fitness and Heart Health. Englewood Cliffs, NJ, CPC International, 1974.

12. Hage P: Perceived exertion: One measure of exercise intensity. Phys Sportsmed 9(9):136–143, 1981.

13. Hickson RC, Rosenkoetter MA: Reduced training frequencies and maintenance of increased aerobic power. Med Sci Sports Exerc 13(1):13–16, 1981.

14. Pollock ML, Gettman LR, Milesis CA, et al: Effects of frequency and duration of training on attrition and incidence of injury. Med Sci Sports Exerc 9:31–36, 1977.

15. Cooper KH: The Aerobics Way. New York, M Evans, 1977.

16. Paffenbarger RS, Wing AL, Hyde RT: Physical activity as an index of heart attacks in college alumni. Am J Epidemiol 108:151–175, 1978.

17. Kearney JT: Resistance training: Development of muscular strength and endurance. In Burke EF (ed): Toward an understanding of Human Performance. Ithaca, NY, Wilcox Press, 1978, 21–24.

18. Clarke DH, Stull GA: Endurance training as a determinant of strength and fatigability. Res Q 14:19–26, 1970.

19. Hickson RA, Rosenkoetter MA, Brown MM: Strength training effects on aerobic power and short term endurance. Med Sci Sports Exerc 12(5):336–339, 1980.

20. Gollnick PD, Hermansen L, Saltin B: The muscle biopsy: Still a research tool. Phys Sportsmed 8(1):50–55, 1980.

21. Saltin B, Henricksson, Nygamd E, Andersen P: Fiber types and metabolic potentials of skeletal muscles in sedentary men and endurance runners. Ann NY Acad Sci 301:3–29, 1977.

22. Smith DM, Khairi MRA, Norton J, Johnston CC: Age and activity effects on rate of bone mineral loss. J Clin Invest 58:518–721, 1976.

23. Smith EL, Reddan W, Smith PE: Physical activity and calcium modalities for bone mineral increase in aged women. Med Sci Sports Exerc 13(1):60–64, 1981.

24. Simpson MT, Olewine DA, Jenkins CD, et al: Exercise-induced catecholamines and platelet aggregation in the coronary-prone behavior pattern. Psychosom Med 36:476–487, 1974.

25. Williams RS, Logue EE, Lewis JL, et al: Physical conditioning augments the fibrinolytic response to venous occlusion in healthy adults. N Engl J Med 302:987–991, 1980.

26. Salten B, Blomquist G, Mitchell JH: Response to exercise after bed rest and training. Circulation 38(suppl 7):1–78, 1968.

27. Kasch FW: The effects of exercise on the aging process. Phys Sportsmed 4(6):64–68, 1976.

28. Nicholas JA: Injuries to knee ligaments. J Am Med Assoc 212:2236–2239, 1970.

29. Grana WA, Moretz JA: Ligamentous laxity in secondary school athletes. J Am Med Assoc 240:1975–1976, 1978.

30. Kirby RL, Simm FC, Symington VJ, Garner JB: Flexibility and musculoskeletal symptomatology in female gymnasts and age-matched controls. Am J Sports Med 9(3):160–164, 1981.

31. Jackson DW, Jarrett H, Bailey D, et al: Injury prediction in the young athlete: A preliminary report. Am J Sports Med 6(1):6–14, 1978.

32. Kalenak A, Morehouse CA: Knee stability and knee ligament injuries. J Am Med Assoc 234:1143–1145, 1975.

33. Marshall JL, Johanson N, Wickiewicz TL, et al: Joint looseness: A function of the person and the joint. Med Sci Sports Exerc 12(3):189–194, 1980.

34. Schultz P: Flexibility: Day of the static stretch. Phys Sportsmed 7(11):109–117, 1979.

35. de Vries HA: Evaluation of static stretching procedures for improvement of flexibility. Res Q 33:222–239, 1962.

36. Moore MA, Hutton RS: Electromyographic investigation of muscle stretching techniques. Med Sci Sports Exerc 12:322–329, 1980.

37. Frisch RE, MacArthur JW: Menstrual cycles: Fatness as a determinant of minimum weight for height necessary for their maintenance or onset. Science 185:951–959, 1974.

38. Frisch RE, Gatz-Welbergen AV, McArthur JW, et al: Delayed menarche and amenorrhea of college athletes in relation to age of onset of training. J Am Med Assoc 248:1559–1583, 1981.

39. Frisch RE: Pubertal adipose tissue: Is it necessary for normal sexual maturation? Evidence from the rat and human female. Fed Proc 39:2395–2400, 1980.

40. Katch FI, Katch VL, Behnke AR: The underweight female. Phys Sportsmed 8(12):55–60, 1980.

41. Vigersky RA, Andersen AE, Thompson RH, et al: Hypothalamic dysfunction in secondary amenorrhea associated with simple weight loss. N Engl J Med 297:1141–1145, 1977.

42. Anderson JL: Women's sports and fitness program at the US military academy. Phys Sportsmed 7(1):83–95, 1979.

43. Dale E, Detlef HG, Martin DE, Alexander DR: Physical fitness profiles and reproductive physiology of the female distance runner. Phys Sportsmed (1):83–95, 1979.

44. Dressendorfer RH, Goodlin RC: Fetal heart rate response to maternal exercise testing. Phys Sportsmed 9(11):91–96, 1980.

45. Hutchinson PL, Cureton KJ, Sparling PB: Metabolic and circulatory responses to running during pregnancy. Phys Sportsmed 9(8):55–61, 1981.

46. Haycock CE, Gillette JV: Susceptibility of women athletes to injury: Myths vs reality. J Am Med Assoc 236:163–165, 1976.

47. Haycock CE, Shiesman G, Gillette J: The female athlete: Does her anatomy pose problems? Presented at the American Medical Association Meeting, June 1977.

48. Gehlson G, Albohm M: Evaluation of sports bras. Phys Sportsmed 8(10):89–97, 1980.

49. Ekblom G: Effect of physical training in adolescent boys. J Appl Physiol 27:350–355, 1969.

50. Dobeln WV, Erikson BO: Physical training, maximal oxygen uptake, and dimensions of the oxygen transporting and metabolizing organs in boys 11–13 years of age. Acta Paediatr Scand 61:653–660, 1972.

51. Daniels J, Oldridge N, Nagel F, White B: Differences and changes in Vo_2 among young runners 10–18 years of age. Med Sci Sports 10:200–203, 1978.

52. Shephard RJ: Program of physical activity for the primary school child—needless or a necessity? In Burke EJ (ed): Toward an Understanding of Human Performance. Ithaca, NY, Monument Publications, 1977.

53. Williamson MR: Anemia in runners and other athletes. Phys Sportsmed 9(6):73–79, 1981.

54. Dressendorfer RH, Wade CE, Amsterdam EA: Development of pseudo anemia in marathon runners during a 20-day road race. J Am Med Assoc 246:1215–1218, 1981.

55. McDonald CA: Enzyme levels after running (letter). J Am Med Assoc 246:40–41.

56. Bloom CM: Effects of exercise on enzyme interpretation. West J Med 128:46–47, 1978.

57. Oliver LR, De Waul A, Retief FJ, et al: Electrocardiographic and biochemical studies in marathon runners. South Afr Med 53:783–787, 1978.

58. Apple FS: Presence of creatine kinase MB-isoenzyme during marathon training. N Engl J Med 305:764–765, 1981.

59. Kielblock AJ, Manjoo M, Booyens J, Katzeff IE: Creatine phosphokinase and lactate dehydrogenase levels after ultra longdistance running. South Afr Med J 55:1061–1064, 1979.

60. Siegal AJ, Siverman LM, Holam BL: Elevated creatine kinase MB isoenzyme in marathon runner. J Am Med Assoc 246:2049–2051, 1980.

61. Roundtable discussion: Proteinuria in the athlete. Phys Sportsmed 6(7):45–55, 1978.

62. Hoover DL, Cromie WJ: Theory and management of exercise-related hematuria. Phys Sportsmed 9(11):91–95, 1981.

63. Upham AT, Cooper WL: Urban Cowboy myoglobinuria. J Am Med Assoc 245:1216, 1981.

64. American College of Sports Medicine: Anabolic–androgenic steroids in sports. Phys Sportsmed 6(3):157–158, 1978.

65. Brief report: Use of anabolic steroids by elite athletes studied. Phys Sportsmed 9(7):22, 1981.

66. Percy EC: Ergogenic aids in athletes. Med Sci Sports Exerc 10(4):298–303, 1978.

67. Ivy JL, Costill DL, Fink WJ, et al: Influence of caffeine and carbohydrate feeding on endurance performance. Med Sci Sports Exerc 11:6–11, 1979.

68. Williams MH: Blood doping: An update. Phys Sportsmed 9(7):59–64, 1981.

BIBLIOGRAPHY

Apple DF, Cantwell JD: Medicine for Sport. Chicago, Year Book Medical Publishers, 1979.

Åstrand P, Rodahl K: Textbook of Work Physiology. New York, McGraw-Hill, 1977.

Cooper KH: The Aerobics Way. New York, M Evans, 1977.

Jenson CR, Fisher AG: Scientific Bases of Athletic Conditioning. Philadelphia, Lea & Febiger, 1979.

Quigley TB, Anderson JL, George F, et al: The Yearbook of Sports Medicine. Chicago, Year Book Medical Publishers, yearly beginning 1979.

Shephard RJ: Human Physiological Work Capacity. New York, Cambridge University Press, 1978.

Wenger NK (ed): Exercise and the Heart. Philadelphia, FA Davis, 1978.

Williams S: Sports Medicine. Baltimore, William & Wilkins, 1978.

6
Cardiovascular Effects and Complications of Exercise and Exercise Training

Richard A. Stein and Andrew B. Rohen

The cardiovascular system responds to exercise in an integrated manner, directed at providing the necessary blood to working muscles. This chapter reviews the significant components of this response and discusses the changes in the cardiovascular system consequent to repeated exercise and exercise training.

PHYSIOLOGIC RESPONSE TO EXERCISE

Shunting of Blood. With exercise the body shunts blood to working muscles and away from nonworking muscles, the hepato-splanchnic organs and, early in exercise, the cutaneous beds.[1] This is effected by a generalized increase in sympathetic tone, causing vasoconstriction that is then overridden in the working muscles by vasodilating metabolic products. Initially blood is shunted away from the skin, but with prolonged exercise, core temperature increases and blood is then redirected to cutaneous beds to facilitate dissipation of heat.

Increase in O_2 Extraction. The amount of oxygen extracted by working muscles from the perfusing bed is increased threefold from 5 ml O_2/100 cc blood at rest to 15 ml O_2/100 cc blood at peak exercise.[2] These two responses (shunting and increased extraction) are significant in that they do not require an increase in cardiac output while permitting increased muscular work. In patients with a fixed cardiac output (e.g., tight mitral stenosis) these represent the extent of their "cardiac reserve."

Increase in Cardiac Output. Cardiac output (CO) increases directly with muscle work to provide an increased supply of oxygen-rich blood to working muscles. This is brought about both by an increase in heart rate (HR) and stroke volume (SV, the amount of blood ejected with each beat).

$$CO = HR \times SV$$

Heart rate increases in the range of 300 percent (e.g., resting rate of 60/minute to peak exercise rate of 180/minute). The increase is directly related to the intensity of work being performed.[3] Stroke volume increases about 35 percent in upright exercise from rest to maximum exercise. With supine exercise, the stroke volume starts off at a higher value and increases only slightly with exercise. Stroke volume increases both because of an increase in heart muscle function (contractility) and due to an increase in diastolic volume (EDV).[4] The ejection fraction (SV/EDV) increases with exercise due to enhanced contractility and the "starling (preload) effect." Nuclear cardiac studies during exercise show that the normal ejection fraction is about 50 percent and increases at least 5 percent with upright exercise.[5]

Oxygen Consumption. Oxygen is increasingly used by the working muscles as exercise progresses, and total body oxygen consumption per minute ($\dot{V}O_2$) increases with increasing exercise loads. At any given exercise level, the $\dot{V}O_2$ reflects the product of the cardiac output and the $A - VO_2$ (arterial–venous oxygen) difference (reflecting oxygen extraction from blood by the working muscles), as seen in the Fick equation[3]:

$$\dot{V}O_2 = CO\,(A - VO_2)$$

As exercise increases so does the $\dot{V}O_2$ representing increases in both CO and the $A - VO_2$ difference. Beyond 50 percent of maximum exercise, the major factor relating to the increase in $\dot{V}O_2$ is cardiac output. With an increase in exercise the $\dot{V}O_2$ increases, but it requires about $1\frac{1}{2}$ to 2 minutes for the $\dot{V}O_2$ to reach its steady-state level appropriate to the exercise load and for heart rate to reach a new value and remain at that level. This is a physiologic "steady state" relative to a given work load. With increasing exercise levels $\dot{V}O_2$ increases until a maximum value is obtained, beyond which further increases in work load do not result in $\dot{V}O_2$ increases. This value (the $\dot{V}O_2$max) represents the maximum effective functioning of the cardiovascular system—the maximum cardiac output and the greatest O_2 extraction:

$$\dot{V}O_2\text{max} = CO\text{max}\,(A - VO_2)\text{max}$$

This value is highly reproducible for a given individual[3] and is easily determined by the product of the volume of expired air and the difference in

O_2 content of inspired (room) and expired air. Its significance is noted later in this chapter.

Myocardial Oxygen Requirements. Although factors such as contractile state and heart wall tension affect myocardial O_2 consumption to some degree, the major determinants are heart rate and systolic blood pressure. Thus it is possible to estimate changes in myocardial oxygen requirements from changes in the "double product" of these two factors (HR × BP). With exercise, the increasing O_2 requirement of the heart is reflected in the increasing "double product." Since the heart is extracting O_2 from its blood supply at near maximum value all the time, the entire increase in myocardial O_2 requirement must be met by an increase in coronary arterial blood flow.

CARDIOVASCULAR EFFECTS OF EXERCISE TRAINING

Exercise training affects the cardiovascular system in terms of both the anatomy of the heart and the parameters of the physiologic response to exercise as reviewed above. The character and extent of these effects reflects the type of exercise used in training, the cardiovascular health of the subject, and the intensity and frequency of the exercise training.

Types of Exercise

Isotonic. Low-resistance (isotonic) exercises such as swimming, running, or cycling are associated with an increase in ventricular and diastolic volume (cardiomegaly), only a slight increase in ventricular wall mass, and no increase in wall thickness. Studies using echocardiography, and more recently "first-pass" nuclear angiocardiography, reveal that the ejection fraction at rest is also somewhat increased with isotonic training. The consequence of this increase in end diastolic volume and in ejection fraction is a greater stroke volume at rest and throughout exercise. Thus at peak exercise and heart rates the trained individual has a higher CO (HR × SV) and a higher $\dot{V}O_2$max (COmax × $A - VO_2$diff). In addition, training improves the peripheral muscle extraction capability thus increasing $A - \dot{V}O_2$ and further increasing the $\dot{V}O_2$max. The physiologic effects of isotonic training are also observed at submaximal exercise: the "trained" heart provides the required cardiac output at relatively reduced heart rates and increased stroke volume. This is important, in that the myocardial oxygen requirement, best estimated by the product HR $\times$ BP systolic, is therefore reduced at given work loads. The "trained" heart is thus more efficient and can provide an enhanced cardiac output at lower cardiac oxygen cost ($M\dot{V}O_2$).

Isometric. Isometric exercise is that done against high or fixed resistance (e.g., weight lifting). It is associated with an increase in peripheral resistance mediated by sympathetic tone. As a consequence, systolic and diastolic BP are increased for a given cardiac output relative to isotonic work, and heart rate increases less than in isotonic exercise. Stroke volume remains essentially unchanged. Training results in an increase in ventricular wall thickness and a modest increase in ventricular volume.

Specificity

Although dilatation or hypertrophy occurs when an individual trains, the major physiologic consequences appear to be related to alterations in the peripheral muscle vasculature of the trained muscles.[6] Thus weight lifting does not appreciably increase running capacity and vice versa. In addition, the increase in cardiac output and $\dot{V}O_2$ seen with training is "specific" for the muscles involved. Studies of individuals trained with right leg isotonic exercise show significantly improved cardiac output and $\dot{V}O_2$max only with right leg exercise—not with left leg exercise. This is termed *specificity*. Some training effects are probably central, however, in that there is some increase (5 percent) in maximal exercise tolerance when trained individuals are exercised using untrained muscle groups. This is termed the cross over effect.

Cardiovascular Health

As reviewed above, isotonic exercise training increases end diastolic volume and stroke volume and increases maximum $\dot{V}O_2$, cardiac output, and $A - \dot{V}O_2$ while reducing heart rates at submaximal

exercise (and at rest). The trained individual thus has an improved exercise tolerance. The patient with coronary artery disease (occult or known myocardial infarction or angina) still attains an improved exercise tolerance and $\dot{V}O_2$, but the physiologic consequences of training are altered.

The patient with coronary heart disease, when trained, manifests an increased $\dot{V}O_2$ that may even exceed the mean maximal value of a nondiseased population. This increase in exercise tolerance and $\dot{V}O_2$ is associated with a fall in heart rate (and therefore HR $\times$ BP product and myocardial oxygen requirement) at submaximal exercise. In this group of patients, cardiac output is reduced at submaximal exercise levels and maximum cardiac output is not increased. Studies using nuclear angiocardiography have shown that stroke volume and ejection fraction remain unchanged with training in the population with coronary heart disease.[6] The major manifestations (increased exercise tolerance and $\dot{V}O_2$max; reduced submaximal heart rates and cardiac outputs) in these patients are mediated by improved O_2 extraction (increased $A - \dot{V}O_2$) by the trained working muscles. Despite this, however, the important clinical phenomenon of a reduced HR $\times$ BP product at given submaximal exercise levels occurs, resulting in a lower myocardial O_2 requirement at given work loads and a consequent reduction in chest pain with exercise.

EXERCISE PROGRAM FORMAT

This section deals with the four major components of an exercise training program: (1) intensity of exercise performed, (2) duration of each exercise session, (3) frequency of exercise (number of sessions per week), and (4) types of exercises and activities that make up the training program.

Intensity of Exercise

In the clinically normal individual, exercise training should, for optimal affect, involve intensities that are between 75 and 90 percent of an individual's maximum.[7] There is only slight improvement in minute oxygen consumption in young and middle-aged individuals who have trained at lower levels of intensity. It is possible to estimate when an individual is in this intensity range by using exercise heart rates. If the individual has a maximum exercise examination, then that individual's maximum heart rate for a given type of activity (e.g., cycling or running) is determined. If this is, for example, 200 beats/minute of running, the individual should, during a running exercise program, achieve heart rates between 150 and 180 beats/minute. Since maximum exercise ECG testing is neither necessary nor available in many instances, the correct intensity can be approximated by estimating an individual's maximum heart rate from the formula of 220 minus age. It must be remembered that these estimations have a standard deviation of ± 10 beats/minute and therefore represent only a gross approximation. However, this is adequate for the estimation of an appropriate training intensity. Remember, though, that for patients with impaired heart rate responses to exercise due to ischemic disease or diabetes, as well as individuals who use drugs that may affect heart rate (such as β blockers), this formula is not appropriate. In such an individual, maximum exercise ECG testing with more precisely defined maximum and submaximum heart rates is required.

For those who are unable to measure their heart rate during or immediately following exercise, exercise can be performed in the laboratory up to training levels and the patient acclimated to the sense of fatigue and dyspnea appreciated at this exercise level; this level can then be approximated in his or her own exercise program. It is also recommended that a 10-second pulse be taken during the immediate 10 seconds following exercise to obtain peak exercise heart rates. A good rule of thumb for the individual who desires to engage in exercise of an appropriate intensity is that it should be associated with moderate breathlessness and a general sense of "working hard."

In special cases where an individual cannot monitor pulse rate but precise exercise intensities are important, a maximal exercise ECG examination using the training activity can be performed. A good example of this is the coronary patient who exercises on a stationary bicycle. In the exercise laboratory the individual can perform increasing work loads until the maximum is achieved. The work load

representing 75 to 90 percent of the maximum exercise capacity can then be determined and approximated by the individual in his or her exercise training program. This avoids the necessity to measure heart rate.

Duration and Frequency of Exercise

Significant improvement in the parameters of a training response are associated with sessions that range from 40 minutes to 1 hour. In the coronary intervention and treatment program that is run at New York City's 92nd Street YMCA/YWCA, sessions last 40 minutes and improvement in maximum exercise capacity is usually seen by 12 weeks of exercise training. Although data suggest that increases in the duration of each exercise program result in increased parameters of a training response, it appears that the maximum improvement relative to time expended occurs in this 40 minute to 1 hour per session range.

Exercise training is most effective when the proper intensity of exercise is performed every other day or three times a week.[7] Studies of exercise frequency in relationship to training have documented that daily training sessions further enhance the improvement of the training response, but studies in an older population have demonstrated an improvement in exercise capacity in patients who would attend an average of only $1\frac{1}{2}$ sessions per week.[8] What is to be emphasized is that, in reasonably fit middle-aged individuals, an exercise training program of less than twice per week is not associated with an improved Vo_2max; at least twice per week is required to achieve training related enhanced minute oxygen consumption and endurance times.

Type of Exercise Used

Exercise should be aerobic in nature; for example, isotonic activities involving large motion against little or low resistance. If one is training for an aerobic exercise sport, then a program should include muscle groups and muscle activities identical to those used in the sport. A runner who wants to increase speed and duration time should use running as a large part of his or her exercise training program; similarly, a cyclist and a swimmer should cycle and swim, respectively. This is based on the physiological concept of specificity, discussed earlier.

Training specificity dictates that a training program aimed at improvement in performance of a given activity (sport) use mostly the muscle groups and activities basic to that sport. Hence, sports that involve upper and lower limb activities should be trained for with programs using upper and lower limb exercises.

The following is a list of activities, easily used in a training program, that train upper and lower limbs for the majority of sports and performance activities:

Upper Extremities	**Lower Extremities**
Swimming using arms (either a crawl or backstroke)	Jumping and kicking calisthenics
Hand ergometry	Cross-country skiing
Repetitive throwing of a medicine ball	Brisk walking of a sufficient intensity and work load (usually uphill) to achieve target training heart rates
Racquet sports (squash, tennis, paddleball, racquetball)	Cycling
Upper extremity calisthenics	

There is still debate as to whether interval exercise or sustained endurance exercise protocols should be used in training programs. *Endurance exercise protocols* are usually based on an individual performing an activity up to the training range and then sustaining that activity for 30 minutes to 1 hour. An example of this would be a runner who, after warm-up, achieved a pace on an incline sufficient to achieve 80 percent of maximum heart rate and then sustained this pace and work load for a full 40 minutes. The other approach that is commonly used is *Interval Aerobic Training,* in which an individual performs activities for from 90 seconds to 5 minutes or more, working up to a level of 80 to 90 percent of near maximum exercise capacity, sustaining this for a brief period of time, and then "cooling down." The cool-down or rest interval allows the heart rate to fall below the training level. During sessions of this nature actual exercise may comprise only 20 to 30 minutes of the total session, but achieved heart rates usually peak above the training level during the maximum exercise and fall below it during the cool-down intervals.

The interval program has an advantage in that exercise can be altered from interval to interval and different muscle groups and activities incorporated into a training program. Furthermore, for the patient who should or must monitor heart rates to ensure that exercise intensity is in the appropriate range, the immediate postexercise cool-down intervals provide several points during an exercise session when heart rate can be easily measured.

Both forms of exercise program have been associated with significant improvement in training response. At present, it seems prudent to incorporate both into a training program—e.g., do interval work for 20 minutes and perform an endurance activity (say, sprinting) for the remaining 20 minutes—since most sport activities may comprise both sustained and sudden intensive exercise.

Exercise Prescription

Perhaps the most useful and reproducible method of recommending exercise is in the form of an exercise prescription. As in the case of medications, such a prescription should include the type, amount, intensity, frequency, and duration of the exercise. In writing an exercise prescription, contraindications and possible side-effects of the activity must be understood.

Most commonly, the prescription involves specific aerobic training recommendations and is based upon the results of a treadmill exercise test. A target heart rate is calculated from the maximum heart rate achieved during the exercise test. This is usually 70 to 85 percent of the maximum rate and should not produce hypertension, symptoms of fatigue, angina, or dizziness, or ST segment displacement. This information should be compared with the individual's usual exercise level and sport preference(s). It is important to individualize the prescription by making an inventory of the athlete's motivational reasons (secondary gain vs training interest vs pleasure) and whether there is a preference for individual or group activities. Finally, the number of "refills" should be stated in terms of number of weeks on a particular program before it is upgraded and the time to next physician visit.

As an example of an aerobic exercise prescription, consider the 54-year-old male who has an $M\dot{V}o_2$ of 20 ml/kg/min. The initial prescription should be for walking 1 mile in 20 minutes three to four times per week for 2 weeks. Thereafter, 2 miles over 40 minutes is begun for another 2 weeks. The prescription for weeks 5 and 6 consists of 3 miles in 60 minutes. If there are no intercurrent symptoms or signs of myocardial ischemia, several minutes can be slowly trimmed from the total time allowed. The walk will slowly evolve into a rapid walk, walking jog, jog, jogging run, and then run. The objective throughout the program is to adjust the prescription sequentially so that the intensity of the training as measured by the heart rate remains 10 beats per minute below the level at which the symptoms or signs of ischemia occur.

The generic nature of the exercise prescription allows it to be applied to the entire spectrum of sports activities as well as competitors. For instance, individuals who are status postmenisectomy or who have significant lumbosacral disease (spondylolysthesis, chronic strains) should have a prescription centered around swimming for aerobic development. The prescription should be an incremental distance three to four times a week achieving 70 to 85 percent of the target heart rate.

Above all, it is imperative that the prescribing physician carefully monitor the individual's performance through personal exercise logs and re-evaluate his or her training level periodically. The monitoring process should be tailored with very close surveillance reserved for cardiac rehabilitation candidates whereas monthly evaluations may be more appropriate for the younger athlete with a chronic problem (e.g., diabetes).

CARDIOVASCULAR COMPLICATIONS OF EXERCISE

Cardiovascular events during exercise are striking, especially when occurring in presumably healthy young people during sporting events or training workouts. In fact, such occurrences are rare. Even when the exercise group is comprised of men with known coronary heart disease who are participating in a cardiac rehabilitation program, the incidence of sudden catastrophic cardiac events is low. The major cardiac complications seen during or immediately after exercise include the following:

1. Acute myocardial infarction
2. Onset of severe persistent angina
3. Persistent cardiac arrhythmias
4. Sudden death
5. Rupture of a mitral valve chordae tendineae

When the exercise activity has potential for chest trauma, there are additional rare complications:

6. Myocardial contusion
7. Traumatic aortic dissection

Patients with coronary heart disease who exercise may report symptoms lasting several hours after exercise, the etiology of which is unclear but which may relate to an impaired cardiac output:

8. Extreme or persistent postexercise fatigue
9. Sleep disturbances on the evening of exercise training

In some cases a careful medical evaluation with appropriate cardiac laboratory examination will detect underlying conditions; in other cases, prompt and capable medical care can ameliorate the consequences. In some instances, however—and most obviously for sudden death in the apparently healthy subject—we, as physicians, have nothing substantial to offer the patient.

Acute Myocardial Infarction

The most common presentation is the sudden onset of severe crushing or pressing chest pain, located in the substernal or precordial area. The pain persists for several minutes to hours and is frequently accompanied by anxiety, nausea, or diaphoresis. Careful questioning sometimes reveals a history of exertional angina in the individual, but often there is no history suggestive of coronary heart disease.

Management involves the rapid transport of the

patient to a hospital emergency room via ambulance if one is promptly available or by car if necessary. Ideal care involves the prompt arrival of an advanced life support ambulance—trained paramedics equipped and able to use IV drugs, oxygen, and an ECG monitor/defibrillator (either independently or via radio hookup to an emergency room physician). Once the subject arrives at the hospital, a 12-lead ECG is obtained and blood drawn for cardiac enzymes. A prudent course is to admit all patients with a good history, even in the face of a normal ECG. Infarct changes in the ECG often require hours to become manifest.

If the ECG remains normal and cardiac enzymes do not rise, a myocardial infarction can be excluded, but it is still incumbent on the physician to exclude underlying coronary artery disease manifesting as acute chest pain during exertion. A maximum exercise ECG exam (followed by exercise nuclear heart studies, if indicated) is appropriate and should be completed prior to allowing the subject to resume athletic endeavors.

Severe Angina

A related condition is the precipitation of a severe ischemic attack by exercise. Most frequently this occurs in the patient with known underlying coronary artery disease (either angina pectoris or a history of myocardial infarction). Severe chest pain, often persisting several minutes into rest, and ECG changes of ST depression and/or T-wave inversion are the hallmark of this condition. Initial management involves excluding a myocardial infarction. Once this is done, the clinical options include:

1. Increased antianginal medication (nitrates, β blockade, or calcium antagonists)
2. Angiography with consequent coronary bypass graft surgery if appropriate
3. Restricting the patient to activities of moderate or lower work levels.

A rational approach involves exercise ECG testing to define the exercise tolerance, followed by a trial of increased medication and repeat testing to assess consequent improvement. If there is not a significant increased tolerance, or if side-effects limit us-

able dosages, then angiography should be performed. Studies have repeatedly demonstrated enhanced exercise tolerance in the successfully coronary-bypass-grafted patient. If the initial exercise test indicates a high degree of coronary obstruction (reduced achieved heart rate with significant ST depression, chest pain, or a fall in blood pressure), then proceeding directly with coronary angiography is indicated.

Arrhythmia

Single or brief episodes of repetitive atrial or ventricular premature systoles are common with near exhaustive exercise. When there is a basic shift to a persistently abnormal rhythm, which is usually sensed by the patient, immediate medical attention is indicated. Proper medical care involves the conversion of the rhythm to normal sinus and the search for underlying conditions which may predispose the subject to exercise-related or spontaneous arrhythmias.

Depending on the arrhythmia, either medication or electrical cardioversion is indicated. Ventricular extrasystolic rhythms can be treated by lidocaine intravenously, but if blood pressure is reduced or mentation impaired (indicating a critical reduction in cardiac output), then immediate electrical cardioversion is mandatory. Atrial arrhythmias (most frequently paroxysmal atrial tachycardia, atrial fibrillation, or atrial flutter) can be treated conservatively if cardiac output is maintained. Digoxin followed by quinidine sulfate is often effective for the latter conditions, but for paroxysmal atrial tachycardia intravenous propranolol is often helpful. Once again, if cardiac output is reduced (by clinical indicators), or if conservative medical therapy is ineffective, then cardioversion is indicated.

Concomitantly with specific therapy, studies to search for these possible underlying conditions should be considered:

1. Myocardial infarction (serial ECG changes and cardiac enzymes elevations)
2. Coronary artery disease (indicated at exercise ECG and confirmed by cardiac nuclear studies or angiography)

3. Cardiomyopathy (indicated on echocardiography or gated nuclear heart studies)
4. Idiopathic hypertrophic subaortic stenosis (an echocardiographic diagnosis)
5. Prolapsed mitral valve (an echocardiographic diagnosis)
6. Pre-excitation syndrome (e.g., Wolf–Parkinson–White syndrome; an ECG diagnosis)

Sudden Death

Sudden death during or immediately following exercise is an uncommon but catastrophic event.[9] Most often it is presumed to be caused by the onset of ventricular fibrillation. In some instances it occurs due to ischemia. In the middle-aged or older population, there is a significance associated with occult coronary artery disease; in the young, congenital abnormalities, including those involving coronary artery circulation, are prominent etiologic factors. In both instances the physician, although unable to minister to the patient, does have a responsibility to family members and associates.

In a case of the young individual tragically dying during or immediately following an athletic event, there is an enormous amount of guilt and fear on the part of family members, coaches, and fellow participants. In most instances there should be no recriminations. Unless significant complaints and symptoms on the part of the young person have been ignored, both the parents and coaches should be reassured that this tragedy was, at our current level of knowledge, both unpredictable and unpreventable. Since the idiology may be congenital in the case of the young individual, an autopsy should always be performed.

Where congenital defects are demonstrated, such as idiopathic hypertrophic subaortic stenosis, noninvasive studies of siblings and parents to detect the condition in close family members should be considered. Certainly for the peace of mind of the parents, other siblings should have echocardiograms, be seen by a cardiologist, and possibly have maximum exercise ECG exams. This allows parents to see their children exercising to exhaustion without symptoms or significant cardiac problems. It is usually only after such an exam that parents allow their youngsters to return to athletic events after the death of a sibling. In the case of coaches or other individuals supervising exercise, this represents a good opportunity to review training practices and discuss the value of warm-ups, cool-downs, and avoidance of extremes of exercise. It also is a good time to review what are significant complaints on the part of youngsters during exercise and what are merely signs of fatigue and muscle weakness, which are part of any athletic training program.

Syndromes that should be considered when reviewing family members after a sudden death during exercise include congenital abnormalities such as idiopathic hypertrophic aortic stenosis, abnormalities of the coronary artery circulation (such as an anomalous origin of the left coronary artery), and electrical conduction abnormalities (such as a pre-excitation syndrome or a prolonged QT interval).

In the case of the middle-aged or older individual who dies suddenly during or following exercise, coronary artery disease with fixed obstruction or sudden and severe spasm of the coronary arteries are often thought to be the etiology. Since the death of a relatively young person does represent a risk factor especially for male children, a review of the patient's serum lipids, if available, should be performed. Cholesterol and tryglyceride studies on male children should be done, as this often may reveal unsuspected risk factors for premature atherosclerosis and lead to early dietary intervention.

Spontaneous Rupture of Chordae Tendineae

The mitral valve is "harnessed" to the papillary muscle of the left ventricular by parachute-like cords—the chordae tendineae. The chordae, necessary to allow apposition of the mitral valves during systole, are thin mesodermal structures that may spontaneously rupture. The incidence of such rupture is greater when there is an underlying tissue abnormality, such as a collagen disease, or a congenital defect of mesodermal tissues as in Marfan's syndrome.

The clinical presentation is usually a severe sharp pain in the precordial area lasting an indeterminate period of time and associated with a nonspecific change in T-wave or ST segments on the electrocardiogram (which may be only brief in duration) and a mitral insufficiency murmur. This murmur is usually a short systolic murmur heard at the apex. Its extent is related to the significance of the loss of the attachments in relationship to the apposition of the mitral valve. In most instances this is not hemodynamically significant in terms of the amount of blood being refluxed into the left atrium during systole and diagnostic evaluation and can be limited to noninvasive studies. The most specific noninvasive study is a two-dimensional echocardiogram, which often shows a flail mitral leaflet and perhaps even loose chordal echoes. Where the rupture is significant or involves the chorda close to the papillary muscle origin, mitral regurgitation may be more hemodynamically important. In this rare instance, atrial enlargement and volume overload of the left ventricle (and consequent ventricular enlargement) may occur, which may ultimately necessitate cardiac catheterization and mitral valve replacement.

Trauma to the Chest During Exercise

Certain kinds of exercise, especially those involving gymnastics, jumping, or contact activities, may result in serious chest trauma. Two significant cardiac complications of such chest trauma are the rare occurrences of aortic dissection and myocardial contusion.

Traumatic aortic dissection usually follows a severe sudden blow to the chest wall. The patient complains of a sharp, tearing midline pain possibly radiating through the chest to the back. The pain is persistent and often the patient is diaphoretic and perhaps hypo- or hypertensive. Depending on the location of the dissection of the intima, the lesion may dissect or travel back toward the aortic valve resulting in aortic insufficiency. If the dissection involves the origin of a major branch artery of the aorta, then a decreased pulse or blood pressure can be noted in that area. (For instance, the left subclavian artery, if involved, would result in a lower blood pressure in the left arm.) Dissection is a serious and emergent medical condition and requires rapid angiography to determine its extent and location. Depending on the location of the dissection and its extent of involvement of the aortic wall,

conservative therapy (usually including a β-blocking drug to decrease the force of contraction of the left ventricle) may be the initial step. Where the dissection is more significant or hemodynamic deterioration is occurring (or is expected), rapid surgical intervention is required.

Another form of injury occurring with trauma is a *direct contusion* of the heart muscle. This is actually a bruise or hematoma in the heart muscle proper and is due to the transmitted force of the chest trauma. The complaints include chest pain, persistent in nature and pressing in character. It can be associated with bruising of the chest wall. The ECG shows changes in acute myocardial infarction evolving to changes of an old myocardial infarction as the contusion is healed. This is similar to a myocardial infarction in that the individual has to be observed for cardiac arrhythmias and hemodynamic deterioration. An occasional serious problem is rupture of the heart wall at the site of the contusion, leading to a spontaneous hemopericardium and, often, death.

In the majority of instances of myocardial contusion, full healing occurs in 10 to 12 weeks. Since ECG changes may mimic those of a myocardial infarction due to coronary artery disease, the individual should be given a copy of his or her electrocardiogram along with an explanation that this represents contusion and not underlying coronary atherosclerotic disease. Such education is important in terms of further care and evaluation of the individual.

Two other complaints related to exercise should be mentioned in this chapter. In our experience, with exercise training of post-myocardial-infarction patients, excessive fatigue lasting hours after the exercise session and sleep disturbances on the night following the exercise training sessions are occasionally noted. The precise physiologic correlates of these two complaints are undetermined. They may relate to a reduced cardiac output response to exercise. We have attempted to treat such complaints with increased use of antianginal medication and, where a low cardiac output was postulated, digitalization. We have not been successful with this approach in the majority of outpatients. In most instances we have alleviated these symptoms by decreasing the intensity of exercise used during the exercise training sessions.

CONCLUSION

Cardiovascular complications ranging from spontaneously reversible chest pain or fatigue to catastrophic events such as sudden death are occasionally seen during exercise. An awareness of these problems is important if one is to be able to detect significant abnormalities on routine pre-exercise evaluations and, where this is not possible, to provide prompt diagnosis and treatment after the event. Further research into the etiology of sudden death during exercise and "clues" as to which individuals are at risk of this catastrophic complication are hopefully forthcoming.

REFERENCES

1. Morse, Robert: Exercise and the Heart. Springfield, Ill, Charles C Thomas, 1972, pp 12–15.
2. Clausen J: Circulatory adjustments to dynamic exercise and effect of physical training in normal subjects and in patients with coronary artery disease, in Sonnenblick E, Lesch M (eds): Exercise and Heart Disease. New York, Grune and Stratton, 1977, pp 39–77.
3. Powell LB: Human cardiovascular adjustments to exercise and thermal stress. Physiol Rev 54:75–159, 1974.
4. Stein R, Michielli D, Krasnow N: The cardiac response to exercise training: A resting and exercise echocardiography analysis. Am J Cardiol 46(2):219–225, 1980.
5. Zaret B, Cohen L: Cardiovascular Nuclear Medicine—Modern Concepts of Cardiovascular Disease. Dallas, American Heart Association, July 1977.
6. Verani M, Hartung G, Hoeptel-Harris J, et al.: Effects of exercise training on ventricular performed and myocardial perfusion in patients with coronary artery disease. Circulation 47:797–803, 1981.
7. Astrand P, Rodahl K: Textbook of Work Physiology. New York, McGraw-Hill, 1977, pp 389–438.
8. Stein RA, Walsh W, Bronz C, Eisenstein B, Frank F, Klier S: The clinical value of exercise training apparently healthy males of 65 years or older (abstr). Arch Intern Med, 1981.
9. Vander L, Franklin B, Rubenfire M: Cardiovascular complications of recreational physical activity. Phys Sports Med 10(6):89–98, 1982.

BIBLIOGRAPHY

Amsterdam E, Wilmore J, DeMaria A: Exercise in Cardiovascular Health and Disease. New York, Yorke Medical Books, 1977.
Astrand P, Rodahl K: Textbook of Work Physiology. New York, McGraw-Hill, 1977.
Goldberger, Emanuel: Textbook of Clinical Cardiology. St Louis, CV Mosby, 1982.
Smith E, Gyton A, Manning R, White R: Integrated mechanisms of cardiovascular response and control during exercise in the normal human, in Sonnenblick E, Lesch M (eds): Exercise and Heart Disease. New York, Grune and Stratton, 1977.

7
Cardiovascular Evaluation for Sports Participation

Richard A. Stein and Ruben S. Cooper

Children and Adolescents

Sports activities have assumed a large role in the daily lives of Americans. Intramural sports competition begins early in elementary schools and is continued in interscholastic and intercollegiate programs. Primary care physicians (i.e., family practitioners, pediatricians, and internists) are frequently asked to "clear" a youngster for competitive school sports activities. Questions such as "What do you think about my youngster playing football in junior high school?" or "Will you excuse my son/daughter from gym class?" are quite common in a daily medical practice. While such decisions cannot be made in a cavalier manner, it is seldom necessary or cost effective to refer every youngster to a pediatric cardiologist.

Pediatric cardiology has generated an overwhelming fund of knowledge and often requires new diagnostic skills, but the essential clinical skills and knowledge needed to make a clinical diagnosis have not changed drastically in the past 30 years. A reasonably accurate clinical diagnosis is often possible with a detailed history, physical examination, electrocardiogram (ECG), and a chest x ray. Nevertheless, newer noninvasive methods such as M-mode, 2-D, and pulse Doppler echocardiography, exercise stress testing, and ambulatory electrocardiographic (Holter) and blood pressure monitoring might be necessary for the proper diagnosis and medical management of both congenital and acquired heart disease in the pediatric and adolescent populations. On occasion these data need to be coupled with invasive hemodynamic and angiographic studies by a cardiac catheterization (i.e., to assess severity of obstructed or insufficient valves) before specific exercise recommendations and proper athletic counseling can be made from a medical and legal standpoint. The purpose of this chapter is to review those congenital and acquired heart problems that may be asymptomatic or clinically silent and pose problems for the physician.

PHYSICAL EXAMINATION

It has been estimated that one in three youngsters including the adolescent population have heart murmurs. Indeed, all of us have intracardiac turbulence that could easily be detected by an intracardiac phonocatheter. Thus it is not surprising that a significant number of the thin-chested pediatric population have audible murmurs. The American Academy of Pediatrics as well as other groups have suggested guidelines in the cardiac evaluation of children prior to sports participation.[1-3] Cardiac evaluation includes assessment of the following[4]:

- Innocent heart murmurs
- Potentially serious heart disease without significant heart murmurs

- Potentially serious heart disease with loud heart murmurs and commonly confused diagnoses
- Arrhythmias (benign and potentially hazardous)

Innocent Heart Murmurs

An *innocent murmur* is a heart sound which has no hemodynamic significance and is identified by the quality of the sound, its timing, and location. There are four types of innocent murmur commonly heard in children and adolescents. These patients have normal blood pressures, heart sounds, electrocardiograms, and x rays:

1. Venous hum
2. Carotid bruit
3. Vibratory or Still's murmur
4. Pulmonic ejection flow murmur

Venous Hum. While innocent murmurs are usually soft and quiet and are heard in early systole, the venous hum is an exception as it is soft in quality and continuous in timing. The murmur is due to venous drainage to the superior vena cava and thus can be abolished in a supine position or by slight neck vein compression or neck rotation. Location is often at the right upper sternal border and neck and on occasion can be heard on the left side if a left superior vena cava is present. The patent ductus arteriosus (PDA) and aortic insufficiency (AI) are in the differential diagnosis.

Carotid Bruit. The carotid bruit, a harsh systolic murmur heard best in the neck, is ejection in quality and mid-systolic in timing. Unlike in the adult population, it is not a sign of an atherosclerotic plaque.

Vibratory or Still's Murmur. The vibratory or Still's murmur is an extremely common murmur and is believed to be produced by vibrations originating from the aortic valve cusps.[5] It is most often heard in the preschool through adolescent period at the lower left sternal border.[6] The murmur is grade 1–3/6, vibratory and medium pitch in quality, and is best heard with the bell of the stethoscope in the supine position.

Pulmonic Ejection Flow Murmur. The pulmonic ejection flow murmur is detected when the patient is undergoing rapid spurts of growth, principally at the preschool and puberty ages. The murmur is an early to mid harsh systolic murmur best heard at the second left intercostal space (pulmonic area) and radiates to the lungs. It is a murmur of relative pulmonic stenosis due to a flow gradient across the valve. This murmur can often mimic mild pulmonic stenosis and an atrial septal defect, but unlike these two conditions the innocent murmur has a normally split second heart sound with a normal intensity of the pulmonic component. The addition of the electrocardiogram, x ray, and echocardiogram differentiates these conditions.

Clearly, we wish to identify those patients who may be at risk for sudden death due to an arrhythmia or a cardiac syncopal episode or who may have clinically silent lesions which may progress; i.e., aortic stenosis (AS), hypertrophic obstructive cardiomyopathy (HOCM), subaortic membranes, and aortic insufficiency.

Potentially Serious Heart Disease Without Significant Heart Murmurs

1. Atrial septal defect
2. Coarctation of the aorta
3. Cardiomyopathies

Atrial Septal Defect. As mentioned earlier, this is often confused with the innocent pulmonic flow murmur. Children and young adults are often asymptomatic. The murmur heard is caused by an increased blood volume flowing across the pulmonic valve and is indeed a murmur of relative pulmonic stenosis. The murmur is often grade 2–3/6 in intensity, is ejection and harsh in quality, and is heard in mid to late systole. The second heart sound is persistently split in all phases of respiration and is usually normal in intensity. A mid diastolic flow rumble at the mid left sternal border is often heard due to a flow gradient across the tricuspid valve in diastole. Two-dimensional and contrast 2-D echocardiography are helpful in visualizing the defect.

Coarctation of the Aorta. This is the most common treatable cause of hypertension in the pediatric population. While the diagnosis is not particularly difficult to make, Stafford et al. recently noted the rather late age in its diagnosis and treatment.[7] Palpation and blood pressure recordings in all four extremities confirm the diagnosis. The murmur is typically grade 2/6 in intensity and is a systolic ejection murmur best heard in the left intraclavicular and left subscapular area. An associated murmur of bicuspid aortic valve stenosis may be present.

Cardiomyopathies. Cardiomyopathies are often silent and may present with clinical features such as easy fatigability, dyspnea, palpitations, dizziness, angina, and syncope. These symptoms are particularly common with all forms of left ventricular outflow tract obstruction. We concentrate on hypertrophic obstructive cardiomyopathy (HOCM), which may include both nonobstructive and obstructive forms of asymmetric septal hypertrophy (ASH).

Asymmetric Septal Hypertrophy (ASH). This is transmitted as an autosomal dominant trait with a high degree of penetrance. There is, however, a broad clinical spectrum ranging from no left ventricular outflow tract obstruction at rest or after provocative maneuvers to obstruction at rest or obstruction only after provocative intervention. There is marked asymmetry of the ventricular septum when compared to the posterior left ventricular free wall and disarray of the muscle cell bundles histologically. On physical exam there is usually an apical lift and a sharp and rapid rising arterial pulse. There is perhaps a palpable thrill along the mid sternal border and a systolic ejection murmur heard along the left sternal border or apex. An associated murmur of mitral regurgitation may be heard as well. The electrocardiogram may be useful if left ventricular hypertrophy with strain or a Wolf–Parkinson–White (WPW) pattern is seen. The chest x ray is not particularly sensitive or specific. Echocardiography, however, is highly reliable by demonstrating the abnormal ratio of septal to left ventricular posterior wall thickness as well as systolic anterior motion (SAM) of the mitral valve leaflet. Mid systolic closure of the aortic valve is often noted as well.

Potentially Serious Heart Disease with Heart Murmur and Commonly Confused Diagnoses

1. Aortic and pulmonic valve stenosis
2. Ventricular septal defect and subaortic stenosis

3. Acyanotic tetralogy of Fallot and ventricular septal defect

Many of these lesions present with loud systolic murmurs and palpable thrills. Coupled with the electrocardiogram, x ray, and echocardiogram, diagnosis is usually not difficult.

Adolescents and young adults enjoy physical activity and competition with their peers.[8] Thus, exclusion or restriction of these activities should be imposed only after thoughtful evaluation of the following factors:

1. Severity of the cardiac problem
2. Physical requirements of the sport in question
3. Type of supervision of the individual by the instructor or coach

Physiologically, exercise can be thought of as either principally *aerobic*, in which there is a decrease of peripheral vascular resistance with exercise, or *isometric*, in which there is an increase in the peripheral vascular resistance. (See Chapter 6 for more detailed discussion.) Clearly, isometric exercise presents the cardiovascular system with a greater burden.

Shaffer, in his review of the adolescent athlete, notes that it is advantageous to classify sports into three groups according to the physical requirements[9]:

1. Body contact (collision) sports: football, basketball, wrestling, hockey, soccer, lacrosse, and rugby.
2. Endurance noncontact sports: track, swimming, tennis, crew, skiing, gymnastics, and volleyball.
3. Leisure sports that require minimal physical requirements: bowling, golf, fencing, and archery.

A number of publications have listed guidelines for disqualifying conditions for sports participation (see Table 7-1).[10–13] Once an accurate diagnosis is reached it is useful to consider the cardiac problems under groupings as classified by The New York Heart Association and also by Neill and Haroutmian for patients with acquired and congenital heart disease (see Tables 7-2 and 7-3).[14]

TABLE 7-1. DISQUALIFYING CONDITIONS FOR SPORTS PARTICIPATION

Cardiovascular Conditions	Contact	Noncontact Endurance	Other
Mitral stenosis, aortic stenosis, aortic insufficiency, coarctation of aorta, cyanotic heart disease, recent carditis of any etiology	x	x	x
Hypertension on organic basis	x	x	x
Previous heart surgery for congenital or acquired heart disease	x	x	

(From Shaffer TE: The adolescent athlete. Pediatr Clin N Am 20:837–849, 1973, with permission.)

1. A functionally normal heart with less than a grade 2 murmur
2. A grade 3 murmur with a heart size or a cardiothoracic ratio of less than 0:60 on the x ray with the right bundle branch block on the cardiogram but no major arrhythmias
3. A heterogeneous group that needs very careful follow-up because of the risk of progression and severity
4. Significantly functionally impaired patients with the major possibility of progressive changes

ARRHYTHMIAS

Disorders in rhythm are best evaluated by palpation of the pulse for a full 60 seconds coupled with a standard 12-lead electrocardiogram. If atrial or ventricular ectopy is noted during the electrocardiogram, a long lead-II rhythm strip recorded following exercise (e.g., sit-ups or deep breathing) is useful. Additional testing studies such as ambulatory (Holter 12 to 24 hour) ECG recording, maximal exercise stress testing, and on rare occasions electrophysiologic study may be necessary. A resting electrocardiogram should always be reviewed for the presence of disturbances in rate and rhythm to include:

1. Congenital or acquired heart block
2. Prolonged QT interval syndromes
3. Multifocal premature ventricular contractions (PVCs)
4. Bradytachy arrhythmias due to:
   A. sick sinus node syndrome (SSNS)
   B. pre-excitation syndrome (WPW—types A, B)

Strong and Linder give some useful guidelines when confronted with ectopy[15]:

1. Atrial or ventricular unifold ectopy is benign and requires no treatment or exercise restrictions.
2. Ventricular ectopy at times may initially increase with mild exercise and cause some concern. In these situations maximal stress testing with maximal heart rates at 140 to 150 per minute may actually abolish the ectopy due to catecholamine supression and clear the patient for sports activity.
3. Supraventricular tachycardia such as paroxysmal atrial tachycardia (PAT) and the pre-excitation syndrome (WPW—types A, B) need not necessarily be restricted but should be referred for Holter recordings and exercise testing.
4. Paroxysmal ventricular tachycardia and multifocal PVCs often need to be treated and require further cardiac evaluation.

Clearly, valvular and subvalvular aortic stenosis including HOCM should be thoroughly evaluated as these lesions can be silent and progress and present with cardiac syncope. Echocardiography as well as exercise testing often aid in the selection of patients who need cardiac catheterization. Patients with documented mild gradients in valvular aortic stenosis need not be restricted from competitive sports.

Abnormal blood pressure responses in postoperative coarctation patients have been documented by a number of investigators.[16–19] This group may need to be restricted even though no gradient is noted at rest. Aortic valve insufficiency is often

TABLE 7-2. FUNCTIONAL GROUPING

GROUP A.	**NORMAL FUNCTIONAL CARDIAC STATUS**
PDA	Postoperative (PO) with no residual defect
ASD	(PO) no residual defect, normal sinus rhythm (NSR)
VSD	(PO) no residual defect, NSR
VSD	Spontaneous closure
TOF	Corrected, no residual defect, NSR
Other	Anomalous subclavian artery, right aortic arch, dextrocardia and situs inversus, other defects of embryologic and possibly genetic significance, but not affecting cardiac function
GROUP B.	**MILD CARDIAC DEFECT**
VSD	Qp:Qs <2:1 with normal PA pressure, NSR unoperated or PO with residual shunt
PSV	RV–PA pressure difference 50 mm or less (unoperated or PO)
COA	(PO) normal blood pressure, arm to leg BP difference <20 mm Hg
ECD	(PO) with mild residual mitral insufficiency
MIC	Congenital mitral insufficiency due to prolapse or other causes; mild, no severe arrhythmia
TOF	(PO) mild residual pulmonic stenosis = insufficiency = small VSD = RBBB
Other	Bicuspid aortic valve (BAV) with mild insufficiency = LV–aorta pressure difference of 20 mm or less: small atrial or other shunts (PO or unoperated) with Qp:Qs 1.5:1 or less; peripheral pulmonic stenosis (PPS) mild
GROUP C.	**MODERATE CARDIAC DEFECT**
VSD	Qp:Qs > 2:1 and/or with aortic insufficiency, pulmonic stenosis or anomalous RV muscle bundle
PSV	RV–PA pressure difference > 50 mm Hg (unoperated or PO)
COA	(Unoperated or PO) with BP differences arms and legs > 30 mm Hg and/or arm BP greater than 150/95
TOF	(PO) with RV–PA pressure difference > 50 mm Hg, grossly dilated or calcified outflow patch, aortic or tricuspid insufficiency or significant arrhythmias
ASV	(Unoperated or PO) with LV–aortic pressure difference 20 mm Hg = aortic insufficiency
TGV	(Postmustard) = residual shunts or arrhythmias
Other	Unoperated (or PO) PDA, ASD, AV canal etc. requiring surgery or reoperation: aortic insufficiency, moderate. Arrhythmias: sick sinus syndrome, other. Cardiomegaly with C/T ratio 60% = with any congenital lesion.
GROUP D.	**SEVERE CARDIAC DEFECT**
Cyanotic	
TOF	Unoperated or with palliative shunt, PO open repair with homograft, prosthetic valve, or with severe arrhythmia
TGV	All not in Group C
SIV	All types with or without prior shunts
TAT	
PVOD	Eisenmenger reaction or primary pulmonary hypertension
Other	Truncus variants, pulmonary atresia with VSD, rare cyanotic lesions
Acyanotic	

Cardiomyopathy including hypertrophic subaortic stenosis (1HS) or following fibroelastosis or ligation anomalous left coronary artery, other

LV outflow obstruction, e.g., subaortic tunnel or other unrelieved aortic stenosis with LV–aortic pressure difference of 80 mm Hg or greater

(From Neill CA, Haroutmian LM, in Moss AJ, Adams FH, Emmanouildes GC (eds): Heart Disease in Infants, Children and Adolescents. Baltimore, Williams & Wilkins, pp 719–724. © by Williams & Wilkins, with permission.)

TABLE 7-3. PROGRESSIVE CHANGES[a]: RISKS[b] AND METHODS OF ASSESSMENT

	Group				Methods of Assessment
	A	B	C	D	
Stenosis or outflow obstruction	0	0	M	H	ECG, vector
Valvar insufficiency	0	0	M	M	Clinical, echo, x ray
Cardiomegaly	0	L	L	M	X ray, echo
Congestive failure	0	0	L	L	Clinical, x ray, echo
Calcification	0	0	L	L	X ray
Polycythemia	0	0	0	M	Hematology, oximetry
PVOD	0	0	L	M	Clinical + radionuclide scanning

[a]Other progressive changes may include systemic hypertension in coarctation.
[b]H, high risk (10% or greater); M, moderate (5–10%); L, low (less than 5%); 0, not observed in series.
(From Neill CA, Haroutmian LM, in Moss AJ, Adams FH, Emmanouildes GC (eds): Heart Disease in Infants, Children and Adolescents. Baltimore, Williams & Wilkins, pp 719–724. © by Williams & Wilkins, with permission.)

difficult to grade clinically, although newer ultrasound methods using Doppler postoperative techniques may prove useful in the future. Until then, those with moderate aortic and mitral insufficiency should be restricted from competitive sports. Always be wary of that great basketball player who may have Marfan's syndrome and runs the risk of a dissection due to an aneurysm of the descending aorta.

CONCLUSION

Heart murmurs are common in youngsters and are often benign. The primary care physician needs to assess the patient's hemodynamic status and couple this with the appropriate exercise recommendations.

REFERENCES

1. American Academy of Pediatrics Committee on the Pediatric Aspects of Physical Fitness, Recreation and Sports: Cardiac evaluation for participation in sports. News Comments 28 (April):2, 1977.
2. Schell NB: Cardiac evaluation of school sports participants. Guidelines approved by the Medical Society of the State of New York. NYS J Med 78:942, 1978.
3. Schaffer TE, Rose KD: Cardiac evaluation for participation in school sports. J Am Med Assoc 228:398–399, 1974.
4. Golinko RJ: Sports medicine—The young athlete: Diagnostic problems and cardiac evaluation. Clinical Symposium, Brookdale Hospital Medical Center, April 9, 1981.
5. Kulangara RJ, Strong WB, Miller MD: Cardiovascular exam of the child. Differential diagnosis of heart murmurs in children. Postgrad Med 72:2, 1982.
6. Castle RF, Craig E: Auscultation of the heart in infants and children. Pediatrics 26:511–561, 1960.
7. Stafford MA, Griffiths SP, Gersony WM: Coarctation of the aorta: A study in delayed detection. Pediatrics 69:159–163, 1982.
8. Starek PJ: Athletic performance in children with cardiovascular problems. Phys Sports Med 10(2):78–89, 1982.
9. Shaffer TE: The adolescent athlete. Pediatr Clin N Am 20:837–849, 1973.
10. American Medical Association Committee on Medical Aspects of Sports: Guide for Medical Evaluation of Candidates for School Sports, Chicago, AMA, 1972.
11. Joint Committee, American Academy of Pediatrics: Competitive athletics for children of elementary school age. Pediatrics 42:703, 1968.
12. American Heart Association ad hoc Committee on Rehabilitation of the Young Cardiac: Recreational activity and career choice recommendations for use by physicians, counselling physical education directors, vocational counselors, parents and young patients with heart disease. Circulation 43:459, 1971.
13. Rose KD: Which cardiovascular problems should disqualify athletes? Phys Sports Med. 3:62–68, 1975.

14. Neill CA, Haroutmian LM: The adolescent and young adult with congenital heart disease, in Moss AJ, Adams FH, Emmanouildes GC: Heart Disease in Infants, Children, and Adolescents. Baltimore, Williams & Wilkins, 1977, pp 719–724.

15. Strong WB, Linder CW: Pre-participation health evaluation for competitive sports. Pediatrics Rev 4:113–121, 1982.

16. Maron BJ, Humphries O, Rowe RD, et al: Prognosis of surgically corrected coarctation of the aorta: A 20-year postoperative appraisal. Circulation 46:119, 1973

17. Simon AB, Zloto AE: Coarctation of the aorta: Longitudinal assessment of operated patients. Circulation 50:456, 1974

18. James FW, Kaplan S: Systolic hypertension during submaximal exercise after correction of coarctation of aorta. Circulation 50:11, 1974.

19. Kutayli F, Taylor A, Webb H, et al: Submaximal standing exercise testing in coarctation of the aorta. Presented at Proceedings, American Academy of Pediatrics, Washington, DC, 1975.

ADULTS

The cardiovascular examination and evaluation performed prior to initiating exercise training for adults must achieve several goals:

1. Detection and assessment of unsuspected cardiovascular disease
2. Evaluation of known cardiovascular disease and of exercise tolerance (with regard to the chosen sport or activity)
3. Education of the individual with regard to prudent exercise practices
4. Evaluation and education regarding coronary heart disease risk factors (it may be one of the few occasions, especially in adult life, when the individual may undergo a history and physical exam)

DETECTION AND ASSESSMENT OF UNSUSPECTED CARDIOVASCULAR DISEASE

History

A careful history regarding cardiovascular symptoms is of paramount importance. These specific areas are to be addressed:

1. Chest pain (ask also about "pressure, tightness, burning")
2. shortness of breath on exertion, and/or orthopnea and paroxysmal nocturnal dyspnea
3. Palpitations
4. Fainting or dizziness at rest or with exertion

Chest pain syndromes should be defined with regard to character, location, and possible precipitating factors (e.g., diet, exercise, or position). If the patient uses nitroglycerin preparations, then the response of the chest pain to sublingual nitroglycerin should be elicited. *Shortness of breath* on exertion is important relative to the exertion level, so care should be taken to define this in terms of activities (e.g., walking, step climbing). *Palpitations* may be single or occasional "thumps" (usually ventricular or supraventricular premature beats, or sustained periods of irregular or rapid heart beats). In addition to current symptoms, the history should screen for indicators of congenital and/or familial cardiovascular disorders. Questions regarding childhood heart murmurs, rheumatic fever, childhood cyanosis, and frequent respiratory infections should be part of this history as should be questions regarding atherosclerotic disease [myocardial infarction (MI) or cerebrovascular accident (CVA)] in parents and siblings, and sudden death in family members.

Physical Exam

Examination of the cardiovascular system must be comprehensive. A full 60-second pulse increases the likelihood of detecting rhythm irregularities, and blood pressure must be obtained. If pressures are elevated, additional blood pressure recordings in the other arm and the legs should be obtained to exclude a coarctation of the aorta.

The cardiac exam should include palpation for thrills and precordial or sternal heaves. Auscultation must, in addition to the standard exam, include listening over the left parasternal area in the sitting position during held expiration (for an aortic regurgitant blowing diastolic murmur), the left parasternal area during Valsalva's maneuver (for the systolic murmur of idiopathic hypertrophic subaortic stenosis), and at the apex or Erbs point while standing (for the click and/or late systolic murmur of a mitral valve prolapse).

Peripheral pulses should be palpated in all four extremities (including femorals, popliteals, dorsalis pedis, and posterior tibial pulses). Carotid arteries should be auscultated for bruits (suggesting atherosclerotic narrowing and possible friable plaque formation). The abdominal exam should include palpation in the midline for a pulsatile mass suggesting an aortic aneurysm.

Laboratory Studies

Suitable laboratory studies relevant to cardiovascular disease include a chest x ray, an ECG, and blood tests for total cholesterol and triglycerides as "first-order" studies, and exercise ECG testing and echocardiography as "second-order" studies. Specific diagnostic problems relating to underlying disease may on occasion necessitate nuclear cardiac studies (thallium 201 perfusion studies and technetium 99 gated nuclear angiocardiography at rest and exercise) or cardiac catheterization and coronary angiography.

The choice of laboratory studies relates to the subject's age, symptoms, and history.

Asymptomatic. Patients presenting with no symptoms should be tested as follows:

1. In premenopausal women and young adults of both sexes without positive historical findings, no laboratory studies are needed.
2. In men over 35, an ECG and a chest x ray are advisable, as is a serum test for cholesterol and triglycerides (regarding risk factor analysis)

3. In men and women over 50 who have been sedentary and are about to initiate an exercise program, a symptom-limited maximal exercise ECG is suggested to screen (with limitations in sensitivity and specificity) for coronary occlusive disease and to evaluate exercise tolerance.

Symptomatic. Patients with symptoms or historical findings clearly require specific laboratory tests to define their etiology and significance. Examples follow:

1. *Heart murmurs:* An ECG is always indicated. An echocardiogram to define chamber size and wall and valve motion is often prudent, especially before labeling a murmur as innocent.
2. *Anginal chest pain:* An ECG is required, as is often an exercise ECG. If the latter is equivocal, then a nuclear cardiac study should be performed to exclude or assess coronary artery disease.
3. *Palpitations:* An ECG is required. A 24-hour ambulatory ECG (Holter) is a good idea to help define the type of arrhythmia and its prevalence. An exercise ECG is indicated if the symptoms are related to exertion.

Evaluation of Symptoms and Findings

Although it is not possible in this chapter to provide an exhaustive review of the prudent evaluations of symptoms and findings, the following areas relevant to young adults and older adults encompass the more common areas of concern.

Young Adults

Chest Pain. Consider coronary artery disease (premature atherosclerosis or, in rare cases, arteritis associated with systemic lupus erythematosis), Idiopathic hypertrophic subaortic stenosis (IHSS), pulmonic hypertension, aortic stenosis (congenital), or anomalous origin of a coronary artery. *IHSS* is suggested by a left parasternal murmur and confirmed by echocardiographic findings of a thickened intraventricular septum and abnormal systolic anterior motion of the anterior mitral valve. *Aortic stenosis* is suggested by the characteristic high right parasternal systolic murmur and thrill and ECG findings of left ventricular hypertrophy. *Anomalous origin* of a coronary artery is associated with an abnormal resting ECG (infarct patterns), as is *pulmonary hypertension* (right ventricular predominance). *Coronary artery disease* is difficult to diagnose in its early stages in the young adult since it is rare and often unsuspected. Exercise ECG studies, nuclear cardiac studies, and perhaps coronary angiography are appropriate diagnostic techniques.

Dyspnea. Dyspnea after only moderate exertion may often be related either to a very untrained state (e.g., recent confinement to bed or a lifestyle that eschews physical exertion) or marked obesity. If the history of exercise intolerance is unclear, an exercise ECG exam can precisely define the range and any limiting factor (e.g., dyspnea, leg fatigue, exhaustion, or chest pain). Pathologic conditions to consider are as follow:

1. Valvular disease (aortic stenosis or regurgitation, mitral stenosis or regurgitation)
2. Septal defects (ASD or VSD) with significant left to right shunting
3. Cardiomyopathy
4. Coronary artery disease

In the last case, exercise-induced ischemia may raise left ventricular end diastolic pressure due to altered diastolic ventricular compliance or reduced systolic function. Another possible cause is mitral regurgitation due to papillary muscle dysfunction. Careful cardiovascular examination and echocardiography can usually define anatomic lesions (valves and septal wall defects) and show ventricular enlargement and reduced function indicative of congestive cardiomyopathy. Ischemia-related ventricular dysfunction is best evaluated by a rest and exercise gated or "first-pass" nuclear angiocardiogram allowing observation of ventricular size and motion and calculation of ejection fraction at rest and during exercise. Ischemia related to papillary muscle dysfunction is diagnosed by the presence of an exercise-induced mitral regurgitation murmur, best observed during the exercise ECG examination.

Palpitations. These commonly include paroxysmal atrial tachycardia, atrial flutter, or atrial fibrillation. Occasionally these represent ventricular

arrhythmias. An ECG and a 24-hour ambulatory ECG should define the arrhythmia. A search for predisposing factors such as mitral valve disease or prolapse, cardiomyopathy, or atrial septal defect involves examination and echocardiography. A pre-excitation syndrome (such as Wolf–Parkinson–White) will be seen on the 12-lead ECG, unless it is intermittent, and may be the predisposing factor. Ventricular premature contractions are usually benign if they are only occasional and occur singly. They may, however, indicate coronary artery disease or cardiomyopathy.

Syncope or Dizziness. Common factors that underlie these symptoms are paroxysmal arrhythmias that interfere with cardiac output. These may be ectopic tachyarrhythmias or may be a heart block causing a bradyarrhythmia. Occasionally these may indicate a congenital AV heart block with a junctional escape rhythm unable to increase in response to exercise. The 12-lead ECG defines this, and a resting pulse below 50 should suggest it as a possibility. Left ventricular outflow tract lesions such as congenital aortic stenosis or IHSS may present with exercise syncope or dizziness.

Older Adults. Many of the same conditions noted above apply to men and women over 50 as well. The likelihood, however, is that an acquired condition is more likely than a congenital abnormality. Coronary artery occlusive disease is more common and must be considered along with pain, dyspnea, and arrhythmias. Calcific aortic stenosis is more frequent in the elderly, with findings related to outflow tract obstruction being common.

EVALUATION OF KNOWN CARDIOVASCULAR DISEASE AND OF EXERCISE TOLERANCE

The more severe and extensive cardiac lesions (arterial occlusive, valvular, or myopathic) preclude the use of all but low levels of activity. However, many patients with cardiovascular disease—and many who have undergone coronary artery bypass grafting, cardiac valve replacements, or anatomic repairs of congenital or acquired abnormalities—can and should engage in regular exercise. The determination of the work load that they may sustain without risk of complication is based on an understanding of the pathophysiology of the specific lesion and on their performance during a symptom-limited, maximum exercise ECG exam.

The patient with coronary artery disease is frequently limited by exhaustion. If this occurs at an appropriate exercise level, it suggests there is no significant degree of ischemia due to coronary artery occlusive disease, and that maximum cardiac output has not been significantly limited by loss of muscle mass from the infarct. Anginal pain as the limiting factor during exercise testing, with or without associated ST depression, indicates coronary artery occlusive disease affecting viable areas of heart muscle. The earlier in the exercise protocol and the lower the heart rate × blood pressure product at which pain occurs, the more significant is the extent of disease.

If exhaustion or dyspnea limits the exercise tolerance at a very reduced level, then limitation of ventricular reserve is indicated, due either to a reduced ability to contract (a low ejection fraction) because of the heart muscle lost at infarction, or to ischemia in other areas of heart wall, associated with exercise, causing a reduction in stroke volume. Nuclear angiocardiography provides an accurate and noninvasive method for determination of ventricular function at rest and during exercise, and thus can precisely define the presence and the extent of ventricular dysfunction.

Studies performed to assess exercise tolerance should all be done in the setting of optimum medical therapy. Patients should continue medication up to the time of testing. Frequently, a repeat test is indicated after an additional drug or increase in drug therapy is initiated. After such testing, exercise is usually prescribed to levels of activity associated with heart rates at 75 to 85 percent of that achieved at the point of termination of the test. If, however, this level of exertion is associated with anginal pain, then either the level of exercise allowed must be further reduced, or a sublingual nitrate can be used just prior to exercise. The presence of significant arrhythmias with exercise indicates the need for antiarrhythmic drug therapy and repeat exercise testing prior to initiating exercise training.

Patients with aortic stenosis usually should not perform strenuous exercise, as the increasing cardiac output required will be associated with significantly elevated left ventricular systolic pressures. On a chronic basis, this might accelerate the development of left ventricular hypertrophy; on an acute basis, it may be associated with chest pain or syncope. Patients with mild valve stenosis (and very low pressure gradients across the valve) and those who have had their valve surgically replaced should be exercise tested. Particular attention to the blood pressure response to exercise is necessary. Exercise levels of the recreation or training activity level must be associated with normally increasing systolic blood pressure and must not be at levels of significant fatigue.

These same guidelines apply to congenital septal defects. Exercise testing to ensure a normally increasing cardiac output (increasing blood pressure and total body oxygen consumption per minute) without excessive increases in pulmonary capillary pressure (manifested by dyspnea) is indicated. An exercise level should be set within the range of normal physiologic responses and freedom from symptoms.

EDUCATION OF THE INDIVIDUAL WITH REGARD TO PRUDENT EXERCISE PRACTICES

The safety, physiologic benefit, and enjoyment of regular exercise is enhanced when the subject has a basic knowledge of areas of concern including:

- Warm-up and cool-down procedures
- Symptoms that should indicate to the individual when to stop exercise and seek medical attention
- A rational program of exercise and activities to meet one's goals
- Adaptations of exercise programs to environmental conditions

Warm-up and Cool-down

Exercise performance is improved when preceded by a period of gradually increasing activity. This appears to be a factor both in muscle mechanics and in cardiovascular response. Individuals perform a given task better (e.g., swim or run faster) following a warm-up. The levels of cardiac oxygen requirement and supply remain in balance in normal individuals with exercise following a warm-up activity as opposed to a sudden burst of strenuous exercise. An effective warm-up has two components: muscular stretching and physiologic preparation.

Stretching. Gradual stretches of the muscle groups to be utilized in the activity should be performed for at least 5 minutes preceding exercise. Running, for example, should be preceded by stretching exercises involving the gastrocnemius, Achilles tendon, quadriceps, and hamstrings.

Physiologic Preparation. This should comprise 5 to 10 minutes of gradually increasing levels of activity, finally arriving at the level to be achieved in the event of sport. It should precede the activity by only a few minutes.

After completing the exercise activity, a cooldown period of gradually decreasing activity (e.g., "walking down" after a run) and a second set of stretching exercises is indicated. These warm-up and cool-down programs reduce the incidence of muscle soreness and strains and enhance enjoyment by improving performance.

Symptoms of Concern

Patients should be advised that any of the following symptoms justify the cessation of exercise and the obtainment of prompt medical care and evaluation:

1. A pressing and/or persistent pain of any nature that is in the chest, throat, or arm that occurs and increases with exercise. This is easily distinguished from the work of breathing chest discomfort associated with the higher levels of exertion.
2. Dizziness, fainting, or blurring of vision, which may suggest a reduced cardiac output
3. Palpitations

4. Recurrent headache
5. Excessive fatigue or weakness occurring during exercise or persisting for hours afterward.

EVALUATION AND EDUCATION REGARDING CORONARY HEART DISEASE (CHD) RISK FACTORS

For both the healthy individual and individuals with coronary heart disease, the pre-exercise evaluation is an excellent opportunity for coronary heart disease risk factor assessment and the development of a CHD risk reduction program. Factors to be assessed include the following:

1. Blood pressure
2. Smoking history
3. Serum cholesterol and triglycerides
4. Diabetes (fasting blood sugar)
5. Gout (serum uric acid)
6. Diet (especially as regards cholesterol and saturated fat content)
7. Obesity
8. Exercise patterns

Careful counseling with respect to the cessation of smoking, compliance with blood pressure mediation, and strict adherence to a low-cholesterol, low-saturated-fat diet are the three major components of a preventive program. In addition, appropriate loss of weight and regular exercise should be advised. Often, "good advice" is not sufficient, and direct physician referral to a cardiac cooking program, weight reduction, and smoking cessation groups are of more value.

CONCLUSION

The role of the physician in the cardiac assessment process prior to initiating an exercise program goes beyond the traditional role of "healer." In addition, it requires the physician to be a thoughtful, inquisitive investigator and an effective counselor and educator.

BIBLIOGRAPHY

Corday E, Dodge HT (eds): Symposium on identification and management of the candidate for sudden cardiac death. Am J Cardiol 39:813, 1977.

Goldberger E (ed): Textbook of Clinical Cardiology. St. Louis, CV Mosby, 1982.

Maron BJ, Roberts WC, Hugh MA, et al: Sudden death in young athletes. Circulation 62:218, 1980.

Rose KD: Which cardiovascular "problems" should disqualify athletes? Phys Sports Med. 3:62–68, 1975.

Schaffer TE, Rose KD: Cardiac evaluation for participation in school sports. J Am Med Assoc 228:398–399, 1974.

Schell NB: Cardiac evaluation of school sports participants. Guidelines approved by the Medical Society of the State of New York. NYS J Med 78:942, 1978.

Vander L, et al: Cardiovascular complications of recreational physical activity. Phys Sports Med 10(6):89–98, 1982.

Wilson P (ed): Adult Fitness and Cardiac Rehabilitation. Baltimore, University Park Press, 1975.

Wolff G: Cardiologic assessment in participants of Pop Warner Junior League Football. Am J Sports Med 8(3):200–201, 1980.

8
Exercise ECG Testing

Richard A. Stein

Exercise ECG testing (stress testing) involves the continuous or periodic recording of blood pressure, heart rate, symptoms (e.g., chest pain, dyspnea, and fatigue), and selected electrocardiographic leads during increasing exercise loads. It is a unique opportunity to record data during exercise and, in the case of the patient with cardiac disease, to reproduce symptoms. Prior to the development of such tests, physicians were limited to examinations and laboratory data obtained in the resting state. Since the major forms of heart disease (coronary artery occlusion and congestive heart failure) first present with chest pain or dyspnea on exertion, a resting evaluation is, by its nature, somewhat limited.

INDICATIONS

Exercise ECG testing is indicated for the evaluation of chest pain. It is one of the pieces of information helpful to the physician in the diagnosis or exclusion of coronary disease. It is also appropriate for the sedentary male over the age of 50 who has major risk factors for coronary artery disease (cigarette smoking, hypercholesterolemia, or hypertension) and is indicated for the patient with known coronary artery disease or angina or who has had a myocardial infarction. In addition, it is useful in the case of patients who complain of reduced exercise capabilities in whom the physician needs to document and quantify this limitation. Other indications include the assessment of cardiac arrhythmias and the effectiveness of antiarrhythmic drug therapy during exercise.

Physiologic Basis of the Exercise ECG

As discussed in Chapter 6, increasing exercise loads are associated with increased cardiac output requirements and concomitant increases in myocardial oxygen requirement ($M\dot{V}O_2$). When myocardial oxygen demand exceeds the supply capability of narrowed coronary arteries, the result is ischemia (imbalance between requirement and delivery of oxygenated blood). The physiologic, clinical, and ECG responses to ischemia are the basis for a "positive test," i.e., one indicative of coronary artery occlusive disease. Exercise tolerance relates to increasing cardiac output and the limited ability of diseased heart muscle to increase the stroke volume with exercise. A limited maximum heart rate will result in reduced maximum cardiac output and thus reduced exercise capacity. Other factors that limit cardiac output are mitral valve stenosis and aortic or subaortic stenosis, which create outflow obstructions. Limited cardiac output may not only reduce exercise capacity, but may also manifest as dizziness, a drop in blood pressure, or visual disturbances.

Suitability for Exercise ECG Testing

Patients should be evaluated prior to exercise ECG testing to exclude those in whom the study is contraindicated due to increased risk. In addition, those in whom the results may not be diagnostic may be inappropriate for testing. The evaluation should include a history with regard to cardiovascular symptoms, in order to exclude patients with:

1. Unstable angina (recent increase or onset of pain)
2. Frequent nocturnal angina
3. Syncope or dizziness on moderate exercise

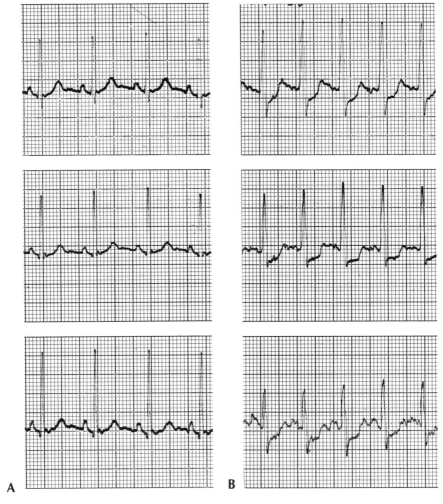

FIGURE 8-1. ECG configurations seen with stress testing. **(A)** Resting ECG. **(B)** Depressed ST segments during treadmill stress test.

A physical examination is performed to exclude the following conditions:

1. Pericarditis (rub on auscultation)
2. Congestive heart failure (rales on auscultation)
3. Significant aortic stenosis (systolic murmur, pulses parvis and tardis)
4. Carotid artery stenosis (bruit over artery)

5. Resting hypertension (above 180 systolic and 120 diastolic)

A resting 12-lead ECG is performed. The following findings are usually contraindications to exercise ECG testing:

1. Heart block (second degree–mobitz II, and third degree)

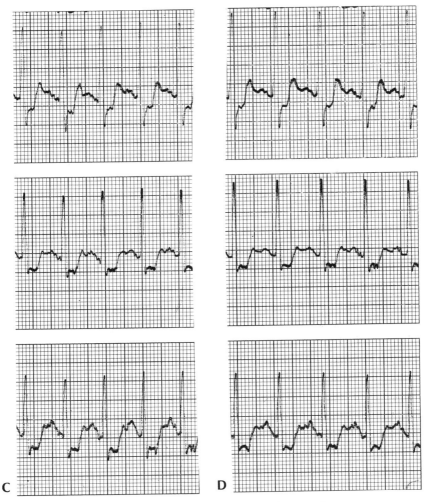

(C) 2 min after exercise. **(D)** 4 min after exercise.

2. Frequent newly noted VPCs or sustained bi-geminy

3. "Recent" infarct pattern that is new or of unknown age (Q wave, inverted T, ST elevation)

4. ECG changes suggestive of significant ischemia (ST depression, significant T-wave inversion)

The following QRS-complex abnormalities of the ECG make the diagnosis of exercise-induced is-chemia from ST depression uncertain, and may therefore represent "relative" contraindications:

1. A pre-excitation (Wolf–Parkinson–White [WPW]) pattern

2. Left ventricular hypertrophy

3. Resting ST depression

4. Left bundle branch block

Psychological factors, relating to fear of a catastrophic cardiovascular event during exercise testing, may limit the exam. To some degree a careful explanation of the procedure, emphasizing the safety precautions and the staff's ability to manage most complications, as well as the patient's ability to terminate the test at any time can overcome this barrier. In the occasional patient, however, the fear and the reaction to it may contraindicate the exam.

EXERCISE ECG PROCEDURE

After a complete description and explanation of the exam, an informed consent is signed by the patient. A history is then obtained, with special attention to current drug therapy (name of drug, dosage, and time of last dose) and any cardiac symptoms occurring within the past 24 hours. The 12-lead ECG is then obtained and reviewed by the physician who will perform the test.

Electrodes are placed on the patient's torso to allow an artifact-free recording of selected leads during exercise. The electrodes are adhesive and are usually placed at the iliac rest (lower extremity limb leads) and over the mid clavicle (upper extremity limb leads). Precordial leads are placed in the usual position. The choice of which leads to monitor is based on the sophistication of the available monitoring and recording equipment and studies of the relative diagnostic sensitivity of various leads. Most (over 85 percent) of depression in the ST segment with exercise is noted in precordial leads V_4 and V_5.[1] The addition of inferior leads (II or aV_F) increases the sensitivity to above 93 percent. Optimum detection may occur with the use of a 12-lead ECG during exercise, which usually requires a three-channel recording system. The selected leads should be obtained at rest (while standing) and during hyperventilation.

Exercise begins with a low-work-level warm-up phase and then proceeds, stage by stage, to greater work levels. Each stage lasts 3 minutes, and recordings of ECG leads and determination of blood pressure and heart rate are obtained in the last 30 seconds of each stage, at which time a physiologic steady state has been reached. At each stage the patient is asked about chest pain, pressure, dizziness, fatigue, and dyspnea. Recordings are also obtained at peak exercise and at 1-minute intervals during a 5- to 10-minute postexercise recovery period[2] (see Fig. 8-1).

Termination of the Test

In the majority of instances exercise ECG testing is "symptom-limited" maximum testing. The normal subject terminates the examination due to excessive fatigue, dyspnea, leg pain, or exhaustion. In the case of chest pain occurring with exercise, exercise should usually be continued until the pain is of "moderate" or greater intensity. At the State University of New York Downstate Medical Center Stress Test Laboratory, patients are asked to grade the intensity of their pain from 1 (barely noted) to 10 (intense). The examination is stopped at grade 6 or 7.

In addition, the test should be terminated if the patient complains of dizziness or blurred vision, or if the patient becomes unable to converse in a cogent manner. An exercise test should also be terminated if the patient becomes cool and clammy or pale. The person performing the test should touch the patient's arm and critically observe the patient frequently. Falling systolic blood pressure, or its failure to rise with an increase in exercise levels, also indicates that the test should be terminated. These findings suggest a limitation in cardiac output. Although ST depression is not usually an indication for terminating an exam, in most instances very deep ST depression (greater than 5 mm) indicates significant ischemia and cessation of exercise testing is appropriate.

Following the termination of the exercise protocol, it is best to allow the patient to "cool down" by walking slowly for 1 to 2 minutes. This minimizes the pooling of blood in the lower extremities and the occurrence of postexercise hypotension and dizziness which is often seen when vigorous exercise is abruptly terminated. This is not ideal if the ECG signal is not interpretable due to motion artifact at peak exercise; in this case, a sudden stop—to obtain a high-quality, peak exercise tracing—is indicated. The patient should be in a sitting position after exercise unless dizziness, nausea, or hypotension is noted, in which instance the patient can be placed in a supine position or with legs elevated. The use of a fully reclining armchair allows this to be done without moving the patient.

INTERPRETATION OF THE EXERCISE ECG EXAM

The exercise ECG exam is interpreted with respect to (1) exercise capacity, (2) symptoms associated with exercise, (3) physiologic response to exercise (heart rate and blood pressure), and (4) ECG changes.

Exercise Capacity

Increasing exercise is associated with an increase in total body oxygen consumption ($\dot{V}O_2$) reflecting increases in cardiac output and $A - VO_2$ difference (oxygen extraction from the blood perfusing the working muscles). $\dot{V}O_2$max, achieved at the point of maximum exercise, reflects the peak performance capability of the cardiovascular system.[3] It is a measurement of fitness and is often termed *aerobic capacity*. In a laboratory setting, the $\dot{V}O_2$max can be measured by collecting and analyzing the last minute of expired air during exercise or can be estimated (within 10 percent of the measured values) from the peak exercise load performed. This value can be compared to a table of normal values[4] for individuals of specific sex and age and the patient's exercise tolerance (or limitation) precisely defined. Values for oxygen cost of various activities are shown in Table 8-1.

Exercise testing is usually performed on a motor-driven treadmill or a stationary bicycle ergometer. In the case of the treadmill, work loads are increased by increasing speed and the angle of elevation. In the case of the bicycle ergometer, work loads are increased by increasing the resistance to pedaling. When a treadmill is utilized, standard protocols (e.g., the Bruce protocol[4]) of increasing speed and elevation every 3 minutes allow for estimation of $\dot{V}O_2$max from total time of the exercise exam. In the case of the Bruce protocol, $\dot{V}O_2$ (ml O_2/kg/ min) is estimated from the following equations[4]:

Men: min of exercise $\times$ 2.94 + 7.65 = $\dot{V}O_2$

Women: min of exercise $\times$ 2.94 + 3.74 = $\dot{V}O_2$

TABLE 8-1. OXYGEN COST OF VARIOUS ACTIVITIES

Oxygen Cost (ml O_2/min/kg Body Weight)	Activities
4.0	Sitting
9.0	Walking, 2.0 mph
16.0	Walking, 4.0 mph, level
20.0	Bicycling, 9.5 mph; manual labor; dancing
29.0	Running, 5.5 mph, level; swimming (breaststroke) 40 yd/min; climbing stairs
38.0	Running, 7.0 mph; swimming (crawl), 50 yd/min; heavy labor

The estimated $\dot{V}O_2$ can then be compared to tables of normals and an individual's exercise performance capability assessed. In the case of the bicycle ergometer, the oxygen consumption for a given ergometric work load is known and the $\dot{V}O_2$max is estimated by dividing the minute O_2 consumption associated with the higher achieved work load by body weight in kilograms (see Table 8-2).

In certain instances, exercise protocols are terminated at specific work loads or heart rates. This is not usually a valid testing procedure as regards evaluation of exercise capacity. $\dot{V}O_2$max can be grossly approximated from these protocols using the ratio of achieved heart rate to predicted maximum

TABLE 8-2. OXYGEN LOST ACCORDING TO BICYCLE WORK LOAD

Bicycle Work Load (W)	O_2 Lost (l/min)
25	0.6
50	0.9
75	1.2
100	1.5
150	2.1
200	2.7
250	3.3
300	3.9

heart rate.[5] The wide error range using this method makes it of little clinical value.

Symptoms

Appropriate feelings during exercise are increasing dyspnea at higher work loads, fatigue, leg soreness, and a sense of exhaustion. Patients may, in addition, note the following, each of which is of diagnostic importance and should be noted in the report form.

1. *Chest pain:* This may indicate exercise-related ischemia and underlying coronary artery disease. The likelihood of this increases if the pain is substernal in location, radiates to the left arm, increases with increasing exercise levels and heart rates, and is relieved by cessation of exercise or nitroglycerin.

2. *Dyspnea at low exercise levels:* This may represent extreme deconditioning (in which case exercise heart rates are increased and physical exam and ECG are normal) or left heart dysfunction due to a myopathic process (ischemic or other), transient dysfunction related to ischemia due to coronary occlusive disease, or valvular dysfunction (insufficiency or stenosis). An additional cause to be excluded is pulmonary dysfunction. Most commonly this represents chronic obstructive pulmonary disease (associated with productive cough and history of smoking) but may be of a restrictive nature. Screening pulmonary function studies should be available in the exercise laboratory to exclude these pulmonary causes of dyspnea on mild exertion.

3. *Dizziness or blurred vision:* These usually reflect a maximized cardiac output in the face of an increasing peripheral muscle demand for blood. They may occur in normal individuals when exercise is carried to and sustained at maximum levels. Occurrences below predicted maximum exertion levels may represent reduced left ventricular function.

4. *Claudication:* This is a cramping or "biting" pain in the calves due to peripheral vascular occlusive disease. It increases with increasing work load and is relieved by rest.

Physiologic Response

Heart rate should increase with exercise in the absence of drugs that inhibit this response (e.g., propranolol). The peak heart rate obtained during the symptom-limited maximum exercise ECG exam varies with the individual's age but should be approximated by the value $220 - age \pm 10$ percent. Where a heart rate response is significantly below this level, the possibility of coronary occlusive disease with global ischemia affecting sino-atrial node function or a sick sinus syndrome should be considered. Other possibilities include diabetes mellitus or other diseases affecting the autonomic nervous system.

Blood pressure response is highly variable. There should, however, be a continuous net increase in the systolic blood pressure and a level or slightly falling diastolic blood pressure in response to exercise. Systolic blood pressure should increase in a range of 50 mm from resting level to peak exercise level.[6] Failure of blood pressure response to increase normally may reflect autonomic dysfunction (as noted above with heart rate) but also may reflect left ventricular dysfunction and an inability to increase cardiac output to meet peripheral muscle demands.

Electrocardiographic Changes

In the normal individual the electrocardiogram remains essentially unchanged during exercise in all 12 leads. A variant of normal is a depression of the J point of the electrocardiogram with a rapidly upward sloping ST segment that reaches the isoelectric line prior to or just at the onset of the T wave. Abnormalities of significance include a change in the QRS complex and a change in the level of the ST segment. The major significant finding is usually a depression of the ST segment in the presence of coronary occlusive disease and resultant ischemia. An ST segment depression of greater than 1.5 mm is considered significant. The specificity of this finding (i.e., its likelihood of representing true coronary artery disease) is greater the larger the amount of ST segment depression and the greater the persistence of the ST segment depression is into the post-exercise recovery. ST segment elevation is a rare finding during stress testing except in the presence of a prior myocardial infarction, in which case ST segment elevation in the leads showing the infarct changes is fairly common and probably represents local ventricular wall dyskinases. Occasionally patients who have histories compatible with variant (Prinzmetal) angina will also show ST segment elevations. In these instances it represents localized spasm in this coronary circulation. T-wave abnormalities are difficult to interpret and in the absence of ST changes are nondiagnostic. Patients who have recent histories of pericarditis or myocarditis and come for an exercise ECG examination with marked T-wave abnormalities preclude the diagnosis of ischemia by virture of ST segment changes.

An additional electrocardiographic finding of significance is the onset of ventricular arrhythmia with exercise. Patients with coronary artery disease and ischemia often have increasing ventricular premature contractions (VPCs) with exercise. This is manifested most frequently in the immediate post-exercise interval when the supressive effect of a rapid supraventricular rhythm is decreasing. When VPCs occur frequently, in groups of three or more in succession, or are manifested as sustained bigeminy, a further evaluation is often necessary. When these occur in the known presence of coronary artery disease, antiarrhythmic therapy is often indicated. In general VPCs are a nonspecific finding and frequently occur singly or in couplets in healthy individuals.

COMPLICATIONS OF EXERCISE TESTING

The major concern with regard to stress testing is the association of an acute myocardial infarction during or immediately after the exercise ECG exam. This phenomenon is rare but it does occur. Rapid availability of medical personnel and equipment to perform a technically excellent resuscitation is essential. It is especially important that a working (frequently checked) monitor defibrillator be on hand in the exercise testing laboratory in addition to cardiac drugs, oxygen, and the other equipment necessary to treat a cardiac arrest successfully. Other complications include sustained hypotension and bradycardia, sometimes reflecting persistent cardiac ischemia and sometimes reflecting a sustained vagal phenomenon seen in normal individuals in the post-exercise interval. Careful monitoring and placement of the patient in a supine or legs-elevated position is the appropriate management of this condition.

In over 3000 stress tests we have seen only two patients who have developed sustained supraventricular arrhythmias [one instance of paroxysmal atrial tachycardia (PAT) and one of atrial fibrillation]. Both of these patients were hospitalized and in neither instance was a myocardial infarction noted. Both rhythms spontaneously reverted to sinus within 24 h. This does, however, make the point that intermittent supraventricular rhythms can occur during exercise ECG testing, and personnel and equipment to treat them should be appropriately on hand.

CONCLUSION

Exercise ECG testing provides the physician with a method of quantitating exercise tolerance and, therefore, of making precise statements about improvement in exercise tolerance after effective training and limitation in exercise tolerance due to disease. In addition, changes in the electrocardiogram or symptoms often suggest the presence of coronary occlusive disease and ischemia; therefore, they may be helpful to the clinician dealing with particular patients. Stress testing is recommended in the majority of patients with a diagnosis of myocardial infarction or a diagnosis (or a high level of suspicion) of coronary artery disease, especially prior to beginning any sort of exercise, work, or activity program. In the case of the normal individual about to begin an exercise program, exercise ECG testing is (in most instances) not required. An exception should be made for people who have either a great fear of a coronary event during exercise (and thus would otherwise be unwilling to be actively involved in a sport or conditioning program) or significant elevation of cardiac risk factors or very significant family history of coronary artery disease.

An additional value of exercise testing for the asymptomatic individual is the ability to demonstrate, by virture of successive tests, an improvement in exercise tolerance. This is valuable as a motivating factor for the patient and provides precise heart rate information that allows the physician and patient to determine whether the exercise intensity used in training is set at effective levels.

Recent advances in nuclear medicine allow the assessment of relative myocardial perfusion (thallium 201 scan) and heart wall motion and left ventricular function (technetium 99 gated scan) at rest and during exercise. These studies, when combined with the physiologic data acquired in standard testing, offer the physician, for the first time, the ability to evaluate the "heart at work."

REFERENCES

1. Blackburn H, Taylor H, Okamoto N, et al: The standardization of the exercise ECG. A systematic comparison of chest lead configurations employed for monitoring during exercise, in Morse R: Physical Activity and the Heart. Springfield, Ill, Charles C Thomas, 1967.
2. Sheffield L, Roitman D: Stress testing methodology, in Sonnenblick E, Lesch M (eds): Exercise and Heart Disease. New York, Grune and Stratton, 1977, pp 145–161.
3. Powell L: Human cardiovascular adjustments to exercise and thermal stress. Physiol Rev 54:75–159, 1974.
4. American Heart Association, Committee on Exercise: Exercise Testing and Training of Apparently Healthy Individuals: A Handbook for Physicians. Dallas, AHA, 1972, pp 15, 32–34.
5. Astrand P, Rodahl K: Textbook of Work Physiology. New York, McGraw-Hill, 1977, pp 189–191.
6. Ellestad, Myrum: Stress Testing. Philadelphia, FA Davis, 1975, p 36.

BIBLIOGRAPHY

American Heart Association, Committee on Exercise: Exercise Testing and Training of Apparently Healthy Individuals, A Handbook for Physicians. Dallas, AHA, 1972.

American Heart Association, Committee on Exercise: Exercise Testing and Training of Individuals with Heart Disease or at High Risk for Its Development, A Handbook for Physicians. Dallas, AHA, 1975.

Ellestad, Myrum: Stress Testing. Philadelphia, FA Davis, 1975.

Sheffield L, Roitman D: Stress testing methodology, in Sonnenblick E, Lesch M, (eds): Exercise and Heart Disease. New York, Grune and Stratton, 1977.

9

Protective Equipment in High-Risk Sports

James T. Marron and James B. Tucker

The use of protective equipment in many of our modern contact sports is a somewhat recent phenomenon, although hockey helmets have been used for the past 20 years and football helmets for the past 40. It is generally accepted that the equipment used must reduce the risk of injury without changing the form and appeal of the sport. Recent experience in the design of football helmet standards points to the great difficulty in defining an acceptable standard that also can be correlated to the realities of the playing field.[1] Despite the inherent limitations, evaluation of equipment and setting of standards can be expected to continue and increase in scope for the years to come. For these reasons it is essential that the sports physician recognize the merits and limitations of various types of equipment and be aware of the expected increase in the number of standards for specific equipment as testing and evaluation continue. In this chapter, equipment is examined on a sport-by-sport basis.

FOOTBALL

Football equipment, particularly for head protection, has received a considerable amount of attention because of the relatively high frequency of head and neck injury in high school and college play.[2] The most frequent cause of brain trauma due to concussive injury is from linear rather than rotational acceleration.[2] Many research efforts have been devoted to designing laboratory models for measuring concussive impact and the protection helmets give from this. Contradictory findings between laboratory and field tests are not unusual.[3] A large study utilizing data from North Carolina indicated that helmets with suspension support, rather than padding or padding–suspension combinations, were associated with fewer concussive injuries, although the data collection in such a study was difficult at best.[4] There were significant differences between injury protection afforded by different helmet makes and models in this study.

Much of the conflicting data in these earlier studies may have merely been an indication of the lack of an acceptable standard against which the performance of helmets was measured. Initial attempts to create a standard were led by the National Operating Committee on Standards for Athletic Equipment (NOCSAE), which was established in 1969. The standard thus devised makes maximal use of available data but, unfortunately, has limitations including questions about reproducibility.[1] The American Society for Testing Materials (ASTM) sometimes ranks football helmets differently than NOCSAE, and the differences could merely reflect differences in test variables.[1] Despite these problems, which reflect the technological difficulties in devising a standard and testing materials according to it, the NOCSAE has been able to effect production of certified helmets that consistently reduce the severity of impact to below prestandard helmet performance.

The question for sports medicine personnel is whether the reduction can be correlated to injury protection. Data gathered through the National Athletic Injury/Illness Reporting System (NAIRS) for the 1975, 1976, and 1977 football seasons could not be used to predict which helmet make and design was safer, but did indicate that no single design was a cause of significant neurotrauma for the wearer.[5] The limitations of this study were due to the great infrequency of significant or catastrophic head injuries in secondary school and college football. Ongoing surveillance is the best method for detecting trends in this type study. It may be too early to tell the effect of the standard for helmets on head injury in football, but it is certain that the example of organizations such as NOCSAE has raised the consciousness of the consumer and manufacturer of football helmets concerning head safety in this sport. The current recommendation is to make sure before purchase that helmets conform to either ASTM or NOCSAE standards. It is hoped that a more definitive response on helmet make and design will be forthcoming from these organizations.

The inclusion of other types of football equipment in our analysis only reflects further that studies on this subject are in their infancy, because the standards for them are in the process of being devised. Shoulder pads are difficult to compare because there are different sizes and structural types for each different specialty player (e.g., linemen, backs, quarterbacks), and because injury rates in both earlier and later studies are not categorized by player position.[4]

Until further information becomes available, advice on the model and size of shoulder, hip, thigh, and knee pads should continue to be based on individual player specifications. The equipment should be *properly fitted to each player* with shoulder pads

covering the anterior, chest, and scapula and extending out over the acromioclavicular and deltoid areas. Hip pads should cover the iliac crests and not ride up inappropriately. Thigh and knee pads work best if the pants in which they are inserted fit properly.

Mouthguards are an essential protective device that should be mandatory for every player in contact sports. The NCAA rules committee requires a two-portion mouth protector, one interocclusal (separating biting surfaces) and the other labial (providing surface between lips and teeth) for contact sports. Ideally these devices should be custom fit to each player.[6] (See Chapter 14.)

Face protectors on football helmets should be constructed to prevent angular forces to the face area and recommendations have been made for full cage protection when possible.[7]

Design of shoes and study of the shoe-surface interface has mainly involved football and soccer equipment in this country. It is first useful to discuss natural versus artificial turf, since this seems to be both a dependent and independent variable in the analysis of football shoe performance.[8] There is little argument that artificial turf becomes warmer than its natural counterpart when ambient temperatures are high, and this is an important factor in considering the possibility for heat injury in the players or sideline personnel. Artificial turf also changes with time; this fact along with second- and third- "generation" turf appearing at different sites makes comparison of injury rates or shoe performance difficult. A number of studies imply that injury rates of all types on artificial turf are significantly higher than on natural turf.[9] A large retrospective study showed no difference in the total number of injuries between artificial turf and grass; however, there was an increased number of scrapes and abrasions on artificial turf, and the study suffered from the usual selection factor bias of a retrospective study.[10] Wet artificial turf may be safer than dry, but this factor is presumably due to the fact that player momentum is decreased by unsure footing.[11]

In summary, artificial turf is probably related to higher injury rates, although significant variations in the composition and condition of different artificial surfaces makes large-scale comparison difficult at best. Potential player overheating and increased abrasions are accepted hazards. An interesting note is that so-called "turf-toe" is almost exclusively related to the use of very flexible shoes on artificial turf. This sprain of the plantar ligament complex of the great toe metacarpophalangeal joint is due to hyperextension of the toe while driving off a fixed foot on artificial turf. Use of stiffer shoes seems to protect players from this malady.[12]

The question of shoe design per se leading to fewer injuries, particularly those of the knee joint, has received increased attention in the past few years. Torg and Quedenfeld[13] found a significant decrease in the incidence and severity of knee and ankle injuries when shorter cleats with a smaller cleat tip surface area were substituted for the larger cleats in vogue at the time of the study. Other studies have supported this and suggested that the swivel football shoe may offer the most protection from high-torque injuries although this protection is minimized with the foot squarely planted when maximum heel-to-ground contact occurs.[14] The failure of the swivel shoe to gain wider acceptance might be related to its greater bulk or cost, since early studies indicated that it did not impair player performance. The use of longer ($^3/_4$-inch) or metal-tipped cleats for soccer or football should be discouraged, because the high torque associated with their use predisposes to knee and ankle injuries.[15]

Sneakers and uncleated footwear have not been examined extensively except for their use in long-distance running. The controversy over whether ankle protection is provided by high-topped sneakers has not been settled by any studies. A review of running footwear requirements[16] notes that cushioning, support, and stability are the prerequisites for good running shoes. The presence of 160 models from various manufacturers suggests that effective marketing techniques, rather than obvious differences in shoe quality and performance, are the factors that determine shoe choice by the recreational runner. The studded outer sole or waffle sole provides more traction and shock absorption. Excessive wear, particularly of the outer sole, should be guarded against since it can result in abnormal heel strike and lower extremity stress.

BOXING, MARTIAL ARTS, AND WRESTLING

Each of these contact sports has its own associated protective equipment. Boxing gloves come in the thumb and thumbless variety with the latter type recently being used on a limited basis in New York State. It is unclear whether the thumbless design will reduce eye injuries as is claimed.

A wide athletic supporter with a metal or plastic cup is standard gear for this group of athletes, as well as high-top laced shoes. Boxing head protection consists of padded devices that offer protection to the eyebrow, forehead, and ear areas and are mandatory in most areas except professional fights. A mouthpiece is standard equipment for sparring and matches. It should ideally be a two-position protector (see section on Football).

Similar to boxing, wrestling headgear is designed to provide maximum protection to ear cartilage. The athletic supporter for wrestlers is of conventional type. The modern mat surface used by wrestlers should keep "mat burns" to a minimum.

Currently only the Amateur Athletic Union mandates the regular wear of mouthpiece and groin cup for non-contact martial arts. The above recommendations should be mandatory at all non-contact meets. Additionally, protective eye, head, hand, and foot gear should be required at all contact matches. No national organization currently endorses these safety practices during martial arts competition.

HOCKEY

The implementation of rules requiring the use of protective face gear in youth and amateur hockey leagues has had a significant impact on the reduction of eye injuries and facial lacerations in this group of sports enthusiasts.[17–19] (See Chapter 14.) Current recommendations include the use of a padded suspension helmet with full face protection employing all wire or wire and polycarbonate face and eye shields, minimally for the goalie, but preferably for all players.[20,21] The use of this equipment is now mandated by the Amateur Hockey Association of the United States and should be encouraged at all levels of play by primary care physicians. Some goalies have led the way in the use of a throat protector attached to the mask, similar to that used by baseball catchers, and this laryngeal protection should become more popular in the future. These recommendations apply not only to traditional ice hockey, but also to roller hockey as well.

An environmental issue in hockey as well as in leisure skating is the identification of high carbon monoxide levels and suspicion of milder forms of carbon monoxide poisoning in skating rinks on the East and West Coasts.[22,23] This is due to the use of gasoline-powered ice conditioners in enclosed rinks and may be lessened by opening these rinks to the outdoors during and immediately after conditioning of the ice, or by using electrically powered ice conditioners.

RACQUET SPORTS

The major hazard in racquet sports is ocular damage[24] and protection by eye guards should be encouraged. Although eyeglasses provide some protection for tennis and badminton players, ricochet from balls striking the racquet (or a partner in doubles) could raise the apparent lower risk that distance provides in these sports. For those who do not wear glasses and for those who play squash, handball, paddleball, and racquetball, the use of industrial safety glasses with polycarbonate lenses or molded plano eye protectors seems prudent. For eyeglass wearers, industrial safety glasses are recommended for the above-mentioned small-ball sports.[25] Currently the National Society to Prevent Blindness, the American National Standards Institute (ANSI), and ASTM are attempting to write a performance standard for racquet sports eye protectors which should help manufacturers create a uniformly acceptable protector.

SKIING

This is another sport where test and performance standards have yet to be devised for bindings. As in other equipment areas, this has as much to do with the technical difficulty of devising a standard as with the difficulties correlating the standard to skiing performance. Lower extremity injuries in skiers occur in a ratio of 2 : 1 to other sites of injury.[26] There appears to be a significant decline in all injuries since 1972 but particularly those in which the ski could have acted as a lever to twist or bend the leg.[27] This has been attributed to continuing improvement in design and adjustment of ski bindings. Current recommendations are that skiers invest in up-to-date, high-quality bindings, which are generally the most expensive in any particular brand line. An expert, preferably one who has attended a ski binding mechanic workshop, must mount and adjust the bindings for the weight of the skier. The shop mechanic should test the bindings on a binding test machine before allowing the skier to use them.[28] The duties of the skier include keeping bindings free from road salt and grit buildup. The binding should be tested before each skiing excursion by a series of slow leans and twists designed to exert a torque on the device and cause release. If lower extremity pain precedes binding release, then readjustment is indicated.

SKATEBOARDING

This relatively new sport has been associated with a number of serious injuries involving mainly the head and upper extremities. The American Academy of Pediatrics noted that there were 25 deaths from 1975 to 1979 and an estimated 300,000 injuries per year.[29] Abrasions, contusions, forearm fractures, and lower leg fractures account for two-thirds of the injuries with head injury being associated with more serious outcome. Illingworth et al. documented 225 skateboard injuries without mortality in 1978. Less than 10 percent of riders had worn any protective equipment (elbow and knee protection and helmet). In the same study, the use of protective equipment did not seem to offer significant injury reduction, although it is difficult to draw conclusions since only 10 percent of the sample wore any.[30] However, this observation implies that prudence in the use of the skateboard may be as important as protection.

The recommendation of the American Academy of Pediatrics is that skateboarding is a sport demanding much skill from the rider and the skateboard is not a toy. Boards must be of appropriate size for the rider. A properly lit, dry, clean surface free of automobiles and obstructions should be used. Protective clothing including long-sleeve shirts, pants, sturdy shoes, knee and elbow pads, and helmets are also strongly recommended.[29]

EQUESTRIAN EVENTS

Knowledge of some of the hazards associated with leisure time horseback riding, as well as competitive jumping, can help the primary care physician's preventive health efforts with this group of sports enthusiasts. It is estimated that over eight million people engage in some sort of equestrian activity in any year with the preponderance of these being females.[31] In a survey conducted by Grossman et al., 110 horseback riders were seen in an emergency room setting. The most common injury was closed head injury and was usually associated with lack of protective headgear. Blunt abdominal trauma with visceral contusion followed by upper and lower extremity injury were the next most common injuries.[31]

The use of a protective helmet with soft visor is currently recommended.[32] The older type of helmet has hard visors that collapse on frontal impact, driving the visor into the frontal bone. It is interesting to note that a number of injuries occur while caring for the horse. These include bites, crush injuries to the ribs and feet, and visceral or extremity injuries from kicks. Reduction in these problems will most likely come from use of common sense when around horses.

Riding boots should be of correct size so that they are easily removed from the stirrup in case of falls; oversized boots or shoes can prevent emergency dismount. People active in equestrian events should have up-to-date tetanus immunization because of the high prevalence of this organism in and around stalls.

Another important measure is for riders to be well aware of their riding capability and avoid competing with "too much" horse under them. This is a commonsense rule which is unfortunately not heeded frequently enough despite its wide acceptance in riding circles.

REFERENCES

1. Calvano NJ, Berger RE: Effects of selected test variables on the evaluation of football helmet performance. Med Sci Sports 11(3): 293–301, 1979.
2. Schneider RC: Serious and fatal neurosurgical football injuries. Clin Neurol 12: 224–236, 1964.
3. Robey James M: Contribution of design and construction of football helmets to the occurrence of injury. Med Sci Sports 4(3): 170–174, 1972.
4. Mueller Frederick O, Beyth Carl S: North Carolina high school football injury study: Equipment and prevention. J Sports Med 2(1): 1–27, 1974.
5. Clarke Kenneth S, Powell John W: Football helmets and neurotrauma: An epidemiological overview of three seasons. Med Sci Sports 11(2): 138–145, 1979.
6. NY J Dent 44(3): 42, 1974 (editorial comment).
7. Rontal E: Facial injuries in football. J Sports Med Phys Fitness 11: 241–245, 1971.
8. Hirata Isao J: Proper playing conditions. J Sports Med 2(4): 228–234, 1974.
9. Garrick James G: Synthetic turf and grass. J Sports Med 2(3): 178, 1979 (letter).
10. Keene JS, Narechania MS, Sachtjen KM, et al: Tartan turf on trial. Am J Sports Med 8(1): 43–47, 1980.
11. Adkison JW, Requa RK, Garrick JG: Injury rates in high school football. Clin Orthop 99: 131–136, 1979.
12. Bowers KD Jr, Martin, R Bruce: Turf-toe: A shoe-surface related football injury. Med Sci Sports 8(2): 81–83, 1976.
13. Torg JS, Quedenfeld TC: Effect of shoe type and cleat length on the incidence and severity of knee injuries among high school football players. Res Q 42: 203–211, 1971.
14. Cameron BM, Davis O: The swivel football shoe: A controlled study. J Sports Med 1: 16–27, 1973.
15. Bonstingl RW, Morehouse C, Benjamin W: Torques developed by different types of shoes on various playing surfaces. Med Sci Sports 7(2): 127–131, 1975.
16. Drez D: Running footwear. Am J Sports Med 8(2): 141–142, 1980.
17. Pashby TJ, Pashby RC, Chishom DJ: Eye injuries in Canadian hockey. Can Med Assoc J 113: 633–666, 1974.

18. Pashby TJ: Eye injuries in Canadian hockey: Phase II. Can Med Assoc J 117: 671–678, 1977.

19. Park RD, Castaldi CR: Injuries in junior ice hockey. Phys Sports Med 8: 81–90, 1980.

20. Vinger Paul F: Sports eye injuries: A preventable disease. Ophthalmology 88(2): 108–113, 1981.

21. Standard ANSI/ASTM F513–77. Philadelphia, American Society for Testing Materials, September 1977.

22. Johnson CJ, Moran JC, Paine SC et al: Abatement of toxic levels of carbon monoxide in Seattle ice skating rinks. Am J Public Health 65(10): 1087–1090, 1975.

23. Spengler JD, Stone KR, Lilly FW: High carbon monoxide levels measured in enclosed skating rinks. J Air Pollut Control Assoc 28(8): 776–779, 1978.

24. Vinger PF, Tolpin DW: Racket sports: An ocular hazard. J Am Med Assoc 239: 2575–2577, 1978.

25. Vinger PF, Hoerner EF (eds): Sports Injuries—The Unthwarted Epidemic, ed 1. Littleton, Mass: PSG Publishing, 1981, pp 138–150.

26. Johnson RJ, Pope MH, Ettlinger CS: Ski binding biomechanics. Phys Sports Med 10(2):49–55, 1982.

27. Johnson RJ, Ettlinger CS, Campbell RJ, et al: Trends in skiing injuries. Analysis of a 6 year study (1972–1976). Am J Sports Med 8: 106–113, 1980.

28. Johnson RJ, Pope MH: Ski binding biomechanics. Phys Sports Med 10(2): 49–55, 1982.

29. American Academy of Pediatrics, Committee on Accident and Poison Prevention and Committee on the Pediatric Aspects of Physical Fitness, Recreation, and Sports: Skateboard Policy Statement. Pediatrics 63(6): 924–925, 1979.

30. Illingworth CM, Jay A, Noble Dilys, et al: 225 Skateboard injuries in children. Clin Pediatr 17(10): 781–789, 1978.

31. Grossman AI, Kulund DA, Miller CW, et al: Equestrian injuries. J Am Med Assoc 240(17): 1881–1882, 1978.

32. Hart R: Personal communication, St. Joseph's Hospital, Syracuse, NY, April 10, 1982. Dr Hart has had much equestrian experience and knowledge of injury prevention.

10
Environmental Factors

James T. Marron and James B. Tucker

Although favorable environmental conditions can positively affect sports by exerting influences on outcome and records in various activities, adverse environmental conditions can present many hazards to the unsuspecting athlete and unprepared physician. The challenges of extremes of heat, cold, humidity and unusual environments such as high altitude and ocean depths are part of the excitement and attraction of some sports; but they can present unique problems, even in the face of a superbly conditioned or prepared athlete. This chapter examines how some natural and artificial environments affect certain sports and the injuries and illness that accompany them.

TEMPERATURE

HEAT

Heat stress, an uncommon cause of significant disease or disability, generally, in the athlete population, can be lethal in its extreme forms. In most cases, prevention is possible when careful attention is paid to fluid replacement and temperature/humidity factors.

Heat buildup occurs in two ways: (1) environmental heat gain from the sun and (2) internal heat production from muscular work. Both factors can produce dramatic increases in body heat which must be dissipated by the exercising athlete. The sun may transmit 100–200 kcal/hour to an exposed person and running fast can add 500–700 kcal/hour. Mechanisms of heat dissipation include radiation, convection, and evaporative cooling. Conduction is not a useful method of heat dissipation in situations where heat injury is more likely, because effective conduction is proportionate to differences between the conducting body (athlete) temperature and ambient temperature. Thus, when skin temperature reaches atmospheric temperature, virtually all heat loss is via evaporative cooling. This system may maximally allow for 1000–2000 ml/hr of sweat production and dissipation of 600–700 kcal/hr in an unacclimatized individual.[1] However, high humidity and low wind speed impair the efficiency of convection losses because much of the sweat produced is not evaporated. The major advantage of the acclimatized individual is the achievement of optimal heat loss with a lower sweat rate.[2] Heat dissipation demands reflex changes causing increase in cardiac output mainly via increased heart rate. People with impairment of myocardial function are at higher risk for both exercise- and nonexercise-related heat injury. Table 10-1 lists predisposing factors to both types of heat injury.[3]

TABLE 10-1. PREDISPOSING FACTORS TO HEAT STROKE

COMMON TO EXERCISE- AND NONEXERCISE-INDUCED VARIETIES
  High ambient temperature and humidity
  Drugs that increase heat production (thyroid
    extracts, amphetamines, LSD)
  Drugs that decrease thirst (haloperidol)
  Drugs that decrease sweating (antihistamines,
    antidepressants, phenothiazines,
    benztropine mesylate, propranolol)
  History of severe heat injury or malignant
    hyperthermia (MH)
NONEXERCISE-INDUCED VARIETY
  Chronic illness, congestive heart failure,
    alcoholism, malnutrition
  Sweat gland dysfunction (scleroderma, cystic
    fibrosis)
EXERCISE-INDUCED VARIETY
  Inadequate acclimatization
  Obesity, large muscle mass
  Potassium, salt, and fluid depletion
  Use of bulky, dark-colored clothing

(From Barcenas CG, Hoeffler HP, Lie JT: Obesity, football, dogdays and siriasis: A deadly combination. Am Heart J 92(2):237–244, 1976, with permission.)

Syndromes of Heat Illness

Heat cramp is a painful disorder characterized by involuntary spasm and tightening of muscles used in vigorous exercise. Oral salt replacement may not be absorbed quickly enough to treat it. Probably the best remedy is prevention, with a relatively high sodium and potassium diet (green vegetables, meat, milk). Adequate fluids are strongly recommended in conditions where vigorous exercise and overheating of muscles may occur. In more severe cases, intravenous fluids and the use of muscle relaxants are sometimes necessary.

Heat exhaustion is a more severe syndrome than heat cramps and may represent a portion of the heat illness spectrum that ultimately leads to heat stroke. This is certainly more common than heat stroke and is caused by a marked deficit in extracellular fluid. It entails progressive lassitude or confusion, some degree of temperature elevation,

usually less than 103°F (39.4°C), and evidence of hypovolemia (tachycardia and postural hypotension). Invariably there is evidence of sweating with cool skin being the rule. The treatment of this syndrome should first include assessment of temperature, since one may be dealing with heat stroke [rectal temperature usually 106°F (41.1°C) or greater]. Removal of the victim to a cool place and replacement of fluid orally is also indicated. Persistence of hypotension or symptomatic hypotension requires intravenous fluid administration and even overnight hospitalization for observation.

Heat stroke is the most severe and life threatening of the heat illness syndromes. It has been suggested that close to 4000 deaths per year (due to exercise- and nonexercise-related heat stroke) occur in the United States, particularly in the South. This syndrome is a true medical emergency and must be promptly recognized and treated. The affected individual has severe central nervous system dysfunction ranging from coma to extreme agitation to psychosis with hallucinations. Skin may be hot and dry or may be sweating. Core temperature is greater than 106°F (41.1°C), and temperatures greater than 110°F (43.3°C) have been recorded. There is circulatory collapse and hypotension with a weak thready pulse. Decreased urine output and subsequent rise in blood urea nitrogen (BUN), due to myoglobinuria from profound muscle damage, may occur. Disorders in coagulation (disseminated intravascular coagulation), hepatocellular necrosis, myocardial necrosis, and profound acid–base disturbances can also be anticipated as well as hypokalemia and hypocalcemia.

The pathophysiology of the true heat stroke syndrome is not entirely clear. Initially vasodilation and increased cardiac output, particularly through the blood vessels of the skin, are the mechanisms by which heat loss is obtained. Later events include evaporation of sweat with loss of salt and water and subsequent intravascular volume loss. As heat load persists, the circulatory system maintains a hyperdynamic state. At some point sweat production fails and a shock syndrome ensues with rapid increase in body temperature and cellular destruction. Sweat gland fatigue is postulated as one pathophysiologic event,[4] although there are clearly cases where sweating has been present with very high core temperatures.

The initial treatment is rapid lowering of core temperature usually in an ice bath. Circulatory resuscitation using rapid infusion of intravenous solutions and support using pressor agents such as dopamine or dobutamine may be indicated. Central pressure monitoring is highly recommended. Vigorous support of continued renal output through use of mannitol has also been recommended.[5] The cellular necrosis seen may take days to appear and serial assessment of muscle and liver enzymes and renal function is indicated.

Prevention of Heat Injury

The key to the management of heat injury is risk awareness and prevention. The primary care physician should keep in mind the predisposing factors listed in Table 10-1 when supervising the athlete who exercises in warm environments.

Adequate fluid and mineral replacement before, during, and after exercise is the most important preventive measure. The body will probably accept a 3 percent weight loss with no symptoms except thirst; with larger losses progressively higher rectal temperatures are expected.[6] It seems reasonable to recommend 400 to 500 ml of fluid before long runs and 100 to 200 ml every 15 to 20 minutes of running if possible.[7] Maximal exercise in warm conditions produces up to 1.5 liters of sweat an hour; this fact should be kept in mind when replacing fluids. Fluid loss is more important than salt depletion in predisposing the athlete to serious heat injury.

Solutions ingested should not contain high concentrations of sugars because these can cause delayed gastric emptying.[8] They also should be hypotonic to promote palatability; alterations in splanchnic blood flow after much vigorous exercise and volume contraction may impair liquid absorption. Thus, use of such replacement early in a race, contest, or practice should be encouraged.[5] Most athletes need to be reminded repeatedly to take adequate volumes of fluid during warm weather, since it has been shown that runners are not able to judge by sense of thirst or other parameters the volume of fluids consumed during competition.[9] Salt tablets

are not the recommended method for replacement because their absorption just before or during competition may be erratic (due to altered splanchnic blood flow).

Careful appraisal of environmental conditions is another facet of heat injury prevention. The wet bulb globe temperature (WBGT) has been advocated as the best measurement of the interaction of heat and humidity, and thus the best predictor of the potential ease for a body to dissipate heat.[10] The WBGT is calculated from three temperature readings:

1. The *wet bulb temperature* (WBT) measures heat and relative humidity.
2. The *dry bulb temperature* (DBT) is the normal temperature out of direct sunlight.
3. The *black globe temperature* (GT) relates temperature and air movement.

The WBGT index is calculated as follows:

$$WBGT = 0.7(WBT) + 0.2(GT) + 0.1(DBT)$$

Minard originally recommended caution at a WBGT of 82°F (27.7°C) and restriction of activity at a WBGT of 85°F (29.4°C) for unacclimatized men.[10] A position statement of the American College of Sports Medicine recommends no distance

TABLE 10-2. SAMPLE PRACTICE TEMPERATURE RECOMMENDATIONS

Sling Psychrometer Temperature	Recommendation
<60°F	No precautions necessary
61–66°F	Alert observation of athletes with heavy weight loss
67–72°F	Insist that water be given on the field
73–77°F	Alter practice schedule to provide a lighter practice routine
>78°F	Postpone practice

(From Murphy RA: Heat illness. Am J Sports Med 1(4):29, 1973, with permission.)

races greater than 16 km (10 miles) when the WBGT exceeds 82.4°F (28°C) and restricts running to early morning or late afternoon when the WBGT exceeds 80°F (27°C).[11] Other authors have stressed that Minard's original recommendations were probably too liberal, particularly for large muscled or obese football players, and have recommended significant curtailment of activities at WBGT greater than 78°F (25.5°C).[1,12] It is probably more prudent to err on the lower WBGT side. The use of the *sling psy-*

chrometer, which measures the wet bulb temperature and thus gives 70 percent of the WBGT, has been advocated.[12] This instrument is less costly and easier to maintain than a full WBGT complement. Table 10-2 gives an example of practice recommendations for a major college football team and can be extrapolated to other sports.[12]

A rare and serious consequence of inhalation anesthesia is *malignant hyperthermia* (MH). It has been suggested by some researchers that the muscle

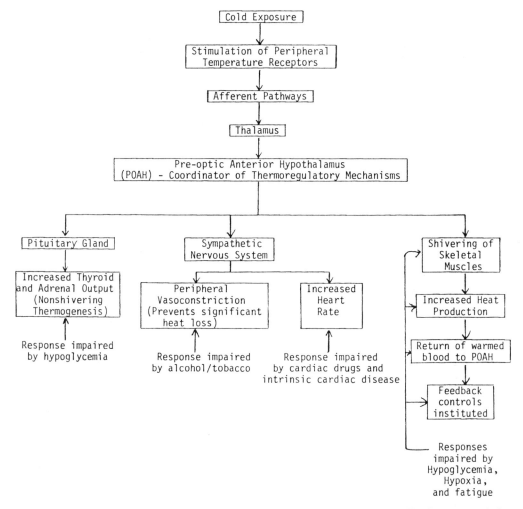

FIGURE 10-1. Physiologic response to cold. Text outside boxes indicates factors affecting expected physiologic response. *(Modified from Dembert ML: Cold injury. Am Fam Physician 25(1): 103, 1982, with permission.)*

defect present in people with MH can also predispose them to heat stroke after vigorous or violent exercise.[13] Heavily muscled individuals with the appropriate genetic predisposition are at greater risk for this syndrome. It is unknown whether some of the cases of heat stroke thought to be due to the more common pathophysiologic factors mentioned earlier are actually secondary to the myopathy present in malignant hyperthermia. Careful questioning about previous hyperthermic reactions to exercise or anesthesia in the prospective athlete (or his or her family) would seem prudent given the autosomal dominant (with variable penetrance) mode of inheritance of this syndrome.

COLD

Hypothermia and cold injury represent common risks to many outdoor sports enthusiasts. The onset may be either subtle, as in the case of the stationary hunter sitting in the field, or obvious and profound as in the case of immersion hypothermia in freezing water. *Hypothermia* can be defined as a physiologic state in which body core temperature falls below 95°F (35°C) from heat loss exceeding heat production.

The basic physiologic response to a cold stress is for heat production to increase by shivering and for core temperature to be maintained by a reduction in peripheral blood flow. A number of different factors can affect this normal response as outlined in Figure 10-1. As seen in this schematic, hypoxia (secondary to altitude), hypoglycemia, tobacco and ethanol use, and fatigue can be common predisposing factors in cold injury or hypothermia of the hunter, hiker, or outdoorsperson. The presence of wind markedly accentuates heat loss through convection and evaporation at any temperature, and the wind-chill factor has been developed to correlate wind speed to temperature. Table 10-3 shows a useful aid for making this determination.

TABLE 10-3. THE WIND-CHILL FACTOR[a]

Degrees Fahrenheit (Dry-Bulb Temperature)

Wind Speed	35	30	25	20	15	10	5	0	5	10	15	20	25	30
	Equivalent Degrees at Indicated Wind Speed													
Calm	35	30	25	20	15	10	5	0	−5	−10	−15	−20	−25	−30
		COLD												
5 mph	33	27	21	16	12	7	1	−6	−11	−15	−20	−26	−31	−35
10 mph	21	16	9	2	−2	−9	−15	−22	−27	−31	−38	−45	−52	−58
			VERY COLD											
15 mph	16	11	1	−6	−11	−18	−25	−33	−40	−45	−51	−60	−65	−70
					BITTER									
20 mph	12	3	−4	−9	−17	−24	−32	−40	−46	−52	−60	−68	−76	−81
					COLD						EXTREME COLD			
25 mph	7	0	−7	−15	−22	−29	−37	−45	−52	−58	−67	−75	−83	−89
30 mph	5	−2	−11	−18	−26	−33	−41	−49	−56	−63	−70	−78	−87	−94
35 mph	3	−4	−13	−20	−27	−35	−43	−52	−60	−67	−72	−83	−90	−98
40 mph	1	−4	−15	−22	−29	−36	−45	−54	−62	−69	−76	−87	−94	−101

[a]Using the wind-chill factor, the equivalent cooling power of various wind conditions is shown. For example, under calm conditions a temperature of 15°F has a cooling power of 15°, but when accompanied by a 10 mile-an-hour wind, the cooling power is equal to a temperature of −2°F.*(Reprinted from Handbook on Emergency Care and Transportation of the Sick and Injured, ed 2. Chicago, American Academy of Orthopaedic Surgeons, 1977, p 310, with permission.)*

The presence of wet skin or clothing dramatically affects heat loss since moisture is a more effective conductor of heat than is dry skin or clothing. If the air between the body and outer clothing remains dry and trapped, a warm layer surrounds the body and prevents heat loss. The great danger of immersion hypothermia is due to the conductivity of the surrounding water (240 times that of air), which facilitates rapid and profound heat loss.

Hypothermia: Symptoms and Treatment

There are a number of clinical presentations of hypothermia that can be correlated to temperature; these are shown in Table 10-4.[1] The most important consideration for sports medicine personnel is to recognize the risk for hypothermia in any given situation. Shivering indicates heat loss exceeding available insulation and heat production. Soon after the onset of vigorous uncontrollable shivering, the loss of judgment and hand–eye coordination occurs [92–95°F (33–35°C)]. The progression through more profound stages of hypothermia soon follows as the body's heat production capabilities are impaired and protective maneuvers become impossible because of decreased levels of consciousness.

Treatment of *moderate acute hypothermia* [91°F (33°C) and above] includes removing the victim from the cold, providing warm fluids to drink, removing wet clothing, and covering with a sleeping bag or blanket. More *severe hypothermia* [less than 91°F (33°C)] usually demands resuscitative efforts aimed at core rewarming by use of a warm bath

TABLE 10-4. PROGRESSIVE CLINICAL PRESENTATIONS OF HYPOTHERMIA[a]

Core Temperature °C	°F	Clinical Signs	Core Temperature °C	°F	Clinical Signs
37.6	99.6	Normal rectal temperature	28	82.4	Ventricular fibrillation possible with myocardial irritability
37	98.6	Normal oral temperature			
36	96.8	Metabolic rate increases in an attempt to compensate for heat loss	27	80.6	Voluntary motion ceases; pupils nonreactive to light; deep tendon and superficial reflexes absent
35	95.0	Maximum shivering			
34	93.2	Victim conscious and responsive with normal blood pressure	26	78.8	Victim seldom conscious
			25	77.0	Ventricular fibrillation may occur spontaneously
33	91.4	Severe hypothermia below this temperature	24	75.2	Pulmonary edema
32	89.6 ⎱	Consciousness clouded; blood pressure becomes difficult to obtain; pupils dilated but react to light; shivering ceases	22	71.6 ⎱	Maximum risk of ventricular fibrillation
31	87.8 ⎰		21	69.8 ⎰	
			20	68.0	Cardiac standstill
30	86.0 ⎱	Progressive loss of consciousness; muscular rigidity increases; pulse and blood pressure difficult to obtain; respiratory rate decreases	18	64.4	Lowest accidental hypothermia victim to recover
29	84.2 ⎰		17	62.6	Isoelectric electroencephalogram
			9	48.2	Lowest artificially cooled hypothermia patient to recover

[a]Presentations approximately related to core temperature. (Reprinted from Dembert ML: Medical problems from cold exposure. Am Fam Physician, published by the American Academy of Family Physicians, 25(1), 1982, with permission.)

[100–106°F (38–43°C)], warm fluids by mouth, ECG monitoring, and intravenous fluids to correct the acidosis, hypovolemia, and dehydration.

Severe profound hypothermia is associated with body temperatures of less than 86°F (30°C) and demands immediate hospitalization. People so affected may show rigidity, no palpable pulses, profound hypotension, and hypoventilation. The mammalian diving reflex is activated by cold water and causes immediate loss of consciousness, apnea, and shunting of blood, exerting a protective mechanism on the central nervous system. Full resuscitative efforts should be made because the lowered metabolic rate may give the appearance of death whereas, in fact, salvage may be possible. The lowered basal metabolic rate and oxygen usage in hypothermic individuals spares them some of the effects of hypoxia and hypotension. Most of the cardiac, renal, and hypotension problems seen in profound hypothermia are appropriate physiologic responses to the condition and will correct if the temperature is raised to normal. Below 86°F (30°C), closed chest massage is not indicated because manipulation of the body below this temperature may predispose to arrhythmias.[14] Defibrillation is essentially useless if core temperature is less than 82.4°F (28°C) and should be withheld until the core temperature reaches this level.[15] Recent evidence indicates that the controversy between active core rewarming (via peritoneal lavage or cardiopulmonary bypass) and passive rewarming (via warm water bath) may not be that significant, since outcome from profound hypothermia depends on the severity of pre-existing disease rather than the type of rewarming or level of temperature.[16] Other associated conditions which may be related to severity of tissue damage from hypothermia include coagulation disorders, renal failure, pneumonia, and gastrointestinal bleeding.

Cold Injury

Cold injury may accompany hypothermia or may occur independently and is due to the effect of cold on the more peripheral body surface areas. There may be actual formation of ice crystals in superficial tissues (true or deep frostbite) or nonfreezing injury (superficial frostbite, "trench foot" or immersion foot). In *true frostbite* the affected part is hard,

white, and devoid of sensation. Treatment consists of hospitalization, correction of hypothermia if present, and controlled rapid rewarming of the injured tissue. The danger of beginning rewarming in the field is based on the fact that recooling may occur on transport and significantly jeopardize the recovery of functional tissue. Warm water [38–42°C (100–108°F)] is used, and rewarming should continue until a hyperemic flushing occurs. Usually, severe pain accompanies the thawing. Ultimately, blistering occurs as well as the demarcation of dry mummified tissue in more severe injury.

Superficial frostbite is similar to deep frostbite except that only the most superficial layers of skin are involved and the deeper tissues retain their resiliency and viability. In immersion foot or "trench foot," the tissue injury is due to prolonged vasoconstriction, hypoxia, and acidosis from local profound cooling. In both of these situations the affected area should be gently rewarmed and development of a hyperemic stage anticipated. In all three cold injury situations, the hyperemic stage may be characterized by warmth, swelling, pain, and if a deep injury occurs, blister formation. Wet gangrene is more commonly associated with immersion foot, whereas dry gangrene is usually associated with deep frostbite. The combination of nonfreezing injury and deep frostbite may also occur. Cigarette smoking and alcohol are not recommended during recovery from frostbite or immersion foot. Decreased tolerance of affected extremities to cold and a predilection to develop vasoconstriction can persist long after the initial problem has subsided. Persistent paresthesias, excessive sweating, and persistent autonomic instability with vasospasm can be seen. In many ways this sympathetic dystrophy mimics Raynaud's disease, and α blockers (phenoxybenzamine hydrochloride) have been tried with some success for these sequelae to local cold injury.

Prevention of Hypothermia and Cold Injury

The most important factor in prevention of this type of injury is anticipation and the use of proper clothing.[17] Careful assessment of anticipated weather conditions helps the outdoorsperson dress appro-

TABLE 10-5. ENVIRONMENTAL RISK FACTORS

Sports	Risk Factors	Prevention
Mountain climbing Hiking Backpacking Snowshoeing Cross country skiing Downhill skiing	Wind and cold Hypoxia (altitude) Hypoglycemia Alcohol use Fatigue Lack of cold adaptation	FOR DRY COLD 　Down garments (particularly about head and 　　trunk) 　Pace group as slow as slowest member 　Waterproof outer garments (parka) 　Cover with several layers of wool FOR WET COLD 　Warm sleeping bags 　Insulated hiking boots or air barrier boots
Water skiing Boating Swimming Scuba diving Skin diving Canoeing Sailing Kayaking	Cold water (less than 60°F) Flailing about in water Fatigue and overexertion Alcohol use Panic Nonswimmer	Wet suits HELP position Life vests Buddy system (in skin and scuba diving)

priately. The risk factors described in Table 10-5 are obvious; if exposure is suspected, the sporting group should stop, make camp, and avail themselves of body heat from companions. Warm liquids, removal of wet clothing, shelter from the wind, and sleeping in tandem in sleeping bags are useful aids. In situations where immersion hypothermia is possible the use of insulated wetsuits is very important. Flailing about in the water potentiates the already rapid heat loss experienced there. In water at 50–59°F (10–15°C), uncontrollable gasping and inability to swim occurs and the use of the heat escape lessening position (HELP) is indicated. In this method the arms are tightly flexed into the anterior axillary line, legs are flexed on the abdomen, and the body is positioned over a life preserver or float in front of the victim. In cases of immersion hypothermia, resuscitative efforts should focus on rewarming and correction of acidosis and hypoxia even in profoundly hypothermic victims.[18]

It is interesting to note that hypothermia has been listed as a frequent cause of death in various shipwreck disasters chronicled by Preston in 1973.[19] He noted that the temperature at which shivering just maintains body temperature is 68°F (20°C), and

any length of time in water at this temperature or less can be associated with hypothermia. Hypothermia may protect vital tissues from the hypoxic effects of subsequent drowning and thus be the basis for the currently accepted principle of vigorous cardiopulmonary resuscitation for 1 hour on people pulled from water of less than 50°F (9.2°C).

REFERENCES

1. O'Donnell TF: Management of heat stress injuries in the athlete. Orthop Clin N Am 11(4): 841–845, 1980.
2. Dasler AR, Flardenbergh E: Decreased sweat rate in heat acclimatization. Fed Proc 30: 209, 1971.
3. Barcenas C, Hoeffler HP, Lie JT: Obesity, football, dogdays and siriasis: A deadly combination. Am Heart J 92(2): 237–244, 1976.
4. O'Donnell T, Clawes G: The circulatory abnormalities of heat stroke. N Engl J Med 287: 734–737, 1972.
5. O'Donnell TF: Acute heat stroke: Epidemiologic, biochemical, renal and coagulation studies. J Am Med Assoc 234(8): 824–828, 1975.
6. Shepard RJ: Environment, in Williams GP, Sperryn PN (eds.): Sports Medicine, ed 2. Baltimore, Williams & Wilkins, 1976, pp 77–97.

7. Kavanagh T, Shephard RJ: On the maintenance of fluid balance during marathon running—Observations on post coronary patients. Br J Sports Med 9: 130–131, 1975.

8. Costell DL, Saltin B: Factors limiting gastric emptying during rest and exercise. J Appl Physiol 37(5): 679–683, 1979.

9. Costell DL, Kramer WE, Fisher A: Fluid ingestion during distance running. Arch Environ Health 21: 520–525, 1970.

10. Minard D: Prevention of heat casualties in Marine Corps recruits. Milit Med 126: 261–285, 1961.

11. American College of Sports Medicine: Prevention of heat injuries during distance running. (Position Statement.) J Sports Med: 3(11): 194–195, 1975.

12. Murphy RA: Heat Illness. Am J Sports Med 1(4): 26–29, 1973.

13. Britt BK: Malignant hyperthermia. Int Anesthesiol Clin 17(4): VIII–XI, 1979.

14. American Academy of Pediatrics, Committee on Pediatric Aspects of Physical Fitness, Recreation and Sports: Accidental hypothermia. Pediatrics 63(6): 927, 1979.

15. Linton AL, Ledingham IM: Severe hypothermia with barbiturate intoxication. Lancet 1(7427): 24–26, 1966.

16. Hudson L, Conn R: Accidental hypothermia. J Am Med Assoc 227(1): 37–40, 1979.

17. Pugh LGC: Deaths from exposure on Four Inns walking competition. Lancet 1: 1210, 1974.

18. Golden F: Recognition and treatment of immersion hypothermia. Proc Roy Soc Med 66: 1058–1061, 1973.

19. Preston SF: Water hazards. Practitioner 211: 209–219, 1973.

UNUSUAL ENVIRONMENTS

WATER

The aquatic environment offers unique challenges to both the sports enthusiast and the primary care physician. (See Chapter 25.) To the latter, these range from the need for accurate evaluations of prospective scuba divers to appropriate counseling concerning water safety in the backyard swimming pool.

Drowning is the most common cause of death due to sporting or recreational activity, with 8000 fatalities per year in the United States and 2000 in Great Britain.[1] Ten percent of these deaths are in children of less than 5 years of age.[2] Drowning exceeded motor vehicle accidents as a cause of death in Queensland, Australia in 1978.[3] Most drownings occur in association with swimming activities in warm water.

There are three basic mechanisms in drowning but, as mentioned earlier, hypothermia can be a significant cause of death in low-temperature water. So-called "dry-drowning" accounts for 10 percent of drowning deaths and is caused by laryngospasm.[4] Salt- and fresh-water drowning kill by profound hypoxia because alveoli become filled with fluid independent of the oncotic pressure of this fluid. In the past, much was written concerning the different pathophysiologic responses to salt and fresh water. Recent evidence indicates that hypoxia is the most significant factor in determining outcome and not electrolyte disturbances or hemoconcentration or hemodilution.[5] Another major cause of death in drowning is from delayed events mainly related to persistent atelectasis and pulmonary infection. This occurs because of surfactant washout and alveoli collapse (particularly in fresh-water drowning).

Individuals who are resuscitated are called "near drowned." The spectrum of "near drowning" can range from minimum unconsciousness to prolonged state of unresponse. Regardless, all "near drowned" victims should be hospitalized for at least 24 hours of observation and have the appropriate studies performed. A standard emergency textbook should be consulted for proper management.

It is useful to note that people who nearly drown in cold water [less than 50°F (9.2°C)] have a much greater chance of successful resuscitation than those who nearly drown in warmer water because of the decrease in cerebral metabolism in the cold and its protective effect from the subsequent hypoxia. As mentioned earlier, the mammalian diving reflex is activated by cold water immersion and consists of cessation of breathing and central redistribution of blood flow. This may exert a protective effect in delaying the gasping efforts that are a prelude to drowning. Thus, as was mentioned in the description of hypothermia resuscitation, efforts should be continued for longer than usual, with 1 hour being the recommended minimal duration. Quick assessment of the drowning victim and environment may lead the rescuer to suspect a diving accident and thus take care to protect the cervical spine. Shallow murky water or an after dark occurrence, facial lacerations or contusions, and the presence of sand or hair in the mouth or eyes may lead one to identify this class of drowning victim. Special care to prevent excessive spine flexion or extension is thus indicated in this group while CPR is begun. In other types of drowning situations, an untrained or unfit person should not attempt rescue since the tragedy may merely be compounded. The time-tested rule of "throw, tow, row, and only then go" should be remembered in water rescue attempts.

Prevention of drowning accidents is an obvious health concern and should be an item for the primary care physician. The awareness that 20 to 40 percent of adult drownings, fully 30 percent of cervical spine diving accidents, and a high percentage of boating accidents are associated with alcohol use should alert the primary care physician to counsel patients accordingly concerning the use of this drug while on or in the water.[6] The obvious measures of continuous supervision of swimming or bathing children and the use of fences around swimming pools are also important preventive measures. The rather marked differences in the incidence of swimming pool drownings between Oahu, Hawaii (low) and Queensland, Australia (high) has been attributed to the law requiring swimming pool fencing in the former locality.[7] Other factors that may be important in preventing drownings include cautioning young children and adolescents as to the hazards of conscious hyperventilation prior to swimming underwater. Craig[8] has shown that this manuever causes a drop in the partial pressure of carbon dioxide (P_{CO_2}) and a resultant delay in the signal to surface for replenishment of oxygen. Subsequent hypoxemia leads to loss of consciousness and a high probability of drowning. All of the victims in his retrospective study who survived (35 out of 58) recalled hyperventilating before entering the water.

The most obvious caution for adults and children who will be on or near the water is to learn to swim. This recommendation as part of the routine pediatric exam may well pay the greatest dividends in prevention of drowning.

Scuba Diving

The underwater environment demands careful attention to certain health and safety factors by both the diver and the physician in order to minimize the risks of this sport. A brief review of physiologic changes associated with undersea diving is a useful starting point.

The ill effects of *barotrauma* are caused by trapped air in body cavities or potential spaces changing volume because of pressure changes in both descent and ascent. For every 33 feet of depth the pressure in these cavities doubles and the volume of air is halved. Conversely, during ascent, the volume of air doubles for each 33 feet of ascent. If the diver holds his or her breath during ascent, alveoli may be distended and rupture, leading to air embolism—theoretically possible at a depth of 4 feet. Embolism to the brain can result in loss of consciousness, hemodynamic failure, and shock, with drowning being very likely. The sudden occurrence of central nervous system symptoms (e.g., confusion, mood changes, cranial nerve palsies, motor paralysis, loss of consciousness, and seizures) suggest air embolism. Mediastinal and subcutaneous emphysema as well as pneumothorax are also potential sequelae to too rapid an ascent or failure to exhale slowly during ascent.

Barotrauma can also cause external and middle ear squeeze. If pressure equalization via the eustachian tube is impossible, perforation of the tympanic membrane is possible at depths of as little as 4 to 17 feet.[9] External ear squeeze from impaction of cerumen against the tympanic membrane is also seen. A rarer complication is inner ear squeeze, due to forceful autoinflation during descent with subsequent rupture of the round or oval window. If perforation of the tympanic membrane occurs, severe vertigo may result, causing panic and too rapid an ascent or even vomiting into the mask with subsequent aspiration. Mucosal squeeze can occur due to increased pressure in the nasal and paranasal sinuses with inability to equalize pressure. Blood blisters in the skin can occur because skin is pinched between the folds of ill-fitting wet suits by the increased external pressure.

Another type of barotrauma occurs because of expansion of dissolved nitrogen in various body tissues. This is usually only an occurrence at depths greater than 33 feet for a long enough duration to allow enough nitrogen to be dispersed throughout tissue spaces (usually greater than 1 hour). Carbon dioxide and oxygen enter into metabolism and respiration and are not a problem. When the diver approaches the surface, nitrogen may coalesce into tiny bubbles in various tissues and the bloodstream producing disabling pain and tissue damage. If the diver performs an activity at altitude after diving, the chance for this decompression sickness is greater.

Decompression sickness may be classified as type I or type II. Type I is a less threatening syndrome in which expansion of the nitrogen bubbles in the skin causes itching and, in the large joints and muscles, aching and pain. If these small bubbles form in the lung, microcirculation, pain, cough, and dyspnea ("the chokes") may ensue. Type II sickness involves bubbles forming in the microcirculation of the spinal cord leading to various paralytic syndromes, asphyxia, or convulsions. These problems usually develop in the first 12 hours after ascent and most commonly in the first hour.[10]

The management and treatment of decompression sickness centers around recompression in a hyperbaric chamber, but its efficacy depends on its use early in the course of the various syndromes. Adjunctive therapy with 100 percent oxygen by mask, hydration, low molecular weight dextran, heparin, and dexamethasone is also used. If air embolism with central nervous system involvement is suspected, the patient should be placed on the left side with head down and high-flow 100 percent oxygen administered after an open airway is established. Location of the nearest decompression chamber or advice on its use may be obtained by calling the U.S. Navy Diving Unit at Panama City, Florida (904) 234-4351 or the U.S. Air Force Decompression Team at San Antonio, Texas (512) 536-3281 weekdays and (512) 536-3278* nights, weekends, and holidays.

A useful mnemonic for this phone number is (512) LEO-FAST.

Other problems in scuba range from dangers of various forms of aquatic life, to the risk of carbon monoxide poisoning secondary to contamination of the air supply by the exhaust from a gasoline-driven compressor. Lipoid pneumonia has been reported due to lubricating oil droplets being suspended in the air tanks and, ultimately, the alveoli of divers.[11] Certain syndromes have been reported that are peculiar to prolonged, deep dives, including excess nitrogen and oxygen dissolution in the bloodstream at depths greater than 125 feet. This excess nitrogen can cause lightheadedness, dizziness, disorientation, and mental instability which can lead to loss of consciousness: the so-called "rapture of the deep." The excess partial pressure of oxygen in the bloodstream occurring at greater depths causes a syndrome similar to oxygen toxicity seen at the surface when pure oxygen is breathed for any length of time. Muscle twitching and convulsion are possible consequences of this complication of deep prolonged dives.[12] Another problem in deep dives is hypothermia, which has an insidious onset and can predispose the diver to fatigue, muscle weakness, and impaired judgment.[13]

Prevention of much of the morbidity and mortality associated with scuba diving involves careful medical examination by the physician and use of good judgment by the diver. *Experienced divers have the highest incidence of fatality.* The statement that "there are many old divers and many bold divers but no old bold divers" is a useful aphorism and points out that lack of judgment is a significant risk factor.[14] The medical exam should include careful assessment of physical fitness, since diving involves heavy exertion and high levels of exercise tolerance are mandatory. All body spaces must equalize pressure readily. Carious teeth, obstructive lung disease with blebs, eustachian tube obstruction, or ear and sinus pathology may predispose the candidate to barotrauma. A perforated tympanic membrane is particularly hazardous. Any conditions leading to even momentary loss of consciousness or orientation such as cardiac arrhythmias, seizure disorder, insulin-requiring diabetes, or episodic vertigo should disqualify a candidate. Personality factors have been mentioned as important considerations since lack of emotional stability or tendency to panic can be disastrous underwater.[15] Encouragement of the novice diver to become certified and dive only with experienced colleagues should also be part of the screening process.

HIGH ALTITUDE

High-altitude illness presents as a disease spectrum associated with recent arrival at altitudes usually higher than 2000 meters.[16] People who are involved in mild recreational activity usually have only minimal discomfort even to heights of 3000 meters. Vigorous activity, such as that seen in mountaineers and athletes, predisposes mountain sickness at lower altitudes. In its milder forms *mountain sickness* is associated with headache, lassitude, irritability, insomnia, lightheadedness, and transient chest, back, and limb pain. There may be also rapid, labored, irregular breathing. Symptoms usually begin soon after ascent (first 36 to 48 hours) and more commonly occur in unacclimatized individuals. Retinal hemorrhage with blurred vision may be a part of the syndrome of acute mountain sickness, since 20 to 30 percent of all persons going higher than 4500 meters have such retinal changes with or without other sickness.[17]

Other manifestations of high-altitude illness are more dramatic and potentially life threatening. High-altitude *pulmonary edema* has been described in both children and adults.[18] (See Chapter 13.) It most commonly affects recent arrivals above 2600 meters. Victims suffer the insidious onset of severe dyspnea, orthopnea, and dry hacking cough, which may produce a frothy blood-tinged sputum. These people may or may not have the other symptoms of acute mountain sickness mentioned above. The syndrome of pulmonary edema is remarkably resistant to diuretics but may be helped by oxygen and morphine sulfate. There probably are many milder cases of high-altitude pulmonary edema that are unrecognized. X-ray findings may show a patchy pneumonic infiltrate but no overt sings of congestive heart failure (CHF). An ECG usually shows right ventricular strain but jugular venous distension or engorgement of the liver are rarely seen. The most effective specific treatment for pulmonary edema is immediate removal to lower altitude, preferably be-

low 1000 meters. There are numerous reports of spontaneous recovery of near moribund victims after such prompt removal.

Another presentation of acute mountain illness is high-altitude *cerebral edema*. This, like the previously mentioned problems, may merely be a separate manifestation of a common pathophysiologic process. There can be a selective neurologic deficit, with the cerebellum being exquisitely sensitive.[19] Increasingly severe headache, mental confusion, emotional liability, hallucinations, gait ataxia, and dysarthria are seen with the syndrome. Coma and death are reported and rapid descent is mandatory. The use of dexamethasone and diuretics has been advocated but their value is open to question.

Acute mountain sickness, high-altitude pulmonary edema, and high-altitude cerebral edema are all results of physiologic responses to hypoxia, with cerebral edema due to increased intracranial pressure and pulmonary edema due to increased pulmonary artery pressure.

Rapid ascent may be a factor more peculiar to our modern society, with rapid transportation systems ferrying people to high altitudes without provision for acclimatization prior to activity. Altitude sickness syndromes are rare under 2000 meters and cerebral edema is rare under 3500 meters. An obvious, though sometimes overlooked, concern is for the rescuers who may ascend to treat people with mountain sickness. Experienced rescuers advise travel in groups of three, with accompanying oxygen (above 2400 meters) and preferably ascent by air to the rescue site. Rescuers, because of rapid ascent and vigorous exercise demands, are themselves quite vulnerable to altitude sickness.[19]

Information on athletes competing at high altitudes has increased greatly since the Olympics in Mexico City in 1968. Such athletes generally do not compete at altitudes where there is great risk for the development of mountain sickness, but the presence of a relative hypoxemia affects performance in both endurance and speed events. The physiologic changes that occur when an individual exercises at a high altitude are in response to the relative hypoxemia experienced. Decreasing oxygen tension stimulates peripheral chemoreceptors to increase ventilation with a subsequent rise in central nervous system (CNS) pH. This factor negatively feeds back on the ventilatory center and limits the amount of hyperventilation. Other physiologic adaptations that have been identified include an increase in hemoglobin and a reduction in blood volume and bicarbonate levels (which allows for maximal hyperventilation). The change in hemoglobin concentration occurs within days, whereas the change in red cell mass takes months.[20,21] The former is probably due to the reduction in plasma volume. The changes of headache, insomnia, and irritability seen as initial manfestations of acute mountain sickness are due to pH (increase), extracellular volume (increase), and intravascular volume (decrease) changes. The most effective preventive measure for acute mountain sickness is gradual acclimatization (e.g., a stay of 2 to 4 days at 5000 to 7000 feet).

The question of whether altitude training can improve performance is dependent on the time the athlete can spend in acclimatization. If an athlete competes within 24 to 48 hours of arrival at altitude, then the effects of intravascular volume loss are minimal.[22] Longer stays usually demand that a 3- to 4-week acclimatization period be incorporated, so that expected reduction in performance can be minimized. Apparently acclimatization is not lost by brief returns to sea level. Another performance factor at altitude is that the less dense air and decreased wind resistance aids speed events. Endurance-related events, where oxygen debt is maximum and sustained, are most adversely affected by altitude.

Regulatory groups have recommended that caution be observed when competition is above 7000 feet (2300 meters) and that competition be prohibited above 10,000 feet (3000 meters) because of the danger of sickness.[23] Others feel that competition above 7600 feet (2500 meters), particularly in events requiring high-intensity (aerobic) activity for greater than 3 minutes, is potentially dangerous because of the risk of altitude sickness.[24]

Acetazolamide has been touted as an excellent prophylactic treatment for mountain sickness, despite the fact that there are no controlled trials of it. Its use is directed at reduction in CO_2 loss from the lungs, but there is a concomitant diuretic effect that enhances the intravascular depletion that is a

later part of mountain sickness. One study has shown that it can decrease symptoms of acute mountain sickness. Its use should be restricted to mountaineers where physiologic compensation can be expected to occur before the effect wears off.[25]

REFERENCES

1. Blonstein JL: Sport and medicine. Proc Soc Med 59(2): 649–652, 1966.
2. Schiefflin TS: A new technique in water survival training for infants and toddlers. Pediatr Ann 6(11): 710–712, 1977.
3. Mulliner N, Pearn J, Guard R: Will fenced pools save lives? Med J Aust 2(9): 510–511, 1980.
4. Vaughn VC, McKay RJ: Nelson Textbook of Pediatrics, ed 10. Philadelphia, WB Saunders, 1975, p 776.
5. Knopp R: Drowning and near drowning. JACEP 7: 249–254, 1978.
6. Dietz PE, Baker SP: Drowning: Epidemiology and prevention. Am J Public Health 64: 303–312, 1974.
7. Pearn JH, Brown J, Hsia EY: Swimming pool drownings and near drownings involving children. Milit Med 145(1): 15–18, 1980.
8. Craig Albert B: Summary of 58 cases of loss of consciousness during underwater swimming and diving. Med Sci Sports 8(3): 171–175, 1976.
9. Becker GD, Parnell GJ: Otolaryngologic aspects of scuba diving. Otolaryngol Head Neck Surg 87: 569–572, 1979.
10. Dembert Mark A: Scuba diving accidents. Am Fam Physician 16(2): 75–80, 1977.
11. Johnston DG, Burger WD: Injury and disease of scuba and skin divers. Postgrad Med 49: 134–139, 1971.
12. Miles S: Medical problems of recreational diving. J R Coll Gen Pract 19: 162–166, 1970.
13. Heatinge WR, Hayward MG, McIver NK: Hypothermia in divers. Br Med J 280(6210): 291, 1980.
14. Landsberg PG: South African underwater diving accidents, 1969–1976. S Afr Med J 50(55): 2155–2159, 1976.
15. Nemiroff MJ, Somers LH, Anderson RE: A five year study of prevention of scuba diving morbidity in a university training program. J Am Coll Health Assoc 24: 95–97, 1975.
16. Houston CS: High altitude illness. J Am Med Assoc 236(19): 2193–2195, 1976.
17. Frayser R, Houston CS, Bryan C: Retinal hemorrhage at high altitude. N Engl J Med 282(10): 1183–1184, 1970.

18. Maldonado D: High altitude pulmonary edema. Radiologic Clin N Am 16(3): 537–545, 1978.
19. Wilson R: Acute high altitude illness in mountaineers and problems of rescue. Ann Intern Med 78(3): 421–428, 1973.
20. Daniels J, Oldridge N: The effects of exposure to altitude and sea level on world class middle distance runners. Med Sci Sports 2(3): 107–112, 1970.
21. Daniels J: Altitude and athletic training and performance. Am J Sports Med 7(6): 371–373, 1979.
22. Shepard Ray J: Environment, in Williams JGP, Sperryn PN (eds): Sports Medicine, ed 2. Baltimore, Williams & Wilkins, 1976, pp 77–97.
23. Sutton JR, Houston CS, Mansell AL, et al: Effect of acetazolamide on hypoxemia during sleep at high altitude. N Engl J Med 301(24): 1329–1331, 1979.
24. Straizenberg E: Exercise at altitude greater than 2000 m. J Sports Med 16: 346–348, 1976.
25. Abamowicz M: High altitude illness. Med Lett Drugs Ther 23(2): 7 (January 23) 1981.

11
Nutrition for the Athlete

Peter M. Hartmann and Eleanor H. Bell

Always searching for anything that provides a competitive edge, athletes have often turned to nutrition to improve athletic performance. Unfortunately, a large number of dietary myths have arisen that are widely believed by athletes. The primary care physician should be prepared to advise athletes about proper nutrition and be ready to dispel these common myths.[1]

Fortunately, the basic principle of nutrition for athletes is simple: The proper diet for an athlete is a normal diet with increased calories to cover added physical activity. This chapter is devoted to elucidating this principle.

THE BASIC DIET

A balanced diet consisting of selections from the basic four food groups should be eaten daily (see Fig. 11-1). This diet assures the athlete of a proper intake of protein, carbohydrates, fat, vitamins, and minerals. Ideally, the athlete should obtain 15 percent of his or her calories from protein, 50 percent from carbohydrate, and 35 percent from fat.[1,2] Additional calories required for intense physical activity should come primarily from carbohydrates, because protein is an expensive source of calories and increased fat intake is atherogenic.

PROTEIN

Many myths surround the role of protein in the athlete's diet. It is not unusual to see athletes consuming large quantities of protein, often in the form of liquid protein supplements, in an attempt to increase muscle size and strength. However, it turns out that the athlete really does not need to increase protein intake beyond the level normally eaten by the average American. A review of protein requirements demonstrates this point.

The average adult American eats 80 to 110 grams of protein daily. The recommended daily allowance (RDA) is 56 grams for a male weighing 70 kilograms and 44 grams for a female weighing 55 kilograms. This recommended allowance of 0.8 grams of protein per kilogram of body weight is nearly double the minimum requirement. For children and adolescents who are still growing, RDA increases to 1.5 grams per kilogram of body weight. This allowance should account for approximately 15 percent of the daily calories consumed.

The above figures certainly allow for a generous margin when the nitrogen losses of adult men are analyzed. In a 70-kilogram man nitrogen losses from urine, feces, skin, and miscellaneous sources translates into 24.5 grams of protein lost daily. If you provide an additional 30 percent of protein intake to allow for variations in the population, plus an additional 7.5 grams of protein for sweat from 4 hours of strenuous activity, you need only 40 grams of protein daily for a 70-kilogram man.[3] Since the average American eats *double* that amount of protein daily there is already an overabundance of protein in the normal diet to meet the needs of the athlete.

The athlete may argue that extra large quantities of protein are needed in order to build in-

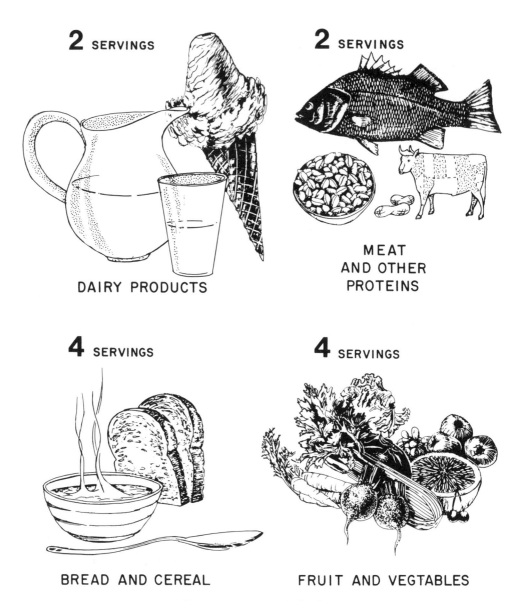

2 SERVINGS

DAIRY PRODUCTS

2 SERVINGS

MEAT
AND OTHER
PROTEINS

4 SERVINGS

BREAD AND CEREAL

4 SERVINGS

FRUIT AND VEGTABLES

FIGURE 11-1. Four basic food groups.

creased muscle mass. Since protein is the building block for muscle, the more protein eaten (the argument would go), the more muscle may be developed. Actually, muscle is only 22 percent protein. An athlete trying to gain an additional 1000 grams (4.4 pounds) of pure muscle in a month would need only 220 grams of additional protein (1000 grams × 22 percent = 220 grams of protein) that month. On a daily basis that adds only 7 grams of protein per day to the diet—an amount represented by an egg, a cup of milk, or an ounce of meat. Since the average American adult eats 40 grams more protein per day than needed for strenuous activity, protein intake already far exceeds that needed to gain this much muscle mass.

Additional protein eaten by the athlete, which is not needed for maintenance and growth, is con-

verted in the liver into carbohydrate and simply acts as a source of calories. However, since protein is an expensive source of calories, protein supplements represent a waste of money. Furthermore, protein-containing foods are usually high in fat, so that a high protein diet is potentially atherogenic.

Optimal provision of protein can be achieved

TABLE 11-1. MEAN HEIGHTS AND WEIGHTS AND RECOMMENDED ENERGY INTAKE[a]

Age (yr) and Sex Group	Weight (kg)	Weight (lb)	Height (cm)	Height (in)	Energy Needs[b] (MJ)	Energy Needs[b] (kcal)	Energy Range in kcal[b]
INFANTS							
0.0–0.5	6	13	60	24	kg × 0.48	kg × 115	95–145
0.5–1.0	9	20	71	28	kg × 0.44	kg × 105	80–135
CHILDREN							
1–3	13	29	90	35	5.5	1300	900–1800
4–6	20	44	112	44	7.1	1700	1300–2300
7–10	28	62	132	52	10.1	2400	1650–3300
MALES							
11–14	45	99	157	62	11.3	2700	2000–3700
15–18	66	145	176	69	11.8	2800	2100–3900
19–22	70	154	177	70	12.2	2900	2500–3300
23–50	70	154	178	70	11.3	2700	2300–3100
51–75	70	154	178	70	10.1	2400	2000–2800
76 +	70	154	178	70	8.6	2050	1650–2450
FEMALES							
11–14	46	101	157	62	9.2	2200	1500–3000
15–18	55	120	163	64	8.8	2100	1200–3000
19–22	55	120	163	64	8.8	2100	1700–2500
23–50	55	120	163	64	8.4	2000	1600–2400
51–75	55	120	163	64	7.6	1800	1400–2200
76 +	55	120	163	64	6.7	1600	1200–2000
PREGNANCY						+300	
LACTATION						+500	

[a]The data in this table have been assembled from the observed median heights and weights of children, together with desirable weights for adults for mean heights of men (70 in) and women (64 in) between the ages of 18 and 34 years as surveyed in the U.S. population (DHEW/NCHS data).

[b]Energy allowances for the young adults are for men and women doing light work. The allowances for the two older age groups represent mean energy needs over these age spans, allowing for a 2 percent decrease in basal (resting) metabolic rate per decade and a reduction in activity of 200 kcal per day for men and women between 51 and 75 years; 500 kcal for men over 75 years; and 400 kcal for women over 75. The customary range of daily energy output is shown for adults in the range column and is based on a variation in energy needs of ±400 kcal at any one age emphasizing the wide range of energy intakes appropriate for any group of people. Energy allowances for children through age 18 are based on median energy intakes of children of these ages followed in longitudinal growth studies. Ranges are the 10th and 90th percentiles of energy intake, to indicate range of energy consumption among children of these ages. *(From Recommended Dietary Allowances, Ninth Revised Edition (1980) with the permission of the National Academy of Sciences, Washington, D.C.)*

with an animal/vegetable ratio of 1:0. It is possible to meet protein requirements on a vegetarian diet: One that includes eggs and milk products poses no problem; one devoid of animal foods is deficient in vitamin B_{12}. The RDA of protein gives a margin allowing for a 75 percent efficiency of utilization if a mixed protein diet, as opposed to a high-quality animal protein diet, is used.

CALORIE REQUIREMENTS

As a result of their increased physical activity, athletes have a need for an increased caloric intake well above their basal requirements. If they do not ingest a sufficient amount of calories to meet this increased need, they lose weight. Conversely, if they consume more calories than they expend, they gain weight in the form of stored fat. Generally speaking, the ideal body fat content should be 5 to 10 percent of body weight for men and 15 to 20 percent for women.[4,5] An athlete may wish to gain or lose fat weight (whichever is appropriate) in order to attain an ideal percentage of body fat. The primary care physician must know how to advise the athlete regarding caloric needs. (See next section.)

Unfortunately, it is difficult to make very accurate determinations of calorie requirements for any individual when first seen because there are large variations in calorie requirements for physically similar individuals. For any random 20 people of the same sex, age, and level of physical activity, one individual can be found who eats twice as much as another yet maintains the same body fat composition.[6] This appears to be due to differences in basal metabolic rates. Therefore, it is necessary to take a careful nutritional history before recommending a particular calorie intake for an individual athlete. The ultimate guide to follow is the athlete's weight and body composition over a period of time while on a particular calorie level diet.

Calorie requirements are calculated for an individual athlete based on nonathletic requirements (basal plus normal activity) plus additional calories for athletic exercise. Child athletes also need calories for growth. The recommended allowances are based on normal intakes of a healthy population,

Method 1
Height in inches × wrist in inches ÷ 3 = IBW

Method 2
First 5 feet = 100 lb for women
        = 106 lb for men
        + 5 lb for each extra inch for women
        + 6 lb for each extra inch for men
(For small or large frames adjust 10 lb either way)

FIGURE 11-2. Formulas to estimate ideal body weight. *(Method 1 developed by Dr. Roger Sherwin of the University of Maryland.)*

but it is important to take a careful diet history before recommending a particular calorie level.

When trying to calculate a calorie level for an athlete, one must determine the nonathletic requirements from standard tables (see Table 11-1) or from formulas (see Figs. 11-2 and 11-3). Next, one should determine the added calorie requirements for the specific athletic exercise and add this to nonathletic requirements to arrive at the total daily requirement.

Method 1
Weight (kg) × 25 for sedentary
        × 30 for moderately active
        × 40 for active
        × 45 for underweight

Method 2
Weight (lb) × 10 = basal energy requirements + activity calories:
a) weight (lb) × 3—for sedentary
or
b) weight (lb) × 5—for moderately active
or
c) weight (lb) × 10—for active

Add basal energy requirements to appropriate activity calories to get total calorie requirements. There is an age adjustment for persons over 25 years (see Older Athletes).

FIGURE 11-3. Formulas for determining calorie requirements. All weights are ideal body weight (see Fig. 11-2).

TABLE 11-2. CALORIC COST OF EXERCISE PER DAY

Short Burst Maximal Effort or 1-min Effort (3400 kcal/day)	1–10 Min Sustained Effort (3000–5000 kcal/day)	1 Min or More of Intense Repeated Effort (4000–5000 kcal/day)	Endurance (3000–5000 kcal/day)
Shotput	Run 880 yd, 2 miles	Football	Run 6 miles
Javelin	Swim 100 yd	Basketball	Soccer
High jump	Wrestling	Ice hockey	Cross-country skiing
Dashes, hurdles	Gymnastics	Lacrosse	
Swim 100 yd			

(From Vitousek S: Is more better? Nutrition Today 14:11, 1979, with permission.)

To determine the number of calories needed for athletic exercise, there are standard tables that can be consulted (see Tables 11-2 and 11-3). In general, 1 hour of strenuous exercise uses 300 to 1000 calories. There are variations depending upon the number and type of muscles contracted, the quantity of contractions, and the level of aerobic activity (the more aerobic the activity, the more calories are needed).[2]

TABLE 11-3. CALORIC COST OF EXERCISE PER MINUTE

Sport	Kcal/min[a]
Long-distance running	19.4
Wrestling	14.2
Swimming	11.2
Basketball	8.6
Bicycle	8.2
Tennis	7.1
Gymnastics	6.5
Gymnastics	5.0
Walking at 3.5 mph	5.2
Baseball	4.7
Volleyball	3.5
Reclining	1.3

[a]Note: There will be obvious variability in these numbers depending on the intensity of exercise and skill of the athlete. The relative order is more significant than the actual numbers. *(From Vitousek S: Is more better? Nutrition Today 14:11, 1979, with permission.)*

LOSING AND GAINING WEIGHT

The preceeding discussion of calorie requirements was directed for the athlete who is already at his or her desired body weight. More or less calories are needed for the individual who wants to gain or lose weight. It should be noted that an increase in muscle mass and strength is obtained by exercising the muscle or muscles in question and not simply through dietary means.

Some athletes desire to lose weight since excessive fat is both unhealthy and may impede athletic performance. However, weight loss is especially important to athletes who participate in sports in which competitors are matched by weight class (e.g., wrestling and rowing). Generally, these athletes want to compete in the lowest weight class possible. It is often the physician's responsibility to determine the minimal safe weight for the athlete.

The ideal competing weight is not the lowest weight that the athlete can attain. Starved and dehydrated athletes (with loss of potassium and muscle weakness) cannot give their best performance.[7,8] The most effective weight for competition is one where there is a healthy and effective level of hydration and electrolyte balance, optimum muscle mass, and no excess body fat.

Excessive weight loss is to be severely condemned. The health of the athlete can be severely impaired by unsafe weight loss programs, especially those that promote dehydration and electrolyte imbalance such as starvation diets, exercising in rubber suits, withholding fluids, frequent spitting before weigh-ins, and the like. Wrestlers have developed nausea, weakness, dizziness, pancreatitis, and thrombophlebitis from such practices. It is also known that calorie restriction in growing individuals results in a shorter stature in adult life.[9–11]

The proper approach to weight loss in the athlete is to determine how much fat weight would need to be lost in order to have the optimum level of body fat. Again, the recommended level is 5 to 10 percent for adult males, 8 to 10 percent for teenage boys, and 15 to 20 percent for women.[4,5] If the athlete is already at this level of fat, there is no need for a weight reduction program.

The usual way to determine the percentage of body fat in the athlete is to measure skinfold thickness using calipers made for this purpose.[12] There are conversion tables supplied with the calipers to allow you to determine percent body fat from the millimeters of skinfold thickness measured. Effective use of skinfold calipers does require some practice. Instruction can be obtained from the dietician at your local hospital or from faculty in the physical education department at a local college.

An even more accurate way to determine body fat content is to perform underwater weighing. However, this is a difficult measurement to obtain and is generally available only to high-level athletes (e.g., Olympic contenders). The following example on how to advise an athlete on how much weight he or she may safely lose may be helpful.

EXAMPLE: A 175 pound college wrestler has 15 percent body fat by skinfold caliper determination. Thus, he has 26¼ pounds of body fat (= 175 pounds × 15 percent). His lean body weight would be 175 pounds total weight less 26 pounds fat = 149 pounds. His ideal weight is his lean weight plus 7 percent = 160 pounds. Therefore, he would be allowed to lose 15 pounds.

The athlete should be advised to lose weight according to the following format:

1. Keep a dietary record.
2. Follow weight loss using skinfold calipers (to be sure loss is fat and not just fluid).

3. Lose 2 pounds per week. (Losses greater than 4 pounds per week result in loss of muscle protein.)
4. Reduce calorie intake by 7000 calories per week (1 pound = 3500 calories, so 7000 calories deficit results in a 2-pound loss).
5. Exercise while losing weight. (One hour of exercise equals 500 calories used up.)

Table 11-4 shows a 2000-calorie weight reduction plan.

TABLE 11-4. 2000-CALORIE WEIGHT REDUCTION PLAN

BREAKFAST
  1 orange *or* 6 oz citrus juice *or* ½ cup melon or berries
  1 cup whole-grain cereal such as shredded wheat or oatmeal
  2 slices whole-grain bread[a] *plus* 2 teaspoons margarine
  1 cup low-fat milk
LUNCH
  3 oz lean meat,[b] poultry, or fish (baked or broiled)
  2 slices whole-grain bread
  1 tablespoon mayonnaise or salad dressing
  Lettuce
  2 fresh fruits (medium apple, pear, peach, etc.)
  1 cup low-fat milk
SNACK (250–300 calories)
  Yogurt and 2 fresh fruits
  or 2 oz cheese and 1 fresh fruit
  or sandwich (2 slices bread or roll and 1 oz meat and 1 teaspoon fat)
  or occasionally 1 small serving of dessert (cake, pie, or ice cream)
DINNER
  3 oz lean meat,[c] poultry, or fish (without added fat)
  1 cup cooked vegetables
  Raw vegetable salad
  2 teaspoons margarine or salad dressing
  1 cup potato, rice, or pasta (plain)

[a]Egg may replace 1 slice of bread.
[b]2 tablespoons peanut butter or ¾ cup cottage cheese may replace meat.
[c]3 tablespoons nuts *plus* 2 tablespoons seeds *or* ½ cup legumes may replace meat.

TABLE 11-5. VITAMINS: SOURCES AND FUNCTIONS

Vitamin/Daily Allowances	Sources	Functions	Deficiency States

VITAMIN A (Retinol) (IU)
Children, 2000–3300
Adult males, 5000
Adult females, 4000
Pregnancy, 5000
Lactation, 6000
	ANIMAL
	  Dairy products
	  liver and liver oils
	  egg yolks
	  fortified margarines
	PLANT
	  Yellow fruits and vegetables
	  dark green leafy vegetables
		Adaptation in dim light
		Maintenance of mucosal and
		  epithelial integrity
			Night blindness
			Xerophthalmia
			Defective bone/tooth
			  development
			Keratinization of epithelium
			  and mucous membranes

VITAMIN B (Thiamin) (mg)
Children under 10, 0.7–1.2
Boys and girls, 1.1–1.5
Adult males, 1.4
Adult females, 1.0
Pregnancy/lactation, 1.3
	ANIMAL
	  Organ meats, poultry, fish, pork,
	  dairy products
	PLANT
	  Whole grain and enriched
	  breads, flour, and cereals,
	  nuts, legumes, green
	  vegetables
		Coenzyme in niacin and energy
		  metabolism
			Beriberi
			Anorexia
			Constipation
			Polyneuritis
			Apathy
			Depression
			Cachexia
			Edema
			Heart failure

VITAMIN B_2 (Riboflavin) (mg)
Children under 10, 0.8–1.2
Boys & girls, 1.3–1.8
Adult males, 1.6
Adult females, 1.2
Pregnancy/lactation, 1.6
	ANIMAL
	  Organ meats, fish, dairy
	  products, eggs
	PLANT
	  green leafy vegetables
		Coenzyme in hydrogen and
		  energy metabolism
			Cheilosis
			Glossitis
			Photophobia
			Loss of vision

NIACIN (mg)
Children under 10, 9–16
Boys and girls, 14–20
Adult males, 18
Adult females, 13
Pregnancy/lactation, 16
	ANIMAL
	  Fish, poultry, meat
	PLANT
	  Legumes, nuts, cereals, whole
	  and enriched grain breads
		Coenzyme for energy
		  metabolism (glycolysis) and
		  fat synthesis
			Pellagra
			Anorexia
			Glossitis
			Dermatitis
			Diarrhea
			Neuropathy

(continued)

111

TABLE 11-5. (Continued)

Vitamin/Daily Allowances	Sources	Functions	Deficiency States
VITAMIN B₆ (Pyridoxine) (mg) Children under 10, 0.6–1.2 Boys and girls, 1.6–2.0 Adult males, 2.0 Adult females, 2.0 Pregnancy/lactation, 2.5	ANIMAL Meat, fish, poultry PLANT Vegetables, whole-grain cereals, bananas, potatoes	Coenzyme in transamination in protein and hemoglobin synthesis; glycolysis	Dermatitis Convulsions Anemia Abdominal pain Lethargy Ataxia
PANTOTHENIC ACID (mg) ?approx 5–10	ANIMAL Egg yolk, organ meats, dairy products, fish PLANT Nuts, legumes, whole-grain cereals, fruits	Coenzyme in hemoglobin fat and carbohydrates energy metabolism	Deficiency seen only with severe multiple B-complex deficits
BIOTIN (μg) ?approx 150	ANIMAL Egg yolk, organ meats PLANT Legumes, nuts	Coenzymes in deamination and carboxylation/ decarboxylation fat and protein metabolism	Deficiency seen only with severe multiple B-complex deficits
FOLIC ACID (μg) Children under 10, 100–300 Boys and girls, 400 Adults, 400 Pregnancy/lactation, 800	ANIMAL Meats, poultry, fish, eggs PLANT Dark green leafy vegetables, whole-grain cereals, mushrooms	Coenzyme for transmethylation synthesis of nucleoproteins and blood cell production	Anemia Tropical sprue
VITAMIN B₁₂ (Cyanocobalamin) (μg) Children under 10, 1–2 Boys and girls, 3 Adults, 3 Pregnancy/lactation, 4	ANIMAL Meats, fish, poultry, eggs, dairy products PLANT None	Nucleoprotein synthesis and blood cell formation	Pernicious anemia Neurologic degeneration

Vitamin/Daily Allowances	Sources	Functions	Deficiency States
VITAMIN C (Ascorbic acid) (mg) Children under 10, 40 Boys and girls, 45 Adults, 45–50 Pregnancy/lactation, 60	ANIMAL None PLANT Citrus fruits, green leafy vegetables, potatoes, melons, tomatoes, strawberries	Synthesis of collagen use and absorption of iron prevent oxidation of folic acid	Scurvy Poor wound healing Poor bone/cartilage development Anemia Capillary fragility
VITAMIN D (Ergocalciferol, D_2) (Cholecalciferol, D_3) (IU) Adults, very small Children, pregnancy/lactation, 400	ANIMAL Fish, liver oil, dairy products, egg yolk, sardines PLANT None MISC. Sunlight	Regulation of calcium and phosphorus absorption Mobilization and mineralization of bone	Rickets (children) Osteomalacia (adults) Tetany (infants)
VITAMIN E (Tocopherol) (IU) Adults, 12–15	ANIMAL Poor PLANT Vegetable oils, wheat/rice germ nuts, legumes, green leafy vegetables	Reduces oxidation of vitamin A, carotenes, and polyunsaturated fatty acids	Anemia Hemolytic disease (infants)
VITAMIN K (Phytonadione, K_1) Allowances unknown	ANIMAL Liver PLANT Green leafy vegetables	Formation of clotting factors (2, 7, 9, 10)	Hemorrhagic disease

For the underweight athlete who wants to gain weight, an increase in calories is required. Generally, an increase in lean body tissue is desired rather than merely increasing fat stores. The following information is helpful:

1. One pound of lean body tissue = 2500 calories.
2. Consume no more than 1500 extra calories daily in order to avoid excess fat.
3. Do 1 hour of muscle training several times weekly.
4. Strive for a 2-pound gain each week. (More than this would be fat, not muscle.)

VITAMINS

Vitamins are easily obtained (although expensive), easily swallowed, and often believed by athletes to possess near-magic properties. It must be remembered that vitamins serve specific functions (see Table 11-5), that they are needed in specific amounts, and that they work together with one another, with minerals, and with carbohydrates, fats, and proteins. It is not difficult to create an imbalance or to consume an overdose.

Yet, when you visit almost any gym or locker room you can overhear athletes proclaiming the merits of megadoses of one vitamin or the other. Some tout vitamin E while others champion B_{15} as a sure way to improve stamina. Unfortunately, there is no scientific evidence for an increased need for vitamins with exercise, and there are no data to show that supplemental vitamins at any dosage improve athletic performance.[13] There is a kind of exception to this rule—the placebo effect. If athletes truly believe they are being helped by supplemental vitamins, they may work out longer and perform better because they expect to.

Vitamin E. One popular vitamin among athletes is vitamin E. Despite its popularity numerous scientific studies have failed to show any improvement in athletic performance from taking extra vitamin E.[14] It does not increase stamina, improve circulation, deliver extra oxygen to muscles, or lower cholesterol. Furthermore, a deficiency of vitamin E is not found because it is so widespread in the diet.[15]

Vitamin B_{15}. Pangamin or B_{15} is the latest rage among certain sports enthusiasts. It is espe-

TABLE 11-6. VITAMIN TOXICITY EFFECTS[a]

VITAMIN A
  Skin lesions
  Blurred vision
  Itching
  Hair loss
  Headache
VITAMIN D
  Weakness
  Anorexia
  Constipation
  Weight loss
  Hypercalcemia
VITAMIN C
  Rebound scurvy
  Oxalate kidney stones
  Decreased copper absorption
  Adverse effects on growing bone
VITAMIN E
  Interferes with vitamin K metabolism,
    causing bleeding diathesis
NIACIN (3 gm)
  Skin changes

[a]There is no evidence that vitamin supplementation enhances athletic performance, and vitamins A, C, D, E, and Niacin have been shown to have toxic effects.

cially intriguing because it is widely used in other countries. However, because it is not acknowledged by the Food and Drug Administration (FDA), it is not available in the United States. Samples of "B_{15}" have been purchased by the FDA and been shown to contain a variety of substances unrelated to the expected content.[16] Even if B_{15} were proven to be of value—which it has not—the athlete is not able to purchase the true product at this time.

Vitamin Toxicity. Vitamins A, D, C, and niacin have all been shown to be harmful when excessive amounts are ingested.[17] Tables 11-6, 11-7, and 11-8 illustrate possible toxic effects and RDAs.

IRON

In both men and women, iron is lost from the body through exfoliated cells from the skin and gut, through hair loss, and (small amounts) in bile. This accounts for a loss of less than 1 milligram of iron per day. Menstruating females also lose iron from menstrual bleeding, which normally accounts for an additional loss of between 1 and 5 milligrams of iron per day of menses. However, only 10 percent of the iron in food is absorbed. Thus the daily iron requirement for men is 10 milligrams, whereas it is 18 for menstruating females. Growing boys require additional iron for growth of lean muscle tissue, so they too need 18 milligrams daily.

Exercise does not substantially increase the need for iron although sweat may have 0.3 to 0.4 milligrams of iron per liter excreted. A normal diet should adequately cover normal needs for the athlete with the possible exception of growing boys and menstruating females. Measurement of the hemoglobin or hematocrit should guide the recommendation for iron supplementation.

Care must be taken in the timing of the measurement of the athlete's hemoglobin or hematocrit. An athlete who has been sedentary for a time and then begins to work out will have physiological "anemia" due to a transient increase in blood volume (dilutional effect). This dilutional anemia resolves in about 2 weeks; thus blood should be tested either before workouts begin or 2 weeks or longer after they do.

Unless the athlete is iron deficient, additional iron does not improve athletic performance and should not be prescribed. Extra iron can cause intestinal upset, worsen certain infections, mask potential anemia caused by abnormal blood loss, and provide an unneeded expense for the athlete. In one study done with Australian swimmers, half were given iron supplements while the other half were not; there was no improvement in performance in the swimmers given iron compared with the control group. Of concern is the fact that one girl developed 20 times the normal iron stores.[18]

In summary, iron supplementation is unnecessary for athletes unless true iron deficiency is present. Measurement of the hemoglobin or hematocrit should be an adequate guide. In the case of menstruating females it is reasonable to routinely place them on additional iron daily since many of them have a deficiency of iron stores.[4]

CARBOHYDRATE LOADING

Since muscle glycogen is an important source of energy for endurance sports, it has been postulated that increasing glycogen stores in muscle may improve performance in endurance sports. Carbohydrate loading is a technique that has been developed to increase glycogen stores. Muscle biopsies show that glycogen increases to 5 grams of glycogen per 100 grams of muscle after carbohydrate loading, compared to 1.5 grams per 100 after a normal mixed diet.

The glycogen loading diet was originally described by Astrand in 1967. It has been reported to enhance the performance of distance running, distance swimming, long-duration cycling, cross-country skiing, rowing, and other endurance sports. Short-term sports derive little benefit from this technique.[19]

There are many variations for the carbohydrate loading diet. Glycogen loading is accomplished by first stripping the muscles of glycogen by exercising the muscle to exhaustion and ingesting a high protein diet for several days. This initial phase is called the *depletion phase* and occurs 4 to 7 days before the competition. Following this, the *loading phase* or supersaturation phase is accomplished by exercising lightly and ingesting a high carbohydrate diet 1 to 3 days before the meet (see Table 11-9).

Care must be taken so that the carbohydrate loading diet is not ketogenic in the first phase, nor laden with simple sugars in the second phase (simple sugars draw water into the intestinal tract and are devoid of vitamins and minerals). Fatigue, nausea, nervousness, and irritability can be avoided in the first phase by not dipping below 100 grams of carbohydrate and by keeping the caloric level equal to that of the second phase. The second or loading phase must have adequate protein, adequate fat, and complex carbohydrate (carbohydrates need not exceed 70 percent of total calories).[19]

PREGAME MEALS

Outstanding athletes are quite variable as to what they prefer to eat before competition. Some eat

TABLE 11-7. RECOMMENDED DIETARY ALLOWANCES, REVISED 1980,ª DESIGNED FOR THE MAINTENANCE OF GOOD NUTRITION OF PRACTICALLY ALL HEALTHY PEOPLE IN THE U.S.A. FOOD AND NUTRITION BOARD, NATIONAL ACADEMY OF SCIENCES-NATIONAL RESEARCH COUNCIL

Age and Sex Group	Weight		Height		Protein (g)	Fat-Soluble Vitamins			Water-Soluble Vitamins		
	kg	lb	cm	in		A (µg RF)ᵇ	D (µg)ᶜ	E (mg α TE)ᵈ	C (mg)	Thiamin (mg)	Riboflavin (mg)
INFANTS											
0.0–0.5	6	13	60	24	kg × 2.2	420	10	3	35	0.3	0.4
0.5–1.0	9	20	71	28	kg × 2.0	400	10	4	35	0.5	0.6
CHILDREN											
1–3	13	29	90	35	23	400	10	5	45	0.7	0.8
4–6	20	44	112	44	30	500	10	6	45	0.9	1.0
7–10	28	62	132	52	34	700	10	7	45	1.2	1.4
MALES											
11–14	45	99	157	62	45	1000	10	8	50	1.4	1.6
15–18	66	145	176	69	56	1000	10	10	60	1.4	1.7
19–22	70	154	177	70	56	1000	7.5	10	60	1.5	1.7
23–50	70	154	178	70	56	1000	5	10	60	1.4	1.6
51 +	70	154	178	70	56	1000	5	10	60	1.2	1.4
FEMALES											
11–14	46	101	157	62	46	800	10	8	50	1.1	1.3
15–18	55	120	163	64	46	800	10	8	60	1.1	1.3
19–22	55	120	163	64	44	800	7.5	8	60	1.1	1.3
23–50	55	120	163	64	44	800	5	8	60	1.0	1.2
51 +	55	120	163	64	44	800	5	8	60	1.0	1.2
Pregnancy					+30	+200	+5	+2	+20	+0.4	+0.3
Lactation					+20	+400	+5	+3	+40	+0.5	+0.5

Water-Soluble Vitamins (cont.) / Minerals

Age and Sex Group	Niacin (mg NE)[e]	B_2 (mg)	Folacin[f] (µg)	B_{12} (µg)	Calcium (mg)	Phosphorus (mg)	Magnesium (mg)	Iron (mg)	Zinc (mg)	Iodine (mg)
INFANTS										
0.0–0.5	6	0.3	30	0.5[g]	360	240	50	10	3	40
0.5–1.0	8	0.6	45	1.5	540	360	70	15	5	50
CHILDREN										
1–3	9	0.9	100	2.0	800	800	150	15	10	70
4–6	11	1.3	200	2.5	800	800	200	10	10	90
7–10	16	1.6	300	3.0	800	800	250	10	10	120
MALES										
11–14	18	1.8	400	3.0	1200	1200	350	18	15	150
15–18	18	2.0	400	3.0	1200	1200	400	18	15	150
19–22	19	2.2	400	3.0	800	800	350	10	15	150
23–50	18	2.2	400	3.0	800	800	350	10	15	150
51 +	16	2.2	400	3.0	800	800	350	10	15	150
FEMALES										
11–14	15	1.8	400	3.0	1200	1200	300	18	15	150
15–18	14	2.0	400	3.0	1200	1200	300	18	15	150
19–22	14	2.0	400	3.0	800	800	300	18	15	150
23–50	13	2.0	400	3.0	800	800	300	18	15	150
51 +	13	2.0	400	3.0	800	800	300	10	15	150
Pregnancy	+2	+0.6	+400	+1.0	+400	+400	+150	—[h]	+5	+25
Lactation	+5	+0.5	+100	+1.0	+400	+400	+150	—[h]	+10	+50

[a]The allowances are intended to provide for individual variations among most normal persons as they live in the United States under usual environmental stresses. Diets should be based on a variety of common foods in order to provide other nutrients for which human requirements have been less well defined.

[b]Retinol equivalents: 1 retinol equivalent = 1 µg. retinol or 6 µg. β-carotene.

[c]As cholecalciferol: 10 µg. cholecalciferol = 100 IU vitamin D.

[d]α-tocopherol equivalents: 1 mg d-α-tocopherol = 1 α TE.

[e]1 NE (niacin equivalent) = 1 mg niacin or 60 mg dietary tryptophan.

[f]The folacin allowances refer to dietary sources as determined by *Lactobacillus casei* assay after treatment with enzymes ("conjugases") to make polyglutamyl forms of the vitamin available to the test organism.

[g]The RDA for vitamin B_{12} in infants is based on average concentration of the vitamin in human milk. The allowances after weaning are based on energy intake (as recommended by the American Academy of Pediatrics) and consideration of other factors, such as intestinal absorption.

[h]The increased requirement during pregnancy cannot be met by the iron content of habitual American diets or by the existing iron stores of many women; therefore, the use of 30 to 60 mg supplemental iron is recommended. Iron needs during lactation are not substantially different from those of nonpregnant women, but continued supplementation of the mother for 2 to 3 months after parturition is advisable in order to replenish stores depleted by pregnancy. *(From Recommended Dietary Allowances, Ninth Revised Edition (1980), with the permission of the National Academy of Sciences, Washington, DC.)*

117

TABLE 11-8. ESTIMATED SAFE AND ADEQUATE DAILY DIETARY INTAKES OF ADDITIONAL SELECTED VITAMINS AND MINERALS[a]

Age Group (Yr)	Vitamins			Trace Elements[b]		
	Vitamin K (μg)	Biotin (μg)	Pantothenic Acid (mg)	Copper (mg)	Manganese (mg)	Fluoride (mg)
INFANTS						
0.0–0.5	12	35	2	0.5–0.7	0.5–0.7	0.1–0.5
0.5–1.0	10–20	50	3	0.7–1.0	0.7–1.0	0.2–1.0
CHILDREN AND ADOLESCENTS						
1–3	15–30	65	3	1.0–1.5	1.0–1.5	0.5–1.5
4–6	20–40	85	3–4	1.5–2.0	1.5–2.0	1.0–2.5
7–10	30–60	120	4–5	2.0–2.5	2.0–3.0	1.5–2.5
11 +	50–100	100–200	4–7	2.0–3.0	2.5–5.0	1.5–2.5
ADULTS	70–140	100–200	4–7	2.0–3.0	2.5–5.0	1.5–4.0

nothing at all whereas others eat large high protein meals. It does not seem to make a great deal of difference what the athlete eats prior to competition as long as it is pleasant and his or her stomach does not feel "full" when competition begins. However, the following guidelines are helpful:

1. *Eat 3 hours before the game.* This amount of time allows for digestion and absorption, but not enough time for hunger to develop. Steak requires 5 to 6 hours for adequate digestion before the game.
2. *Enjoy the meal.* This is very important. Psychologic factors and preferences have more to do with performance than the composition or size of the meal.[20]
3. *Keep fat and protein at reasonable levels.* Too much fat delays emptying of the stomach. Too much protein compromises hydration since high protein intake shunts blood flow to the kidneys.
4. *Drink 2 or 3 cups of fluid.* This helps prevent dehydration. Fruit juices are preferable to sugary drinks, which may draw water into the stomach. Ices and popsicles are considered liquids.
5. *Include bouillon or broth.* This helps compensate for salt lost in sweating.

6. *Ensure adequate carbohydrate intake.* Carbohydrate ensures glycogen and glucose stores necessary for immediate energy and a good blood glucose level.
7. *Drink another cup of water $1^{1}/_{2}$ hours after the meal.* This provides added protection against dehydration.
8. *Avoid very salty foods.* Potato chips, ham, cold cuts, pickles, hot dogs, and the like all tend to cause thirst.
9. *Avoid gassy foods.* Carbonated beverages and beans are a problem for almost everyone. Athletes with lactose intolerance may have difficulty with milk.
10. *Avoid caffeine-containing beverages.* Caffeine increases urine production and may contribute to dehydration. It also may cause jitteriness and/or hyperacidity.
11. *Avoid alcoholic beverages.* Alcohol is a central nervous system (CNS) depressant and adversely affects coordination. It also promotes dehydration through its diuretic effect.
12. *A liquid pregame meal may be ideal for many athletes.* Liquid meals are easily digested, leave the stomach promptly, and can be taken up to within a few minutes of competition. They are convenient when traveling. It helps those who

	Trace Elements[b]			Electrolytes		
Chromium (mg)	Selenium (mg)	Molybdenum (mg)	Sodium (mg)	Potassium (mg)	Chloride (mg)
0.01–0.04	0.01–0.04	0.03–0.06	115–350	350–925	275–700
0.02–0.06	0.02–0.06	0.04–0.08	250–750	425–1275	400–1200
0.02–0.08	0.02–0.08	0.05–0.1	325–975	550–1650	500–1500
0.03–0.12	0.03–0.12	0.06–0.15	450–1350	775–2325	700–2100
0.05–0.2	0.05–0.2	0.1–0.3	600–1800	1000–3000	925–2775
0.05–0.2	0.05–0.2	0.15–0.5	900–2700	1525–4575	1400–4200
0.05–0.2	0.05–0.2	0.15–0.5	1100–3300	1875–5625	1700–5100

[a]Because there is less information on which to base allowances, these figures are provided here in the form of ranges of recommended intakes.
[b]Since the toxic levels for many trace elements may be only several times usual intakes, the upper levels for the trace elements given in this table should not be habitually exceeded. *(From Recommended Dietary Allowances, Ninth Revised Edition (1980), with the permission of the National Academy of Sciences, Washington, DC.)*

TABLE 11-9. CARBOHYDRATE LOADING FOOD PLANS

Food	Depletion Phase (Days 7–4 Before Event)	Loading Phase (Days 3–1 Before Event)
Meat, poultry, cheese, fish, & eggs	12–18 oz	6–8 oz
Bread & cereal	4 servings	8–16 servings
Vegetables	2 servings	4 servings
Fruits & juices	2 servings	4 servings
Fats & oils	4–12 T	2–4 T
Milk	2 servings	2 servings
Desserts	1–2 unsweetened (no artificial sweetener)	2 sweetened
Beverages	Unsweetened, unlimited kcal : 0	Sweetened, unlimited to kcal level
Water	8 or more	8 or more
TOTAL KCAL	2550–4080	2640–3980

(From Forgac MT: Carbohydrate loading—a review. Copyright the American Dietetic Association. Reprinted by permission from the Journal of the American Dietetic Association, Vol 75:42, 1979.)

are nervous before competition and suffer gastrointestinal (GI) tract anxieties.[5,9] One must avoid choosing a formula that is too high in protein or too low in calories, such as some weight reduction formulas and liquid breakfasts. Sustagen, Sustacal, and Ensure are acceptable brands. They are lactose free—an aid to the 60 percent of blacks and 90 percent of Orientals who cannot tolerate milk.

POSTGAME MEALS

What is eaten after an athletic event is even less important than what is eaten pregame; individual preference is the main consideration. However, in general, most athletes feel better if they ingest only liquids during the immediate postgame period.

After an hour or so, the athlete may wish to begin eating solids, and a well-balanced meal is recommended. Most athletes have a large appetite at this time, so that large portions should be made available. Athletes who drink large quantities of beer to replenish lost body fluids should be actively discouraged: alcohol acts as a diuretic. Also, this practice is not consonant with an athlete's desire to promote healthful behavior for the sake of his or her body.

AGE-RELATED REQUIREMENTS

Child Athletes

Nutritional requirements are special for child athletes, because children require calories and nutrients for normal growth and development in addition to requirements for maintenance and exercise. In general, the child athlete needs 60 kcal/kg ideal body weight for growth and development of lean body mass. Inadequate nutrition will result in decreased stature as an adult.

For child and adolescent athletes who desire to lose weight, a careful dietary regimen must be followed. In general, calorie restriction should cause minimal weight loss but rather permit the youth to "grow up to his or her weight."[21] It is necessary to

make serial measurements of the athlete's height to be certain that growth continues normally while on the weight loss program. Fasting and unbalanced diets are to be condemned because they can retard normal growth.

During puberty, when the athlete is at the peak of a growth spurt, he or she can be expected to gain 5 to 18 pounds of fat-free weight in a year. Therefore, a high school wrestler should gain 2 to 4 pounds of lean body weight during the course of a wrestling season. Thus, a wrestler or other athlete in a sport classed by weight who does not gain weight during the season is compromising normal growth.

The fact that child athletes are growing also increases their requirement for iron. Supplemental iron may be needed if their diet is marginal. This is more likely in children from lower socioeconomic groups.

Older Athletes

The older athlete also has special nutritional concerns. Although calorie requirements vary considerably from person to person, in general, persons aged 25 to 35 need 50 calories less per day, and persons aged 35 to 55 need 150 calories less per day, than they did when younger. Since calorie requirements decrease with age, it is necessary for the older athlete to gradually reduce calorie intake over the years in order to avoid weight gain. One should not gain weight with age; the ideal body weight remains about the same after age 25.

Carbohydrate loading is probably unwise in older athletes since the heart is a muscle and may not tolerate the diet as well as younger athletes' hearts.[22] Also, sucrose intolerance is more of a problem in this age group since intestinal enzymes lose effectiveness with age. Because undigested sugars cause abdominal discomfort, distention, and gaseousness, these simple sugars are best avoided just before competition by these athletes.[23]

Adult athletes, who are more likely to consume alcohol than younger ones, need to realize that alcoholic beverages are a poor source of energy for sports. Alcohol must first be converted into glucose by the liver, a process that goes on very slowly.

Exercise does not hasten the metabolism of alcohol. Also, the caloric consumption from alcohol can be sufficient to trigger a weight problem.

SUMMARY

There are no special diets that give athletes a competitive advantage with the *possible* exception of carbohydrate loading for endurance sports. The athlete requires only a balanced ordinary diet with extra calories, and some modifications on the day of competition.

The optimal diet for the athlete and for the population in general is one in which 15 percent of the calories are derived from protein, 35 percent from fat, and 50 percent from carbohydrate. Vitamin, mineral, and protein supplements are not advised except for iron in menstruating females. Nutritional requirements for athletes can be met entirely by food from the four basic groups.

REFERENCES

1. Serfass RC: Nutrition for the athlete. NY State J Med 2:1824–1825, 1978.
2. Vitousek SH: Is more better? Nutr Today 14:10–17, 1979.
3. Dornin JV: Protein requirements and physical activity, in Pariykova J, Rogozkin VA (eds): Nutrition, Physical Fitness and Health, International Series on Sports Sciences, vol 7. Baltimore, University Park Press, 1978, pp 53–60.
4. Smith NJ: Gaining and losing weight in athletics. J Am Med Assoc 236:149–151, 1976.
5. Buskirk ER: Diet and athletic performance. Postgrad Med 61:229–236, 1977.
6. Miller DS: Food intake and energy utilization, in Parizkova J, Rogozkin VA (eds): Nutrition, Physical Fitness and Health, International Series on Sports Sciences, vol 7. Baltimore, University Park Press, 1978, p 3–8.
7. Hursh LM: Food and water restriction in the wrestler. J Am Med Assoc 241:915–916, 1979.
8. Tipton CM, Tcheng T: Iowa wrestling study: weight loss in high school students. J Am Med Assoc 214:1269–1274, 1970.
9. Smith NS: Nutrition and the young athlete. Pediatr Ann 7:49–63, 682–689, 1978.
10. Croyle PH, Place RA, Hilgenberg AD: Massive pulmonary embolus in a high school wrestler. J Am Med Assoc 241:827–828, 1979.
11. Buskirk ER: Weight loss in wrestlers. Am J Dis Child 132:355–356, 1978.
12. Tower J: The physician and optimum body weight for junior high and high school wrestlers. Alaska Med 20:60–62, 1978.
13. Huse DM, Nelson RA: Basic, balanced diet meets requirements of athletes. Phys Sports Med 54:52–56, 1977.
14. Sharman IM, Down MG, Norgan NG: The effects of vitamin E on physiologic function and athletic performance of trained swimmers. J Sports Med 16:215–225, 1976.
15. American Academy of Pediatrics, Committee on Nutrition: Nutritional aspects of vegetarianism, health foods and fad diets. Pediatrics 59:460–464, 1977.
16. Wright JE: Vitamin B_{15}, wonder substance or waste of money. Muscle Fitness 42:38–88, 1981.
17. Slater AR: Vitamins: Their use and abuse. Nutr MD 1(11):1–4, 1975.
18. Fitch K: Medicine and asthma, in Erikson B (ed): Swimming Medicine IV, Proceedings of the Fourth International Congress on Swimming Medicine. Baltimore, University Park Press, 1978, pp 1–421.
19. Forgac MT: Carbohydrate loading—a review. J Am Diet Assoc 75:42–45, 1979.
20. Fair JD: Effects of three pre-competition meals upon subsequent performance in a two-mile run. MS thesis, Univ North Dakota, 1974.
21. Newmann CG, Jelliffe DB (eds): Symposium on nutrition in pediatrics. Pediatr Clin N Am 24:117–122, 1977.
22. Smith NS: Food for Sport. Palo Alto, Calif, Bull Publishing, 1976, pp 1–188.
23. Blair S, Sargent R, Davidson D, et al: Blood lipid and ECG responses to carbohydrate loading. Phys Sports Med 8:69–75, 1980.

12
Field Management of Athletic Injuries

Burton L. Berson and Stuart Cherney

The prompt, accurate evaluation and treatment of the injured athlete is essential. In the case of a severely injured athlete the first aid measures administered by the field physician can be lifesaving. The diagnosis of many injuries is often best made immediately at the time of injury, with subsequent treatment therefore hinging upon the initial field examination. The physician must make an unhurried, thorough assessment and, depending on the nature of the injury, determine the following:

1. Can the athlete return to play?
2. Does he or she require sideline observation or more thorough evaluation in the training room?
3. Is immediate hospital evaluation required? If doubt exists as to the severity of the injury, it is better to err on the side of conservatism in order to avoid converting a mild injury to a moderate or severe one.

MEDICAL ORGANIZATION

It is strongly recommended that a physician be in attendance at all contact as well as certain noncontact sport competitions (large track and field events, martial arts, etc.), although this is not always practical. Because a significant percentage of injuries occur during practice sessions, there should be a clearly understood protocol established to handle such injuries.[1] The on-call physician, emergency

transportation unit, and admitting hospital must be arranged prior to each event. Standardization helps decrease confusion at times of injury. (See Chapter 2 for more details.)

The assigned field physician must always assume with equanimity the leadership role in handling an injured athlete. This includes orchestrating the roles of trainers, paramedics, coaches, and others at the scene and providing and arranging necessary follow-up care. All coaches and trainers should be formally instructed in basic first-aid measures and cardiopulmonary resuscitation techniques.

Adequate space should be provided at the school arena or stadium so that a thorough physical examination can be performed. It must be large, quiet, well lighted, and include an examination table. No athletic practice or competition should take place without immediate access to a telephone and knowledge of its location. A two-way radio system may also be used to summon medical aid.

Transportation is most safely carried out in a well equipped emergency vehicle with a paramedic staff. Paramedic attendance at high-level competition is strongly advised due to their expertise in advanced life support measures and in moving the injured. A well equipped emergency vehicle allows rapid stabilization and sophisticated treatment at an early stage.

Medical field equipment and useful instruments are discussed as is appropriate throughout this chapter. A list of recommended physician supplies and field equipment is provided in Appendix A.[2]

PRINCIPLES OF INITIAL INJURY EVALUATION

Prompt treatment of the seriously injured athlete is the major function of a field physician. Decisive and lifesaving action may be necessary. It is the obligation of the physician to have thorough knowledge of advanced cardiopulmonary resuscitation techniques and be familiar with the handling of the common and idiosyncratic injuries of the sport event being covered (Chapters 14 to 20).

A seriously injured athlete is considered a multiple trauma victim, and evaluation and treatment should follow established guidelines. As always, a history must be obtained; if the athlete cannot verbalize, the mechanism of the injury can usually be described by physician, coach, players, or spectators. Prior injuries and significant medical problems should also be elicited. The physical examination should proceed after historical information is gathered. *Do not move* the athlete until properly evaluated for possible spine injury. Carefully remove or cut away any part of uniform or equipment which interferes with the examination or treatment.

Athletic injuries can be divided into three levels of priority. The first level includes those from which death may be imminent. The second level consists of those which are potentially fatal, can increase in severity with time, or require further emergency evaluation. The third level comprises nonprogressive, nonurgent conditions that typically respond well to good first aid. An outline of conditions in each of these levels is given below:

1. *First priority:* Immediate threat to life (death within minutes)
   a. Respiratory arrest (upper airway obstruction, acute respiratory failure, acute pulmonary edema, pneumothorax)
   b. Cardiac arrest
   c. Anaphylactic shock
   d. Uncontrolled hemorrhage/hypovolemia

2. *Second priority:* Urgent (potentially fatal) threat to life
   a. Severe head injury (see also Chapter 14)
   b. Neck and back injury (see also Chapters 14 and 15)
   c. Visceral injury (see also Chapter 16)
   d. Facial injury (see also Chapter 14)
   e. Myocardial infarction (see also Chapter 7)
   f. Seizures (see also Chapter 21)
   g. Burns
   h. Musculoskeletal trauma (see also Chapters 17 and 18)
   i. Heat stroke/hypothermia (see also Chapter 10)
   j. Near drowning (see also Chapters 10 and 25)

3. *Third priority:* Not urgent
   a. Abrasions
   b. Lacerations
   c. Skin blisters/bullae
   d. Puncture wounds

First-priority injuries are discussed thoroughly in Chapter 13. The remainder of the present chapter deals with second- and third-priority injuries.

SECOND PRIORITY INJURIES

Head Trauma (see also Chapter 14)

Head injuries and altered states of consciousness are routinely encountered in many contact sports. Alteration in the athlete's behavior is probably the single most important clue of intracranial injury. In all instances, especially in the unconscious athlete, examination and treatment must assume the possibility of concomitant cervical spine injury. Cervical immobilization and minimal head motion must be used in these cases (face masks can be removed with a bolt cutter). Maintenance of the airway is of prime importance and any necessary life-sustaining measures should be instituted.

Cerebral concussion is an immediate, limited impairment of neural function after head trauma. The spectrum ranges from a "ding"—briefly dazed with full recovery in seconds to minutes—to unconsciousness lasting several minutes with residual effects lingering for days to weeks. Usually, no focal neurological changes are found on physical examination. Symptoms include headaches, visual disturbances, nausea, vomiting, and retrograde amnesia.

Cerebral contusion—actual bruising of the brain—is associated with longer periods of unconsciousness. Focal neurological findings may be present. *Acute subdural hematoma* is the leading cause of death from trauma in contact sports. The patient usually remains unconscious and develops rapid onset of focal neurological signs. Immediate neurosurgical evaluation is imperative. *Epidural hematoma* is classically described as a brief loss of consciousness followed by a lucid interval before a rapid onset of neurological focal signs, though this is not always the case. Surgical treatment is mandatory as soon as the diagnosis is made.

The physical examination begins with evaluation of the athlete's state of consciousness. Orientation, recent memory, and other higher integrative functions (calculation, general behavior, etc.) should be tested. Next, the head is carefully palpated for depressions and lacerations. The ears and nose are examined for blood and cerebrospinal fluid. Pupils are tested for equal size and response to light—unequal pupils may indicate localized intracranial pressure or injury or direct ocular trauma. Ocular movements should also be assessed. All cranial nerves should be tested following the initial evaluation. Gross motor and sensory function of all extremities should be checked next. Equilibrium can be tested on the sidelines by finger-to-nose, heel-to-shin, or straight-line walking.

An athlete who has had a concussion (and may or may not have lost consciousness) should not be allowed to return to a game or match. Unconsciousness lasting several minutes requires transfer for hospital evaluation, x rays, and 24 to 48 hour observation. Likewise, persistent retrograde amnesia or symptoms of concussion should be observed in the hospital. All athletes not hospitalized following injury should be given a "head trauma sheet" instructing the athlete and family to seek immediate medical care for severe headache, visual disturbance, projectile vomiting, or change in sensorium. It is in the best interests of the primary care physician and athlete that follow-up examination for all head injuries be made in 1 or 2 days.

The physician's three highest priorities in treating a serious craniocerebral injury on the field are (1) maintenance of airway, (2) stabilization of the cervical spine, and (3) speed in transfer to a hospital facility and neurosurgical evaluation.[3,4] An IV line should be started in all potentially serious head injuries using crystalloid at a low flow rate in order to avoid potential cerebral edema.

Neck and Back Injuries (see also Chapters 14 and 15)

Cervical spine injuries, with or without neurological damage, are rarely associated with fatality. However, initial management is crucial to preventing, creating, or exacerbating any spinal cord injury. If any suspicion at all exists regarding cervical spine injury, the athlete is treated as a *definite* cervical spine injury; this especially includes the unconscious athlete and severe head trauma victim.[5,6] The athlete is not moved until a determination is made.

Assessment begins with determination of the mechanism of injury (i.e., direct or indirect force). The practice of "spearing" (face blocking) has been implicated in cervical spine injury in football. First, ask if the athlete has neck pain or numbness anywhere. If the response is "yes," a cervical spine injury must be presumed. Next, see if the patient can actively flex and extend hands, arms, ankles, and knees. Failure of any motor function indicates the presence of serious spinal cord injury. No attempt should be made to change the position of head or neck during this initial evaluation.

Stabilization of the cervical spine is mandatory once the possibility of injury has been confirmed. A cervical collar is carefully placed. All attempts to move the patient should be made with the neck in neutral position. At least three, preferably five, people are needed for transferral: one at either side and one at the head. With each hand under a shoulder, the head and neck are stabilized between the elbows of an experienced person stationed at the patient's head (Fig. 12-1). In situations where the athlete is not initially supine, an additional experienced individual should stabilize the head during turning. This is done by holding the head firmly in both hands and maintaining a neutral position with

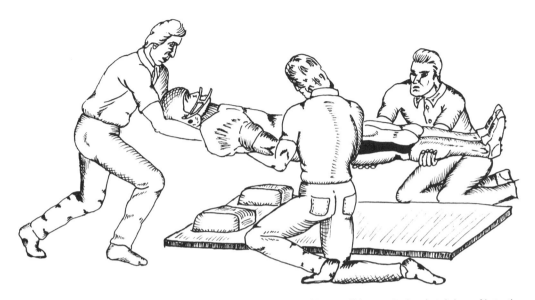

FIGURE 12-1. The proper method of moving an athlete with possible cervical spine injury. Note the stabilization of the spine in the neutral position.

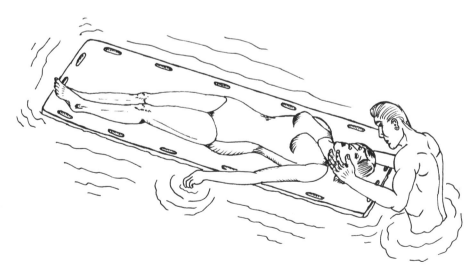

FIGURE 12-2. A rigid object such as a spine board should be floated under an injured athlete who has suffered a potential neck injury.

gentle traction.[5] Once supine, further critical care can be initiated if necessary. In cases of respiratory arrest, the esophageal obturator airway or "blind" nasotracheal intubation are recommended because they require the least amount of cervical spine manipulation. Helmets should *not* be removed unless absolutely necessary. Transfer to a cervical stabilization–traction board should be made as quickly as possible.

After a potential diving injury, a spine board should be floated underneath the athlete prior to transfer from the water (Fig. 12-2). If an efficient commercial unit is not at hand, any rigid board can be used. Sandbags, folded towels, or similar items are placed on either side of the head; the head, shoulders and waist are then strapped to the board. The victim can then be transferred to a stretcher for emergency transportation. Hospital evaluation and treatment should include x rays and thorough neurological examination.

Back injuries caused by direct trauma usually are associated with soft tissue contusion. Pain, swelling, spasm, and stiffness are common complaints. Stable spine fractures are often difficult to distinguish from contusions. Initial treatment consists of ice packs and rest. X rays should be taken in cases of persistent pain and spasm.

Lower spine injuries associated with neurological deficits are treated as unstable. Any lower extremity weakness, sensory loss, or radiculopathy following back injury requires careful log roll transfer to a full-length spine board. The athlete is then secured to the board with head-to-toe strapping (Fig. 12-3).

Visceral (Abdominal/Urological) Injury (see also Chapter 16)

Athletic injuries to the abdomen and retroperitoneal organs are almost always due to blunt trauma. Potentially life-threatening situations can occur if hemorrhage or viscus organ rupture occurs. The physician should be able to recognize such conditions and arrange immediate transfer to a general surgeon's care.

A commonly encountered phenomenon is *temporary cessation of respiration* following a blow to the epigastrium. "Having the wind knocked out" of an athlete is a respiratory reflex following stimulation of the celiac (solar) plexus, which is a part of the sympathetic chain in the aortoceliac artery region. This condition is treated by resting the athlete in a supine position, loosening his or her uniform around the chest and waist, and offering reassurance; within moments spontaneous breathing will resume. The athlete may return to competition upon complete recovery, which may take several minutes. If more than 5 minutes are required, the athlete should be carefully observed before allowing return to the game.

Blunt trauma to the abdomen or flank can cause serious injury to underlying organs. Rupture of the spleen, liver, intestine, and mesentery occur in a decreasing order of frequency.[7,8] Pancreatic and duodenal injuries are rare. Bladder rupture and renal contusion or laceration are possible genitourinary system injuries. After such injuries the athlete may complain of severe, persistent abdominal pain which may radiate or may be asymptomatic for a variable period. Nausea and vomiting may be present. These

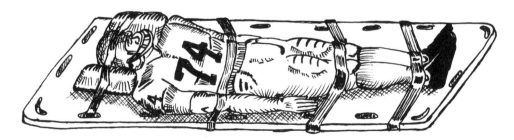

FIGURE 12-3. Proper stabilization on a spine board consists of sandbags or towels around the neck and firm anchoring of the head, trunk, and extremities.

symptoms are related to underlying peritoneal irritation. Diaphoresis and faintness are seen with impending shock. Physical examination should take place in an appropriate examination room and vital signs recorded periodically.

A *ruptured spleen* occurring without trauma is rare. When it occurs, it is almost always associated with splenomegaly—the underlying cause of which is usually infectious mononucleosis.* Splenic rupture from other traumatic causes, such as CPR procedures, seat belts, and deceleration injuries, may also confront the sports physician.

Early evaluation of splenic rupture is crucial as it can be a fatal condition. Any trauma to the left flank followed by signs of shock, abdominal pain and rigidity, nausea and vomiting, left chest pain and sharp left shoulder/arm pain, and difficulty in full ventilation of the lungs may indicate that the spleen has ruptured.[10]

If a ruptured spleen is suspected, prompt evacuation to a medical facility for complete evaluation is indicated. Keep a high index of suspicion as a visceral injury occurs most often to the spleen. The hemorrhage location (free peritoneal cavity, retroperitoneal space, or into the spleen itself) may modify the clinical picture. Generally, the intensity of the symptoms, shock, and degree of hematocrit fall correlate with the urgency of treatment. Abdominal x rays may be of some help. Computed tomography is a possible future modality of diagnostic aid.[11] The treatment is usually total splenectomy.[12] Some

Infectious mononucleosis is primarily a disease of young adults and hence quite common in athletes. There is much apprehension about it in sports circles because of misinformation about its effects. The physician is concerned with the general manifestation of the disease but more importantly with the enlarged spleen that carries a risk factor for possible rupture.

A herpes virus, Epstein–Barr virus (EBV), is the etiology of infectious mononucleosis. It is the cause of all heterophile-positive and most heterophile-negative cases. The virus is present in multiple organ sites but most prevalent in the throat, B lymphocytes, and in the bloodstream.

The common pathophysiology is one of pharyngitis, tonsillitis, adenitis, and hepatitis, and occasionally there is carditis, pneumonitis, and encephalitis. The spleen enlarges. The trabeculae and capsule (of elastic nature) are engorged with round cells.[9]

effort is being made to preserve the spleen or parts thereof by surgical means.

Prevention is very possible in most cases of splenic enlargement from infectious mononucleosis. Rupture usually occurs in the second to third week of the disease. Avoidance of all possible sports trauma as long as there is splenomegaly is the rule in preventing this serious problem. Physical signs of splenic rupture that require immediate transfer to a surgical facility are (1) marked abdominal tenderness, (2) loss of bowel sounds, (3) abdominal rigidity, and (4) unexplained shock. If shock is present, intravenous crystalloid infusion should begin at once through several large-bore catheters preferably above the diaphragm.

Flank pain and tenderness are seen more often in a retroperitoneal process. Kidney injury can occur in any contact sport, especially boxing or the martial arts. Bladder rupture results from a direct blow to the full bladder and presents as lower abdominal pain and tenderness which may initially be mild. Gross hematuria on initial postinjury voiding demands immediate urological investigation. Inability to void is also suggestive of genitourinary injury and requires emergency evaluation. Testicular contusion is managed with ice packs and elevation. Torsion should always be considered and ruled out. If pain persists in the face of testicular swelling, a laceration requiring surgical repair may be present.[13]

Injuries About the Face, Eyes, Ears, and Throat (see also Chapter 14)

Face. Common injuries about the face are contusions and lacerations. Simple contusions are treated with ice packs and pressure. Lacerations should be thoroughly cleansed with sterile saline. Small lacerations can be sutured in a field training room if sterile instruments and drapes are available. Larger lacerations are best handled in an emergency room where adequate light, assistance, instruments, and sterile conditions ensure optimum results. The critical item in the repair of facial lacerations is careful, accurate apposition of tissue margins. Return of an athlete with a facial laceration must be tailored to the extent of the injury and the importance of return to competition. An acceptable temporizing measure prior to definitive suturing includes thorough cleansing, reapproximation of skin edges with sterile adhesive strips, and sterile dressing.

Facial fractures should be suspected when severe pain, swelling, deformity, or bleeding are present. Nasal fractures are usually associated with all of the above findings. Anterior nosebleeds are treated by rest, gentle compression of the nostril by pinching for a full 10 minutes, and local ice packs. If bleeding persists, as in the case of posterior bleeds, nasal packing may be required—an emergency room procedure. Displaced mandibular and maxillary fractures are marked by loss of normal dental occlusion.

Throat. Blunt trauma to the throat may result in laryngeal or tracheal injury. Edema and hematoma formation can develop insidiously with resultant airway compromise. The athlete with persistent or progressive difficulty speaking, pain, hoarseness, dyspnea, or hemoptysis requires immediate evaluation and referral to an emergency facility with the airway stabilized.[14]

Ear. Swelling of the outer ear following blunt trauma is caused by underlying hematoma formation. Repetitive insults result in massive fibrotic scarring—the wrestler's "cauliflower ear." Initial treatment includes ice packs and compression dressings. Large hematomas should be aspirated under sterile conditions. Bleeding from the ear canal in the absence of serious head trauma is most likely due to tympanic membrane rupture. Careful aspiration and otoscopic examination should confirm the perforation. Pack the outer ear loosely with sterile cotton pending definitive treatment. Liquids or fluids (antibiotics, peroxide, etc.) should not be placed in the canal.

Eye. Commonly encountered eye injuries are superficial foreign bodies and corneal abrasions. Thorough irrigation of the eye with a sterile ophthalmologic solution (sterile water or normal saline) represents good initial management. The undersurface of the eyelids are examined and any foreign material is removed with a sterile swab. A 0.5 percent solution of topical tetracaine may be instilled for pain relief during examination. After the contest the athlete should be reevaluated and more thoroughly examined. Follow-up is mandatory. Direct trauma to the eye (as seen in boxing, hockey, or racquetball) often causes contusion, the results of which vary in severity (hemorrhage, lens dislocation, retinal detachment). A direct orbital blow can cause a blow-out fracture of the infraorbital margin. Further specialist evaluation is indicated for (1) persistent pain, (2) change in visual acuity, (3) change in visual fields, or (4) double vision.[15] A dry sterile eye patch is used to cover any seriously injured eye. In penetrating injuries, *both* eyes should be patched to decrease eye motion and no drops of any type (steroid or antibiotic) should be placed in the eye. Lastly, if any severely injured athlete is wearing contact lenses, the lenses should be removed.[16] After adequate hydration, hard lenses are easily removed by a rubber bulb suction device; soft lenses can be manually extracted.

Myocardial Infarction (see also Chapter 7)

A myocardial infarction occurring during athletic participation is an ever present possibility. One of the reasons is the great number of middle-aged men participating in strenuous physical activity (i.e., distance running and singles tennis) after many years of living a sedentary life. The probability of a male having developed some degree of coronary atherosclerosis during those sedentary years is great.[16] Another reason is the return of middle-aged men to sports participation after a myocardial infarction. This is generally controlled by the physician in charge of the patient and is a minimal hazard. In any case, it is imperative that the primary care physician be aware of the exercise risk potential, be astute in the clinical diagnosis, and be proficient in the immediate management of a myocardial infarction.

The diagnosis of a myocardial infarction occurring or a strong possibility of same is in most instances made by the physician from the individual's history. Severe angina or "intermediate" coronary insufficiency syndrome is generally less of a diagnostic differential in physically conditioned athletes. Precordial chest pain with radiation to the left arm, shoulder, neck, jaw, or back strongly suggests myocardial ischemia. If it is unrelieved by nitroglycerine, infarction must be suspected. The clinical picture of sweating and shortness of breath that is often part of the myocardial infarction picture may be confused with the perspiration and "windedness" associated with exercise. The bradycardia of the "athletic heart" may be confused with the parasympathetic overtone bradycardia of a myocardial infarction. Premonitory and prodromal symptoms suggestive of coronary artery disease heightens the suspicion of myocardial damage occurring. The physical findings of an acutely ill person with low blood pressure, faint heart sounds, and a paradoxically split second sound reflect compromised left ventricular performance. The presence of an S_3 (gallop) and moist rales in the lung bases indicate a degree of left ventricular failure. If the history or the physical findings are suggestive of a myocardial infarction, the presumptive diagnosis should be made.

Pathophysiologically, myocardial infarction refers to the death of heart muscle (tissue), which results primarily from an interruption of the blood supply. This interruption causes an acute oxygen deficiency and muscle cell death. The circulatory catastrophe is usually the result of an acute obstruction of a coronary artery or its segment. This obstruction, which can be relative or absolute, in most cases is caused by a thrombus superimposed upon an atherosclerotic plaque. Localized hemorrhage into a plaque, arterial spasm, and emboli are less frequent causes of coronary artery obstruction.[17]

Athletes with an actual or suspected myocardial infarction should be hospitalized immediately. The urgency is for treatment of complications: shock, arrhythmias, and congestive heart failure. A less urgent reason for hospitalization is to establish a definitive diagnosis if there is only suspicion of a myocardial infarction having occurred.

The emergency management of a myocardial infarction is reasonably standardized (Table 12-1). The primary care physician must do what he or she is equipped to do while considering the acuteness of the problem, expeditiously facilitating definitive care as outlined and planning for hospitalization as soon as possible.

Primary care physicians are most active in the

TABLE 12-1. EMERGENCY CARE OF MYOCARDIAL INFARCTION

Dx:	History, PE, ECG
Rx:	IV, 5% D/W, O_2, Morphine 2–10 mg IV (pain)

Monitor & observe for & Rx:

Shock:	Dopamine 1–10 µg/kg
CHF:	Furosemide 40 mg IV
	Morphine 2–4 mg IV
	Rotating tourniquets

Arrhythmias:

Bradycardia: Atropine 0.5 mg (IV)
Ventricular irritability: Lidocaine 50–100 mg (IV bolus)
Asystole ———— Epinephrine 0.5 mg IV

CPR

Ventricular ———— Electrocardioversion
fibrillation   (200–400 W/s)

area of prevention of myocardial infarctions by careful medical screening and supervision. Exercise prescriptions based on the physical status of the athlete and the frequency, intensity, and duration of exercise are a useful tool of prevention.[18] Overall risk assessment includes: the athlete (presence or absence of coronary artery disease), the environment (presence or absence of high heat and humidity), and the sport (cardiac output demands). A useful tool for preparticipation screening has been the "stress test" electrocardiogram for determining presence or absence of ischemic coronary artery disease in a person with symptoms or risk factors (metabolic, familial, hypertensive, smoker, and to some degree age) (Chapter 8). The primary care physician must screen whenever possible for existing coronary artery disease. When significantly present, it is a definite risk for myocardial infarction especially documented in running and soccer.[19,20]

Seizures (see also Chapter 21)

Epilepsy manifesting as grand mal convulsive seizure is an infrequent problem in the accomplished athlete. If seizures are uncontrolled, participation to accomplishment is unlikely. If controlled by medications, the possibility of becoming uncontrolled by athletic participation is ever present. The primary care physician should be familiar with the problem and know how to handle it.

The pathophysiology of a clinical convulsive seizure involves aggregates of neurons that depolarize synchronously.[21] If there is an aura, the type of sensation is a manifestation of a focal discharge which helps localize the lesion (i.e., odor indicates temporal lobe).

The etiology of a sports-occurring convulsive seizure may be a convulsion as a result of a simple prolonged vasovagal syncope. On the other hand, it may be a seizure precipitated by hyperventilation of sports participation. Head trauma may precipitate a seizure but indeed must be quite severe.

The diagnosis of a convulsive seizure usually is not difficult. There are generalized major motor convulsions (tonic–clonic) with loss of consciousness. The so-called minor seizures, psychomotor and petit mal, do not present as an urgent problem. Status epilepticus presentation of hysterical conversions have been documented but are unlikely to be a problem in the athletic population.

In the treatment of a convulsive seizure, hypoxia and self-injury are the major concerns. An open airway must be maintained. A plastic (*not* rubber) airway may suffice. Most of the time, all that is needed is to prop the mouth open with a wooden stick, the diameter of which is placed between the molars. This prevents tongue laceration by the teeth and provides an airway. Protecting the patient from injury is accomplished by removal of sharp objects from the vicinity and forcefully limiting the tonic–clonic excursions to a safe range. Treatment of continuous convulsive seizures (status epilepticus) requires intravenous drugs (initial doses: phenytoin, 50 mg/min up to 1 gm; *or* phenobarbital, 150–200 mg; *or* diazepam, 5–10 mg).

Prevention of seizures in athletes can be accomplished through screening and forestalling the participation of persons who are known to have uncontrolled epilepsy. This is truly a difficult decision to make when one considers the psychological benefits of sports participation for a youngster with this problem. Obviously, the severity of the malady influences this recommendation, so all cases must be individualized. Therapeutic control of the seizures and participation in a "safe" sport are to be encouraged.

Burns

Burns in a healthy adult engaging in athletics occur most frequently in machine sports. The auto race driver is at the highest risk. Lightning injury (burn) occurs most frequently to the golfer but can occur in other field sports during a thunderstorm.

The auto race driver is at high risk for burns from burning fuel, usually ignited by a crash. The role of the physician in organization of an emergency system including fire equipment and trained personnel, medical personnel, and medical vehicles for transport to a designated burn care center is extremely important. The responsibility of minimizing all hazards and creating safety in the environment is indeed of equal importance.[23]

Protective equipment for the driver consists of protective underwear, socks, gloves, shoes, face mask, helmet, and racing suit. These are all fire resistant and are warm while racing. Safety equipment in the automobile includes roll bars, seat belts, contoured seats, fire extinguishers, and fuel bladders to prevent fire if a tank ruptures.

One extremely important mechanism of minimizing the hazard of burns is the prevention of the accident. This is accomplished by avoiding the compromised performance of the driver because of an intercurrent illness. Annual and abbreviated (event-related) health exams are helpful. Drugs and alcohol are to be avoided. Personal (sport-unrelated) stress should be recognized and evaluated. Stress can come from such diverse areas as domestic pressures and a subtle but fundamental fear of racing.

Burns from lightning injuries are prognostic signs of death (leg burns, 30 percent and cranial burns, 37 percent). The highest mortality is in the usually unburned lightning-struck victim who suffers cardiopulmonary arrest (76 percent).[24] The overall mortality from lightning injury is estimated very roughly to be about 20 to 25 percent.

The athletic activity with the greatest hazard for lightning injury is golf. This is played in the season of electrical (thunder) storms and the golf course is an open, exposed area.

Lightning is caused by charged particles and electrical fields between the clouds and the earth. When the charges reach a certain potential difference, a flow of electrical current takes place. This flow is along conductors of lesser resistance than air. On a golf course, these are trees, people, metal golf club shafts, and metal flag sticks.

Treatment of those lightning-struck persons who appear to be dead should probably include vigorous resuscitation efforts: the respiratory arrest often lasts longer than the asystoli, leading to death by hypoxia, not by cardiac arrest.[25] External burns are a later manifestation and require no immediate treatment.

As always, prevention is a major interest of the primary care physician. Officials of organized golf tournaments, such as those conducted by the Professional Golfers Association and the United States Golfing Association, require play to stop when they deem the risk of lightning injury is great. Unfortunately, these organized tournaments represent only a small portion of the golf played. For the vast unsupervised group of athletes, education in safety principles is the best alternative. In simple terms, the participant should avoid being a conductor of electricity. The hazards increase by standing under a conductor (tree) or holding one (golf club or flag stick) when there is an electrical charge in an overhead cloud.

Musculoskeletal Trauma

General Considerations. The major concern regarding the athlete with an extremity injury is his or her health and safety. Decisions to return to play are made frequently but are not always easy or objective. Common sense dictates that no athlete should be allowed to compete if the examining physician is uncertain of the nature of the injury. One must bear in mind that fractures and severe sprains may not always be obvious, especially in younger athletes. Basic signals of significant injury are (1) persistent, severe pain, (2) deformity, (3) swelling, (4) instability, and (5) loss of function. Generally, extremity trauma can be broken down into contusion, strain, sprain, fracture, and dislocation. The principles involved in their diagnosis may be applied to almost any part of the anatomy.

Contusion refers to a blunt injury that leaves the integument intact and damages only soft tissues. Diagnosis is based on local tenderness and slight swelling with little disability. Severe contusions may result in hematoma formation. Treatment consists of RICE: *R*est, *I*ce packs, *C*ompression bandaging, and *E*levation for at least 48 hours. Significantly large or expanding hematomas should be aspirated only under sterile conditions in order to facilitate rapid rehabilitation and remove a possible nidus of infection.

Strain is an injury to the musculotendinous unit (i.e., muscle and/or tendon at any location from origin to insertion). The severity of injury is divided into three degrees:

1. First-degree strains involve damage without loss of anatomical continuity in the muscle–tendon unit. Diagnosis is based on local pain, tenderness, swelling with pain on active flexion or passive stretching. There is no loss of strength

or motion. Emergency treatment involves the RICE regimen.

2. Second-degree strains involve partial disruption that results in loss of strength as well. In addition to rest and ice, definitive splinting (tape, plaster, etc.) is required.

3. Third-degree strains involve complete disruption. A snap or pop may be heard and the affected muscle–tendon unit is functionless. Palpable defects may be present to help localize the injury. Surgery is usually indicated, with best results following early repair.

Sprain is the term given to ligamentous injury. Since ligaments stabilize joints, any interruption of continuity may result in joint instability, which includes joints of little motion such as the acromioclavicular and proximal tibiofibular. Sprains are also divided into three categories:

1. First-degree sprains are ligamentous injuries without loss of gross anatomical integrity. Mechanism of injury, point tenderness, pain on passive stress, and no instability confirm the diagnosis. Treatment is symptomatic (RICE) and return to play may be allowed.

2. Second-degree sprains are partial ligamentous disruptions.

3. Third-degree sprains are complete ligamentous disruptions.

Second- and third-degree sprains are associated with more pain, swelling, and disability. If examined before reflex spasm sets in, the amount of instability may be accurately determined. The differentiation between these levels of injury often requires thorough evaluation, which consists of stress x rays, examination under anesthesia, and arthroscopy or arthrography. In any event, ice, compression, immobilization, and x rays are mandatory.

Fractures should be suspected when there is gross deformity, swelling, instability over a bone shaft, crepitus, or severe pain and disability. Osteophony may be useful on the field to evaluate the presence of a fracture. If a fracture is suspected, the extremity is splinted until x rays and definitive orthopedic evaluation have been completed. The

presence of pulses and motor and sensory functions should be noted. Open fractures are treated similarly after a sterile dressing is applied to the wound.

Dislocation is a complete separation of the opposing joint surfaces. These injuries are often easy to diagnose on physical examination (e.g., shoulder, fingers). First aid involves immobilization and evaluation of distal neurovascular status. Reduction of dislocations on the field is not advised if emergency room evaluation can be carried out in a reasonable period of time. By carrying out reductions in an emergency room after x rays are done, the exact nature and extent of the injury can be determined (since fractures frequently accompany dislocations) and any problems arising during reduction are more easily handled in that setting.

Upper Extremity Injuries. (see also Chapter 17) Examination of the upper extremity injury is aided by knowledge of the mechanism of injury. Actual examination on the field should be limited to determining the extent and location of the injury. Stabilization of the extremity is then achieved manually or with splints before the athlete is taken to the sidelines. Definitive examination should take place on the sidelines or in the training room. All equipment and uniform is carefully removed or cut away (always freeing the uninjured side first). The sling and swathe is adequate immobilization for most upper extremity injuries, but from the elbows down, additional rigid splinting is necessary (Fig. 12-4).

Start the examination with inspection of the upper extremity, looking for swelling, ecchymosis, and deformity. One-finger palpation of point tenderness can often best ascertain the location of the injury. Once it is determined, complete the examination of the entire extremity—occult injuries may be detected. Begin at the sternoclavicular joint. Look for deformities and angulation and palpate for point tenderness. Clavicle fractures may be immobilized in a sling or figure-of-eight strapping after assessing distal neurovascular status. Joint instability may be determined bimanually but stress x rays are valuable in diagnosing the severity in acromioclavicular sprains ("AC separations"). These sprains commonly result from a fall on the point of the shoulder, and grade III sprains are easily diagnosed when

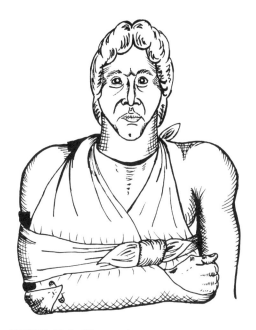

FIGURE 12-4. Sling and swathe is used for immobilization of upper extremity injuries.

there is significant upward displacement of the distal end of the clavicle.[26] Shoulder sprains or spontaneous reductions usually affect the anterior capsule. By abducting and externally rotating the shoulder, a positive "apprehension" is elicited: the athlete tenses and refuses any further passive motion. Glenohumeral dislocations are noted by loss of deltoid contour and fullness anteriorly, severe pain on forced abduction, and an adducted internally rotated arm which is often held to the chest by the athlete's uninjured arm.

Acute *rotator cuff tears* are uncommon but can be detected by weakness of shoulder abduction and tenderness along its course (supraspinous fossa to greater tuberosity of humerus). Rupture or strain of the long head of biceps may occur, noted by weakness and tenderness over the bicipital groove.[26]

Injuries about the *elbow* include sprains (usually 2° hyperextension), strains, fractures, and dislocations. Acute swelling may be present, along with stiffness. Diagnosis is not complete without x

rays. Posterior dislocation, marked by loss of anatomical landmarks, demands immediate emergency room reduction. Forearm fractures should be immobilized in a rigid splint and sling during transportation.

Falls on the outstretched hand may result in *wrist injury*. The same mechanism may produce concomitant fractures or dislocations in most parts of the upper extremity. Severe swelling, pain, and difficulty moving the wrist are indicative of underlying fractures. The distal radius, scaphoid, triquetrum, and pisiform are susceptible to fractures. Dislocations can involve the entire carpus, lunate, or perilunate bones. Rigid splinting is required.

The *hand* is very susceptible to injury in many sports. Fractures of the metacarpals and phalanges are common. An attempt should be made to reduce interphalangeal and metacarpophalangeal dislocations on the field before swelling and pain become excessive. It is absolutely essential that all dislocations, whether reduced spontaneously or by the primary care physician, be x rayed after the contest to ensure proper relocation and assess the presence or absence of a fracture. Collateral ligament sprains, especially of the thumb metacarpophalangeal joint (gamekeeper's thumb), are considered significant if lateral instability exists. Tendon injuries may be of the closed or open type (seen with lacerations). Inability to flex the distal finger joint after grabbing a jersey signals rupture of the flexor digitorum profundus tendon and requires surgical repair. The "baseball" or mallet finger follows direct impact to the tip of the finger which causes an avulsion of the extensor tendon. It is marked by inability to extend the distal phalanx and a flexed attitude. Avulsion of the central slip of the extensor tendon at the middle phalanx results in a boutonniere deformity. When a tendon is lacerated, the wound should be cleansed and covered with a sterile dressing. The injured athlete should then be referred to a hand surgeon. Subungual hematomas may be evacuated acutely by piercing the sterilely prepared fingernail with a needle or hot paper clip. Ice should be applied. A malleable metal splint may be used for temporary stabilization of the finger until x rays are taken. *All* hand injuries should be x rayed to determine the nature and extent of the injury.

Lower Extremity and Pelvis. (see also Chapter 18) *Pelvic injuries* most commonly encountered are contusions, avulsion fractures, and fractures of the pubis or ischium following straddle injuries. The football player's "hip pointer" is a contusion of the iliac crest resulting in swelling and pain. Ice and rest usually suffice as treatment. Avulsion fractures, rather than the more common hamstring strains, may occur in younger athletes. Forced hip flexion with the knee extended can cause ischial tuberosity avulsion, marked by local tenderness at that location. Forced hip abduction can cause adductor strain or avulsion of their attachments at the ischiopubic rami. Severe swelling and a palpable defect following hamstring or adductor strain indicate complete disruption. In these cases surgery may be indicated.

The forces required to dislocate or fracture the hip are rarely encountered in sports. *Hip fractures* are accompanied by severe pain, inability to move the limb, and shortening of the extremity with rotation. An athlete with any suspected hip fracture is placed on a spine board where both the trunk and limb are immobilized. Contusion to the greater trochanter is treated with ice compresses. Iliopsoas strains or lesser tuberosity avulsions occur after forced hip extension. The hip is held in flexion, adduction, and external rotation and the athlete complains of severe groin pain. Rest and cold are the initial management requirements. Persistent pain and swelling in the younger athlete with strains about the hip call for x-ray evaluation to rule out avulsion fractures.[27]

Thigh injuries can result in massive hematoma formation with treatment as outlined. Fracture of the femur is unusual but all field physicians should be able to recognize and immobilize a femoral fracture. Pain, deformity, gross motion, and swelling are the hallmarks. Shock may occur. If available,

the Thomas splint carried by emergency squads is very easy to use. One person applies gentle longitudinal traction to the ankle while the splint is positioned and thigh and leg are lashed to the frame. A hitch is placed around the ankle and attached to the end of the splint. Additional traction is then applied by tightening the ankle strap in a "windlass" fashion (Fig. 12-5). An IV should be started with crystalloid.

Injuries about the *knee* have always been of great concern to the sports physician. The complexity and disabling nature of knee injuries mandate special concern to this anatomical area. In recent years, diagnosis and management of knee trauma has been changed by better understanding of biomechanics and the role of the cruciate ligaments. Arthroscopy has advanced the ability to diagnose knee disorders. The physician, therefore, must become familiar with a thorough physical exam of the knee. Any significant knee injury can be managed on the field with a compression dressing, ice, and use of a commercial knee immobilizer. The athlete is kept non-weight-bearing and should be transported off the field on a stretcher.

Dislocations of the tibiofemoral joint require rigid splinting and immediate transfer to an emergency facility for reduction. Damage to the popliteal artery is a catastrophic and limb-threatening complication. Absent pulses, coldness, severe pain in the lower leg, paresthesias, or motor/sensory deficits indicate vascular compromise. A knee may reduce spontaneously after vascular injury has already occurred. Any suspicion that vascular insult has occurred merits expeditious transfer and emergency vascular evaluation.

Lateral dislocation of the patella follows valgus stress to the knee combined with external rotation

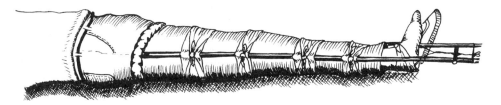

FIGURE 12-5. An example of the Thomas splint providing longitudinal traction following femoral fracture.

of the tibia. This may be reduced by extending the knee and gently pushing the patella medially. If spontaneous reduction has occurred, there will be swelling and tenderness along the medial retinaculum. Ice, compression bandage, knee immobilization, and x rays are recommended management. Quadriceps and patellar tendon ruptures result in an inability to extend the leg against gravity.

Specific examination of the injured knee begins on the field. The mechanism of injury, "snaps" or "pops," giving way, or previous knee injuries must be ascertained. Before moving the athlete to an examination area a brief physical examination should be performed on the field in an attempt to chart any instability before muscle spasm and guarding set in. Point tenderness over the medial and/or lateral ligaments help to localize the damaged ligament. The knee is then placed under varus and valgus stresses in extension and 30° of flexion. Instability of a stressed ligament in extension suggests posterior cruciate ligament rupture in addition to collateral ligament disruption, whereas instability in flexion suggests injury limited to the collateral ligament and possibly the anterior cruciate ligament. Several tests are used to test anterior cruciate injury. A positive anterior drawer test (knee in 90° of flexion) or Lachman test (knee in 20° flexion) indicate anterior cruciate insufficiency. Pivot shift and flexion-rotation-drawer tests indicate old anterior cruciate ligament injury. The posterior drawer test and sag test reflect posterior cruciate damage. These tests can be done in a few minutes' time. The athlete is then taken to an examination room, remaining non-weight-bearing. After removing any obscuring clothing, the knee is inspected for deformity, ecchymoses, and effusion. Range of motion is measured to detect locking or hyperextension. Meniscal injuries are associated with a valgus external rotation stress. Locking is commonly associated with bucket handle tears. Any or all of the physical examination should be repeated if the athlete is not in great discomfort. If pain is severe or deformity noted, further examination should be deferred until x rays are completed. A bulky dressing and knee immobilizer is placed on the knee and ice packs are applied.[26,27]

Marshall outlined the following six criteria,

any of which prevent a player's return to a game[27]:

1. Acute swelling of the knee
2. Acute instability in any plane
3. Dislocated patella
4. Dislocated knee
5. Excessively limited motion or locked knee
6. Severe pain.

The safety and future health of the athlete with an injured knee should always come first. An accurate diagnosis at the time of injury can help achieve this goal.

Leg injuries present several unique problems. Gross, unstable fractures are easily diagnosed and placed in a rigid splint extending above the knee. Stress fractures of the tibia or fibula most commonly present as chronic pain syndromes. Serial x rays usually make the diagnosis clear. *Shin splints* are believed to be caused by a periostitis at the origin of the tibialis muscles, generally seen in poorly-conditioned athletes. Rest, stretching, resistance exercises, and training on softer surfaces often provide sufficient relief. *Compartment syndrome* is a relative ischemia of an enclosed fascial compartment of the leg. Pain persisting after a direct blow or running has stopped, cramps, paresthesias, decreased motor, or sensory function signal ischemia. Rest and elevation are tried first; if there is no response, then hospital observation is required and fasciotomy may be indicated.[28]

Ankle injuries are extremely common. Once again, the injury's mechanism helps elucidate its nature. Lateral sprain of the ankle is associated with lateral swelling and tenderness over the anterior talofibular or calcaneofibular ligaments. If significant instability to varus stress or anteroposterior drawer stress is present, then a grade II or III sprain has occurred. Tenderness over the deltoid ligament indicates medial collateral ligament sprain. Concurrent medial and lateral ligament sprains result in marked ankle instability. Severe swelling, deformity, crepitus, or instability point towards fracture. All ankle injuries, except for the mildest sprains, should be immobilized in a compression splint, elevated, have ice packs applied, and be x rayed. An athlete who cannot demonstrate 100-percent mobility on the sideline following ankle injury should not be allowed to re-enter a game.

Achilles tendon rupture results from forced plantar flexion of the ankle. A snap may be heard. The average age of occurrence is 42, and it tends to occur in the poorly conditioned athlete. A palpable defect may be found, and with the knee flexed there is no plantar flexion when the calf is squeezed (Thompson test). A simple compression dressing and no weight bearing is sufficient prior to definitive therapy.

Foot injuries can be very annoying to the athlete. Sprains of the ligaments of the foot are generally treated by adhesive strapping. Fractures or dislocations produce disabling pain as a rule. Severe foot pain accompanied by swelling is reason to order a radiologic examination. Stress fractures of the metatarsals present as chronic pain and an x ray or bone scan is used to make the diagnosis.[28] Toe fractures are treated by buddy-taping and rest, whereas toe dislocations are easily reduced and require no specific treatment afterward.

INJURIES IN YOUNG ATHLETES
(see also Chapter 20)

The entire spectrum of athletic injuries can occur in any age group. However, the growing individual has certain musculoskeletal properties that result in different patterns of injury than the adult. Longitudinal bone growth occurs at the epiphyseal growth plates at both ends of the bone. These growth plates are cartilaginous and, therefore, not as strong as the surrounding bone. Stresses that may cause ligamentous injury in adults often result in fractures across the growth plate in children. Other areas of bony growth in the body also have bone separated from bone by a cartilaginous plate (e.g., apophyses of the pelvis). The diagnosis of epiphyseal injuries is made by x ray.[29]

In children with severe knee injuries, epiphyseal fractures across the distal femoral epiphyseal growth plate are frequently found. The capital femoral epiphysis may "slip" following hip trauma and can present as hip or knee pain, external rotational deformity, and limited internal hip rotation. These growth plate injuries have been classified by Salter

and Harris into six basic types. The possibility of growth plate fracture requires that x rays be taken routinely after injuries.[29,30] Upper extremity injuries may follow different patterns in young athletes. In the shoulder, epiphyseal fractures of the proximal humerus are prone to occur in gymnastics and contact sports. Remodeling of the bone is seen with growth. Elbow injuries may result in a supracondylar fracture of the humerus. Neurovascular compromise is a serious complication.

Another fracture that has a higher incidence in the young athlete is the avulsion fracture. Mechanisms that produce muscle or tendon strains in the adult may often only avulse the growing bone at the origin or insertion in the child. Examples are (1) ischiopubic avulsion fractures instead of adductor strains, (2) ischial tuberosity avulsion instead of hamstring pull, and (3) lesser trochanter avulsion instead of iliopsoas strain.

THIRD PRIORITY INJURIES

In the less-than-urgent category of injuries fall a variety of annoying conditions that, although not life threatening, can hamper continued play (Appendix B).

Abrasions (loss of superficial skin) are common in many sports and can be due to falls, friction from uniform or sports gear (groin cup), or trauma from an opponent or a piece of equipment (*shinai* in Kendo). An abrasion is best treated with a vigorous soap and water scrub as soon as possible in order to remove embedded dirt particles, which can serve as a nidus of infection and cause later discoloration. A sterile dressing is recommended though antibiotic/iodine ointments are of questionable value. If the abrasion is extensive, analgesic medications are recommended.

Lacerations can occur from impact on sharp or dull objects. Therefore, it is important to assess the width and depth of even small lacerations with particular consideration for foreign bodies. Thorough soap and water cleansing is imperative. Minor clean lacerations can be closed with benzoin and adhesive bandages and the athlete returned to the game *if* there is no further danger of injury. More often than not, a minor laceration is likely to be repaired ringside, with the athlete returning to the match only to have the wound widened/deepened and eventually requiring sutures. All contaminated lacerations that are not minor should be thoroughly debrided and referred for suturing. On-site suturing is not to be recommended since proper equipment is usually not available; the physician cannot observe further play; and the athlete should not be returned to the game even sutured as the wound will open up on repeated impact. Tetanus prophylaxis is mandatory.

Puncture wounds, although uncommon, can occur in some sports—skiing, martial arts, and track. Careful exploration, debridement, and cleansing are imperative. Some puncture wounds can reach the bone and this fact should be kept in mind. Tetanus immunization status should be assessed.

Skin vesicles (blisters) and *bullae* result from frictional forces generated in footwear and other sports wear. It is best to leave the lesion intact, letting it burst spontaneously. Good hygiene and sterile gauze go far in hastening healing and preventing infection. Blood-containing vesicles or bullae should be carefully monitored for infection.

REFERENCES

1. Cahill BR, Griffith ER: Exposure to injury in major college football. Am J Sports 7:183–185, 1971.
2. Mayne BR: A team physician's bag. Phys Sports Med 5:85–87, 1981.
3. Gurdjian ES: Acute head injuries. Surg Gynecol Obstet 146:805–820, 1978.
4. McCown IA: Boxing safety and injuries. Phys Sports Med 7:43–51, 1979.
5. Cloward RB: Acute cervical spine injuries. CIBA Clin Symp 32(1):1–32, 1980.
6. Kewalramani LS, Taylor RE: Injuries to the cervical spine from diving accidents. J Trauma 15:130–142, 1975.
7. DiVincenti FC, Rives JD, LaBorde EJ, et al: Blunt abdominal trauma. J Trauma 8:1004–1013, 1968.
8. Davis JJ, Cohn I, Nance FC: Diagnosis and management of blunt abdominal trauma. Ann Surg 183:672–678, 1975.
9. Ryan AJ (moderator): Infectious mononucleosis in athletes. Phys Sports Med 2:41–49, 1978.
10. Hahn B: Ruptured spleen: Implications for the athletic trainer. Athletic Training 13:190–191, Winter, 1978.
11. Druy EM, Rubin E: Computed tomography in evaluation of abdominal trauma. Comput Asst Tomogr 3:40, 1979.
12. Requarth Wm H: Acute abdominal emergencies, in Scheenwind John H (ed): Medical and Surgical Emergencies, ed 3. Chicago, Year Book Medical Publications, 1975, chap 10.
13. Smith DR: General Urology. Los Altos, Calif, Lange Medical Publications, 1981, pp 244–261.
14. Nahum AM: Immediate care of acute blunt laryngeal trauma. J Trauma 9(2):112–125, 1969.
15. Vaugn D, Asbury T, Cook R: General Ophthalmology. Los Altos, Calif, Lange Medical Publications, 1980, pp 318–323.
16. Bassler TJ: Marathon running and immunity to heart disease. Phys Sports Med 4:77, 1975.
17. Hancock E: Ischemic heart disease: Acute myocardial infarction, in Scientific American Textbook of Medicine. New York, Scientific American, 1981, vol X-I.
18. Berg C: Exercise prescription: A practitioners view. Phys Sports Med 2:98–104, 1978.
19. Waller B, Roberts W: Sudden death while running in conditioned runners aged 40 years or over. J Cardiol 45:1292, 1980.
20. Smodlaka V: Cardiovascular aspects of soccer. Phys Sports Med 7:66–70, 1978.
21. Cutler RW: Epilepsy, in Scientific American Textbook of Medicine. New York, Scientific American, 1981, vol XII, pp 1–6.
22. Toone BK, Roberts J: Status epilepticus: An uncommon hysterical conversion. J Nerv Ment Dis 167:548–552, 1979.
23. Schanz LK: Auto racing medicine. Phys Sports Med 6(5):118–122, 1978.
24. Cooper M: Lightning Injuries: Prognostic signs for death. Ann Emerg Med 9:134–138, 1980.
25. Tausigg HB: "Death" from lightning—and the possibility of living again. Ann Int Med 68:1345–1353, 1968.
26. Hoppenfeld S: Physical examination of the spine and extremities. Englewood Cliffs, NJ, Prentice-Hall, 1976.
27. Marshall JL, Rubin RM: Knee ligament injuries—A diagnostic and therapeutic approach. Orthop Clin North Am 8:641–667, 1977.
28. Detmer DD: Chronic leg pain. Am J Sports Med 8:141–144, 1980.
29. Tachdjian MD: Pediatric Orthopedics. Philadelphia, WB Saunders, 1972, pp 1532–1767.
30. Zariczny B, Shattuck LJ, Mast TA, et al: Sports-related injuries in school-aged children. Am J Sports Med 8:318–324, 1980.

BIBLIOGRAPHY

American Red Cross: Advanced First Aid and Emergency Care. Garden City, NY, Doubleday, 1979.

Craig TT: Comments in Sports Medicine. Chicago, American Medical Association, 1973.

Edmonson AS, Crenshaw AH (ed): Campbell's Orthopedics, ed 6. St. Louis, CV Mosby, 1980.

Meislin HW: Priorities in Multiple Trauma. Germantown, Md, Aspen Systems Corporation, 1980.

O'Donoghue DH: Treatment of Injuries to Athletes. Philadelphia, WB Saunders, 1976.

Rockwood CA, Green DP: Fractures. Philadelphia, JP Lippincott, 1975.

Ryan AJ, Allman FL: Sports Medicine. New York, Academic Press, 1974.

Sabiston DC (ed): Textbook of Surgery, ed 10. Philadelphia, WB Saunders, 1972.

Zuidema GD, Cameron JL, Sabatier HS: The Management of Trauma. Philadelphia, WB Saunders, 1979.

APPENDIX A

EMERGENCY EQUIPMENT

Physician's Bag

Sterile swabs
Sterile tongue blades
Sterile gloves
Sterile suture set
Sterile 4 × 4s
Sterile ABD pads
Sterile roll gauze
Sterile scalpel
5- and 10-cc syringes with 22-gauge needle
Lidocaine 1 percent plain
14-gauge intercaths
Eye patch (× 2)
Safety pins
Padded tongue blade
Adhesive bandages
Povidone–iodine
3-0 and 6-0 nylon sutures
1 and 2-inch adhesive tape
Tape adherent (benzoin)
4-inch cast padding (× 4)
Malleable metal finger splints (× 2)
3- and 6-inch elastic bandages (× 6)
Heavy duty bandage scissors
Flashlight
Stethoscope
Sphygmomanometer
Ophthalmoscope/otoscope
Contact lens suction cup

Field Equipment

5-gallon water containers
Assorted felt
Assorted foam rubber
Arm slings (× 4)
Towels
Ambulance
Heavy blanket (× 2)
Adjustable crutches (2 pair)
Ice pack with plastic bags
Spine boards (1 long, 1 short)
Cervical collar
Field stretcher or scoop
5-pound sand bags (× 2)
Splints—inflatable and cardboard
Thomas ½ ring splint
Bolt cutter or screwdriver (to remove faceguard from helmet in emergency)

CPR Equipment

Oral airway (adult and child sizes)
Disposable laryngoscope (adult and child sizes)
Endotracheal tube or esophageal obturator airway (adult and child sizes)
Ambu bag (adult and child sizes)
50-cc syringe with nasotracheal suction tube
5- and 10-cc syringes with 22-gauge needles
Ringer's lactate
IV tubing and catheters
Meperidine
Dexamethasone
Atropine
Phenytoin
Diazepam
Epinephrine
Lidocaine
Sodium bicarbonate

APPENDIX B

BASIC FIRST AID

Abrasion: Superficial skin loss. Treatment: soap and water, antibiotic or iodine ointment, sterile dressing.

Lacerations: Full-thickness disruption of skin. Treatment: irrigation, suturing, tetanus prophylaxis.

Blisters: Superficial skin bullae. Treatment: sterile gauze.

Puncture wounds: Caused by penetrating object. Treatment: remove foreign body; do not close skin; debride skin edges; tetanus prophylaxis.

Anaphylactic: Severe, acute allergic reaction (e.g., insect bites). Treatment: epinephrine 1:1000 0.5 cc subcutaneously every thirty minutes.

Heat-related condition: See Chapter 10 for details.

	Heat Exhaustion	Heat Stroke
Body temperature	Normal	106°F
Skin	Cold, clammy, pale	Hot, red, dry
Pulse	Rapid	Rapid
Level of consciousness	Faint or normal	Decreased
Symptoms	Weak, dizzy, nauseous	Weak to unresponsive
Cause	Salt and water depletion	Sweating mechanism failure
Treatment	Lie flat in shade	Ice or alcohol baths
	Loosen clothing	Start intravenous treatment
	Sips of salt water	
	Cool towels	

Heat cramps are related to salt and water depletion and treated with salt water sips and massage.

13
When an Athlete's Life Is in Danger

M. William Voss

The conditions (factors) that create life threatening situations for an athlete usually fall into at least one of four areas:

1. The athlete
2. Characteristics of the sport
3. Environmental factors
4. Climactic conditions

The athlete's predisposing characteristics (physical and psychological) include genetic factors, functional limitations, acute (or insidious) disease, and pathology from previous disease. Risk factors characteristic of the sport itself have long been recognized and handled by officially enforced safety rules (and penalties) and equipment and machine (vehicle) safety design requirements. Environmental factors (arena, stadium, field, area) have been minimized by standards and safety requirements for types of surfaces, lighting, object hazards, and fixed equipment design and material (Chapter 9). Climactic conditions (weather hazards) are to a certain degree modified by seasonal participation in particular sports and the indoor/outdoor location (Chapter 10). Regarding the remainder of risk modification, it is the responsibility of either the athlete or the officials to judge the danger involved in the existing climactic conditions (i.e., rain, snow, extremes of temperature, lightning) and make the decision to continue or suspend competitive play.

Life-threatening situations do occur in most recreational and competitive athletics and are major concerns of the responsible physician (as well as coach and trainer). Fortunately, the overall incidence of mortality is low. Tackle football played as an organized sport (approximately two deaths per 100,000 participants), machine racing (i.e., auto, airplane, power boat), and organized boxing have the most publicly visible and reported deaths due to trauma. Mortality from drowning is a very significant number, but many are accidental and not related to water sports. Reliable mortality rates from the numerous other athletic activities are not available.

The basic principles of organization, diagnosis, prompt management, and treatment of the athlete with a life-threatening medical condition are the same as for any injured athlete and are outlined in Chapter 12. Heavy reliance for diagnosis is placed on the history and physical examination. For an athlete whose life is in danger, these are usually accomplished under emotional and rushed circumstances. Physician equanimity is crucial, though very difficult to retain under competitive-sport conditions.

Take an accurate history from everyone, especially those closest to the event and those with the most knowledge of the patient, even if you yourself were a witness. Learn to rely on the player, the coach, teammates, and even spectators. Avoid jumping to conclusions.

The physical examination of an athlete whose life is threatened is best performed in a stepwise, systematic sequence: (1) vital signs, (2) head and neck, (3) chest, (4) abdomen, and (5) skin and extremities. Evaluate the gravity of the situation. These are excellent rules to follow:

1. Never think totally in terms of diagnosis
2. Never ignore positive findings

The primary care physician responsible for the medical care of the athletes is in reality both a sports medicine physician and an emergency physician. As such, he or she should be able to recognize and deal appropriately and expeditiously with all conditions that are a threat to the athlete's life. First priority injuries are outlined below:

First-priority: Immediate threat to life (death within minutes)*

1. Respiratory arrest
   a. Upper airway obstruction
   b. Acute respiratory failure
   c. Acute pulmonary edema
   d. Pneumothorax (may include open chest wound)
2. Cardiac arrest
3. Anaphylactic shock
4. Uncontrolled hemorrhage/hypovolemia

IMMEDIATE THREAT TO LIFE

Respiratory Arrest
Causes of respiratory arrest are airway obstruction, head trauma, maxillofacial injury, drowning (Chapter 10), stroke, and myocardial infarction (Chapters 7 and 12).
   Airway Obstruction. This is a common cause of respiratory arrest though it is a relatively infrequent occurrence in organized sports competition. Considering the wide range of athletic participation (organized and individual) and the diverse nature and hazards of the activities, however, it continues to become a more common and important injury. In most instances, it can be treated successfully and

---

There are many undetected (or known) medical conditions that constitute a threat to life if strenuous athletic activity and/or severe environmental stresses are superimposed. See also Chapter 12 for second-priority injuries.

the life saved. It can occur as a result of an unconscious state, a foreign body, obstruction by blood, mucus, or saliva or traumatic deformity of the larynx.[1] Central nervous system (CNS) depression following head trauma is a major cause of respiratory failure.[2]

1a. Upper airway obstruction
   i. When unconscious in supine position and becomes apneic, the tongue falls back and occludes the airway
      Treatment: Establish an airway by supporting the neck and tilting the head back
   ii. Foreign body (rare in athletes)
      Diagnosis: Cannot breathe or talk; gives "choke" sign
      Treatment: Heimlich maneuver
   iii. Trauma to neck (larynx)
      Treatment: Cricothyroid cannula (only if physician is experienced—very rarely needed in sports medicine)

The adequacy of breathing and circulation must be determined immediately in the unresponsive, injured athlete. Airway obstruction is characterized by exaggerated respiratory efforts with little or no air flow felt from the patient's mouth or nose. The accessory muscles of respiration are seen to retract in the intercostal, supraclavicular, and suprasternal areas. Snoring, stridor, or wheezing may occur. In contrast, respiratory failure is associated with little or no respiratory effort. Breath sounds are absent, diminished, or characterized by adventitial noises, such as rales and rhonchi. Cyanosis may become increasingly apparent. When an athlete is unconscious in a supine condition and becomes apneic, the tongue has probably fallen back and occluded the airway due to the relaxation of the oropharyngeal musculature and force of gravity on the tongue. In contrast, a foreign body is usually aspirated, becomes lodged in the larynx or trachea, and obstructs the airway. The classical triad for diagnosis is present when the athlete cannot breathe (is cyanotic), cannot talk, and gives the "choke" sign (hand to neck—often with voluntary protrusion of the tongue). General guidelines[3] for foreign body upper airway obstruction include the following:

1. *Complete* airway obstruction is almost silent.
2. *Incomplete* upper airway obstruction can be made worse by probing the hypopharynx with a finger or by turning the athlete upside-down.

Many techniques are available for the establishment of a patent airway. The specific technique used varies according to the experience of the physician or first aid rescuer and equipment available. If cervical spine injury is suspected, the athlete must be placed in the supine position (as outlined in the section on neck injuries, Chapter 12; see also Chapter 14). Protective mouth pieces, chewing gum, or other objects (blood, teeth) must be manually removed. An oropharyngeal or nasopharyngeal airway should be inserted and the presence of spontaneous respiration reassessed. The head-tilt into extension and forward chin lift can also be used to open the upper airway. In cases of potential cervical spine injury, neck extension should be avoided and a forward jaw thrust without head-tilt is used.[3,4]

The treatment of upper airway obstruction due to a foreign body is as follows:

1. If the athlete has acute and complete obstruction, four back blows with the patient upright or horizontal followed by four abdominal thrusts compressing the upper abdomen just below the diaphragm—the Heimlich maneuver.[3] If unsuccessful, emergency tracheostomy or cricothyreotomy may be necessary.
2. If the athlete has partial obstruction and appears to be moving adequate amounts of air, keep in the sitting forward position with neck extended until endoscopy can be performed.
3. If the airway is stable, arrange a referral where x rays of the neck and chest can be obtained to determine location and size of the foreign body.

When a patent airway is not established using the described methods, there are these alternatives:

1. Esophageal obturator airway
2. Nasotracheal or endotracheal intubation
3. Transtracheal catheterization/cricothyreotomy

The *esophageal obturator airway* (EOA) is inserted blindly through the mouth into the esophagus. A distal balloon is inflated with air to obstruct the esophagus and the patient is ventilated via multiple air holes in the pharyngeal portion of the tube. The advantages of the EOA are speed, blind insertion without manipulation of the cervical spine, and the prevention of aspiration. Its use is contraindicated in foreign body upper airway obstruction and posterior pharyngeal bleeding. In addition, the location of the obturator balloon should be checked since inflation can cause tracheal obstruction if it is too proximal.

Endotracheal intubation requires training and confidence in its use. It offers the best control of the patient's airway. "Blind" *nasotracheal insertion* is a refined technique which does not require manipulation of the cervical spine and, therefore, is an excellent choice in cases of suspected or proven cervical spine injury. The tube is carefully advanced to the larynx through the nasopharynx and is pushed quickly and atraumatically through the vocal cords when air flow is felt at the proximal end.

Once the airway is established, artificial breathing techniques are started if spontaneous respiration is absent. Mouth-to-mouth (with nostrils pinched), mouth-to-tube, bag-valve-face mask, or bag-valve-tube are acceptable options, although mouth-to-mouth breathing is most effective. Adequate ventilation should be continued until arrival at an emergency room facility. Tubes should not be removed outside of an emergency room even in an alert patient because of the possibility of vomiting, aspiration, or loss of adequate resuscitative frequency (i.e., one breath every fifth chest compression). Adequate bilateral ventilation can be confirmed by auscultation though this method may be unreliable in children and young adolescents.[3]

A *direct blow (trauma) to the larynx* that fractures or deforms the anatomy in such a way as to impede the flow of air is fortunately rare in sports medicine. Such obstruction is usually incomplete at onset; however, the anatomical site has a great propensity for rapid edema formation which is additive, often completing the airway obstruction and prohibiting the use of standard endotracheal intubation or EOA. The treatment is to establish an airway surgically by performing a cricothyreotomy.

There is disagreement among sports medicine physicians concerning the use of cricothyreotomy. (Tracheostomy is strictly a hospital procedure). Opponents of its use cite the rarity of the requirements and the lack of experience by practitioners. Proponents of the procedure state that with the great diversity and magnitude of risk taking in very-high-velocity sports, the need for the procedure is becoming more frequent. They also state that the procedure is not too complicated for the sports medicine practitioner. Some simple guidelines for the use of cricothyreotomy are as follow:

1. Use it only as a last resort.
2. Insert a No. 14- or 16-gauge needle into the cricothyroid membrane to maintain airflow until more satisfactory airway control can be gained. If ineffective, then:
3. Surgically enter the trachea at the level of the second or third tracheal ring and insert a temporary makeshift rigid or semirigid airway (pen barrel or stethoscope hose) if a commercial airway is not available. Secure with adhesive tape.

Standard cricothyreotomy kits are available from several sources and the primary care physician may elect to have one on hand for such emergencies.

Acute Respiratory Failure. Acute respiratory failure in an athlete can be very deceptive. On the one hand, it is obvious and dramatic; on the other, subtle and insidious. One athlete might be gasping and struggling for breath while another is somnolent and quiet with shallow respirations and a silent chest, but both could be equally in great danger from acute respiratory failure. The signs of such failure are those produced by hypoxia and hypercapnia upon the circulatory and central nervous system, including tachycardia, hypotension, mental aberrations, cyanosis, and unconsciousness.[5]

By definition, respiratory failure exists when arterial oxygen tension has fallen below 50 mm Hg. The first cellular consequences of the hypoxia are in the biological sequences that require high oxygen tension; specifically, synthesis, degradation, and detoxification. Another impairment is generation of adenosine triphosphate (ATP) in the mitochondria. This causes a shift to anaerobic glycolysis which is $1/18$ as efficient as oxidative phosphorylation in

meeting the high energy needs of the heart and brain. Its end product is lactic acid, which is accumulative and can be fatal.[6]

1b. Acute respiratory failure
   i. Syncope (most common).
      Psychophysiologic reaction: Athlete becomes hypotensive, pale, nauseated, and loses consciousness—often with a period of apnea and occasionally a convulsion.
      Treatment: Establish airway only and observe. Breathing usually resumes. If necessary, start rescue breathing.
   ii. Craniocerebral injuries may cause apnea.
      Etiology: a. Transient paralysis of oropharyngeal musculature.
      b. Respiratory arrest.
      Treatment: Airway; rescue breathing

The most common type of acute respiratory failure seen in sports medicine is caused by simple *syncopal apnea.* This psychophysiological reaction leads to pallor, nausea, hypotension, and coma—with a period of respiratory arrest. A seizure may occur. Usually the condition is self-limiting and breathing resumes normally. While the athlete is unconscious the physician may ensure an open upper airway by pulling the jaw forward.

Respiratory arrest has many causes—metabolic, traumatic, toxic, neurologic, and vascular. Treatment precedes defining etiology and an airway should be established immediately. If apnea persists for more than a minute or two, mouth-to-mouth resuscitation should be instituted. Insertion of a plastic oropharyngeal airway in the unconscious patient is advisable. Prolonged ventilatory support may be accomplished with manually operated bag and mask.

Acute Pulmonary Edema (see also Chapter 10). Occurring at high altitude, acute pulmonary edema is a perplexing and poorly understood entity when associated with exercise in a completely normal individual. It is much exaggerated and occurs at lower altitude and with less exercise in the presence of abnormalities in the cardiovascular–pulmonary axis. (An example is the absence of the right pulmonary artery in skiers.) It has been reported to be fatal in at least one case and occurred

in three other cases at altitudes of only 2000 to 3000 feet.[7] Thirty-three cases of high-altitude pulmonary edema in climbers resulted in nine deaths (27 percent).[8] This condition occurs in people who live in the lowlands and travel to high altitude, and in people who live at high altitude on their return home after a visit to the lowlands. There is an apparent 10 percent recurrence in susceptible individuals.

Exposure to high altitude (8000 to 24,000 feet) in exercise sports continues to increase rapidly. Sports most common at these altitudes are skiing and mountain climbing. Acute pulmonary edema occurs most often in climbers. The winter Olympic Games are usually conducted at moderate altitudes. In one case, the summer Olympics were conducted at Mexico City, which is at an altitude of 6000 feet above sea level. In addition to the exercise at rarefied atmosphere, the cold temperatures predisposed athletes to acute mountain sickness and possible pulmonary edema. Sickle cell trait disease increases the risk of sickle crisis at high altitudes. The primary care physician therefore most be alert to the chronic as well as the acute problems of exposure to high altitude.

The clinical features and pathophysiology of high-altitude pulmonary edema in the unacclimatized individual begins with hypoxia. Cerebral edema and pulmonary edema are the undesirable consequences. The body adapts initially by tachypnea (increase minute volume) and tachycardia without a significant increase in cardiac output. The rapid mouth breathing of dry air results in dehydration and respiratory alkalosis. The medullary respiratory centers become depressed as a result of the alkalotic cerebral spinal fluid and respond less well to hypoxia. The hyperventilation then becomes hypoventilation with profound hypoxia and hypercarbia. Cerebral edema, increased pulmonary artery pressure, cyanosis, and coma develop. If full-blown high-altitude pulmonary edema ensues, death often occurs. The precise pathophysiology, which may be similar to neurogenic pulmonary edema resulting from massive sympathetic responses, is unknown. There is no evidence of decreased cardiac output or left ventricular heart failure as shown by normal pulmonary wedge pressure. The pulmonary edema of high altitude has features of excessive permeability and hemodynamic factors common to the two main types encountered.[9] The individual acclimatized (average, 4 days) to altitude has, through erythropoietic stimulation of bone marrow, increased the red cell mass and hematocrit. The plasma volume also increases. The changes of long-term adjustment to high-altitude living are pulmonary hypertension and right heart strain.[10]

The initial clinical symptoms of altitude sickness are headache, insomnia, dyspnea, light-headedness, confusion, nausea, malaise, and fatigue. These are unpleasant although not serious. Progression of symptoms to chest pain, cough, confusion, lethargy, and sleepiness is more serious. The symptoms of acute pulmonary edema are profound dyspnea and orthopnea with cyanosis.

The treatment of high-altitude pulmonary edema must be prompt and specific. Oxygen (up to 100 percent) should be given along with rest and rapid descent to a lower altitude. A sitting position improves ventilation. If these measures are immediately impossible or ineffective, diuretic therapy may be instituted. Furosemide 4 mg IV every 12 hours is recommended.[11] Acetazolamide has been proposed in prevention of high-altitude pulmonary edema. Morphine sulfate 5 mg IV to decrease pulmonary blood volume and aminophylline 250 mg IV or by suppository may be given to reduce continued respiratory distress. Digitalis and antibiotics have specific indications for their use. In the hypoventilation phase there may be a place for medroxyprogesterone acetate as a respiratory stimulant.

Prevention of high-altitude pulmonary edema is difficult because of the unpredictability of its occurrence. Medical discretion seems to indicate that modification of the extremes of exercise and altitude, the elimination of intercurrent illness (i.e., cyanotic congenital heart disease, primary pulmonary hypertension, and sickle cell disease), attaining adequate rest, hydration, and adequate nutrition, while avoiding overeating and the use of alcohol all have a beneficial effect.

Pneumothorax. This condition is associated with shortness of breath, tachycardia, and pleuritic chest pain. Occasionally, only a cough of recent onset will indicate its presence. Breath sounds are

decreased, and hyperresonant percussion is present on the involved side. *Open pneumothorax* refers to the presence of a sucking chest wound, over which a sterile dressing should be applied. If an occlusive dressing is applied, the patient must be observed for development of a *tension pneumothorax*—a life-threatening condition in which increasing intra-pleural pressure is caused by a one-way "ball-valve" leakage of air into the pleural space. Physical examination may reveal shift of the trachea to the opposite side, distended neck veins, and subcutaneous emphysema in addition to hyperresonant percussion. The high intrapleural pressure may be equilibrated to atmospheric pressure by inserting a needle percutaneously into the intrapleural space at the second right interspace in the midclavicular line. The condition of the athlete should improve immediately and the needle should be left in place pending more definitive treatment. The danger of untreated tension pneumothorax is lower airway obstruction, great vessel compromise, and cardiovascular collapse. *Hemothorax,* or *hemopneumothorax,* may be associated with any of the above findings, but there is typically dullness to percussion. This condition is treated as above. Hypovolemic shock is a potential outcome, as each hemothorax can contain up to 3000 milliliters of blood.

Flail chest is caused by segmental fractures of three or more ribs. Paradoxical motion of the involved segment is seen during respiration. Stabilization of the flail segment with a hand or sandbag is usually adequate, followed by immediate transport to the hospital.

Cardiac Arrest

Cardiac arrest occurring during or within 1 hour after exercise usually results from one of these three conditions:

1. Cardiovascular collapse
2. Ventricular fibrillation
3. Ventricular standstill (asystole)

In the general population, cardiovascular disease is a cause of sudden death in 90 percent of cases in males and 50 percent in females.[12] The remaining causes are most related to diseases of the respiratory tract, the central nervous system, the gastrointestinal tract, and the genitourinary system. When an athlete suffers a nontraumatic or non-drowning sudden death it is usually from cardiovascular causes and in a male under 50 years of age. In the presence of ischemic coronary artery disease, strenuous exertion alone or combined with other factors (i.e., extreme climactic conditions or infection) can lead to sudden death.[13] The risk is often enhanced by lack of regular exercise, smoking, and in some cases by the element of competition. This health hazard is difficult to determine because the physician has no definite way of identifying asymptomatic persons who are at risk—although systolic blood pressure tends to be higher in the ischemic heart disease group.

Sudden death from ischemic causes other than atherosclerotic coronary artery disease is due to a variety of causes. The most perplexing of these is death with a normal lumen of the coronary arteries (no or minimal atherosclerotic changes) and presumably from arterial spasm.[14-16] Prinzmetal's angina is a vasospastic phenomenon that can cause infarction.[17] It is often difficult to assign the etiology of sudden death to vasospasm alone when other factors are present (e.g., climactic: high humidity and high temperature). It is well documented that heat stroke can cause significant cardiovascular damage, manifested as congestive heart failure and transient repolarization (ECG) abnormalities.[18]

The sine qua non for protecting athletes from sudden death due to cardiac causes is prevention. Every effort should be made to impose proper exercise restrictions on persons participating in both recreational physical activity or competitive sports. The greatest graded restrictions should be placed on individuals with aortic valve disease (stenosis and insufficiency), congestive heart failure from any cause, and recent myocarditis or any etiology. All myocardiopathies—congestive, hypertrophic,[19] and restrictive—are high risk factors. Mitral valve disease (mitral stenosis and mitral insufficiency) are high risk factors especially when associated with secondary changes such as ventricular hypertrophy and ECG changes of left ventricular strain (mitral insufficiency) or atrial fibrillation (mitral stenosis). Tricuspid and pulmonary artery disease appear to

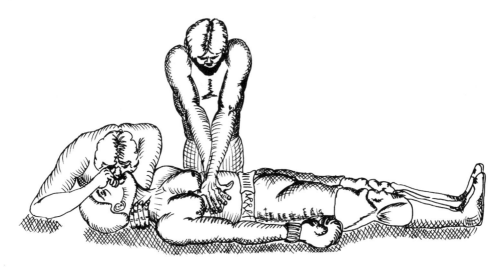

FIGURE 13-1. Cardiopulmonary resuscitation (CPR).

have a lesser risk factor than the valves on the left side (high pressure) of the heart. Congenital heart disease, with shunting particularly at the ventricular level (ventricular septal defect) and beyond (patent ductus arteriosus), is high risk for strenuous athletic competition.

The least serious of the congenital lesions is the atrial septal defect unless associated with pulmonary artery hypertension and right-to-left shunting. Cyanotic congenital heart disease has its physiologic limitations and thus presents as a formidable risk factor. Prosthetic valve replacement probably is a risk factor due to the valve's functional and mechanical limitations, its placement vulnerability to trauma, and the high probability of associated diseases. Marfan's syndrome, although primarily a risk factor from aortic media disease (rupture), has frequent valve cusp and septal deformities.[20] Electrical (ECG) abnormalities that impose risk are Wolf–Parkinson–White (WPW) conduction pattern (if associated with paroxysmal atrial premature second- and third-degree atrioventricular conduction defects), multifocal premature ventricular contractions, and premature ventricular beats that increase in frequency with exercise.[21]

The role of a "cardiac warm-up" appears to have significant implications especially when as-

sociated with some cardiac pathology. It is known that the adaptation of coronary blood flow to a rapid increase of cardiac work is not instantaneous and can lead to ischemia.[22,23]

Placing exercise restrictions on an athlete is difficult. The decision is, of course, made by the athlete (or coach) on the recommendations of the physician, who should first ascertain the following:

1. What is the lesion?
2. What currently is known about the lesion's risk potential?
3. What is the sport and associated cardiac strain?
4. How does the athlete respond to psychological stress of competition?[24]

Treatment of cardiac arrest suffered in a sports event is on-the-spot cardiopulmonary resuscitation (CPR) (Fig. 13-1), performed principally according to recommendation of the American Heart Association.[25] The indications as recommended by the American Heart Association for basic life support are as follow:

1. Respiratory arrest
2. Cardiac arrest, which can result from:
   a. Cardiovascular collapse (electromechanical dissociation)

b. Ventricular fibrillation

c. Ventricular standstill (asystole).

The steps leading to use of CPR evaluate (1) airway, (2) breathing, and (3) circulation. The treatment procedures are artificial ventilation and artificial circulation. After the airway has been stabilized, the circulatory system is evaluated. The diagnosis of cardiac arrest is made when there is no discernible heartbeat on physical examination (palpation of carotid or femoral pulses and auscultation of the precordium) and the patient has lost consciousness. Treatment should begin immediately after recognizing the need. If circulatory failure accompanies respiratory failure, artificial circulation techniques must be instituted in addition to respiratory resuscitation.[3]

The first aid treatment of cardiac arrest is *artificial circulation*. If the arrest is witnessed, a "precordial thump" (a sharp blow to the precordium with the fleshy portion of a clenched fist) is performed. This maneuver may generate a small electrical stimulus and restore a cardiac beat in cases of asystole due to block or reversing ventricular fibrillation of recent onset. If no response occurs external cardiac compression is begun at once with the victim supine and on a firm surface (Fig. 13-1). Effective external cardiac compression in the adult requires depression of the lower one-third of the sternum by 4.0 to 5.0 cm ($1\frac{1}{2}$ to 2 inches). Care should be taken to avoid applying compression over the xiphoid. Compression rate should be 60 per minute with each stroke sustained for 0.5 seconds. Artificial respirations should be timed to occur on the upstroke after each fifth compression. Counting each stroke out loud facilitates coordination of efforts (1001, 1002, . . .). Effectiveness of the external compressions is determined by the presence of the carotid or femoral pulse.

When to begin and when to terminate CPR if ineffective in restoring spontaneous circulation and ventilation is a medical decision. Efforts should continue until the physician in charge decides to terminate the resuscitation, which should be in a hospital setting. Once a spontaneous pulse returns, the external compressions should stop.[3] When the procedure is in progress, the physician should be planning the next move, should it be necessary. Some elements of advanced life support may be instituted by the primary care physician if available. It is unlikely that a primary care physician at a sporting event or practice will have available more than epinephrine [1:10,000 (0.1 ml/kg) diluted to 0.3 to 2 ml] for transthoracic intracardiac injection and supplemental oxygen with a bag-valve-mask device for ventilation. The latter requires special proficiency for operation. Although beyond the scope of this book, drug therapy for the arrest situation should be understood by all physicians involved with sports.

Transfer to trained personnel with available necessary equipment should be prompt and efficient. Full life support in a back-up ambulance is ideal. Essentials should include a full range of cardiac drugs, a defibrillator, telemetered ECG capability, and voice communication with the hospital's emergency room.

Basic cardiac life support courses are offered throughout the United States. Any physician at attendance of a sporting event should be currently certified in advanced cardiopulmonary life support techniques. Every year, the *Journal of the American Medical Association* publishes the current standards for cardiopulmonary resuscitation and emergency cardiac care based on the American Heart Association guidelines.

Anaphylactic Shock

Anaphylaxis is an immediate hypersensitivity reaction manifested locally as urticaria and angioedema or systemically as bronchospasm and profound hypotension (shock). When fatal, the cause of death is cerebral hypoxia. Systemic anaphylaxis (the more serious) can be caused by insect stings or by injection of drugs or serums.

In the general population of the United States about 50 percent of deaths from venomous creatures are from the order *Hymenoptera* (stinging insect) hypersensitivity. The known remainder are largely from bites of snakes, spiders, and possibly the fire ant.[26]

The primary care physician is most often presented with the stinging insect type of hypersensitivity. The most frequent cases are joggers, golfers, and tennis players. An unknown number of cases occur in campers, fishermen, and hikers. The *Hymenoptera* has three families of interest to the sports physician: Aphidae (honeybees); Bombidae (bumblebees); and Vespidae (wasps, hornets, and yellow jackets). Formicidae (ants) are of lesser concern.[27] The most common cause of anaphylaxis is the yellow jacket. Most cases occur in males under the age of 20.

The pathophysiology centers around the production of IgE by an antigen that sensitizes the mast cell or basophil.[28] Subsequent exposure to the antigen causes a cell-attached IgE-antibody and antigen complex. This disrupts the mast cell or basophil membranes releasing mediators of anaphylaxis such as histamine, kinins, prostaglandins, the slow reacting substance of anaphylaxis, and heparin chymase. Eosinophils attracted to the area produce a number of enzymes which neutralize these mediators.[29] Mediator release by mast cells is modulated by the cyclic nucleotides cAMP and cGMP. A high local tissue level of cAMP which depends upon β-adrenergic activity inhibits histamine and other mediator release from the mast cells. On the other hand, α-adrenergic receptors decrease levels of cAMP. This reduction accompanied by cholinergic receptor increase of cGMP serves as a potent stimulator of mediator release.

Other mechanisms not triggered by IgE are known to facilitate release from mediators of immediate hypersensitivity from mast cells. One such mechanism is through the classical complement pathway, generating the anaphylatoxins C3a + C5a which can stimulate the release of mast cell mediators. Another method may be by physical stimuli. Exercise-induced anaphylaxis has been described.[30] It is not known, however, whether hypothermia or hyperthermia are causative factors in this entity.

Rarely is there a history suggestive of anaphylaxis from an insect sting. More often the history is noncontributory. A positive history of anaphylaxis in a blood relative increases the risk.

The clinical picture involves feeling faint, itching of the skin, difficulty in breathing, tightness in the chest, wheezing, abdominal cramps, and collapse. The diagnosis is made by the history of an insect sting and the characteristic allergic reaction.

The treatment is immediate injection of 0.5 ml of 1:1000 epinephrine subcutaneously in adults (0.01 ml/kg of 1:10,000 epinephrine in children) if only pulmonary symptoms are present. If the patient is hypotensive, inject it intravenously or into the base of the tongue. Repeat at intervals of 10 to 20 minutes as needed. If the sting is on an extremity, a tourniquet should be applied to limit absorption. Oxygen should be given by mask if available and there is no upper airway obstruction. CPR may be necessary.

Evacuation to a hospital should be prompt and with medical attendance. Therapy for anaphylaxis is difficult at best in a hospital. It is usually quite impossible beyond tourniquet and epinephrine therapy on an athletic field.

The sports medicine physician's most effective role in anaphylaxis is prevention. Hypersensitive athletes should wear a medication condition identification tag. They should also be instructed in the use of a prescribed commercial bee-sting kit. Decreasing outdoor exposure to stinging insects is difficult for the athlete who wears a definitive uniform and participates in a specific area. The wearing of scented cosmetics and lotions attract insects, as does dark or floral clothing. The wearing of shoes affords protection. Immunotherapy with insect venom is more effective than whole-body extracts in preventing anaphylaxis.[31]

Uncontrolled Hemorrhage/Hypovolemia

Massive external bleeding is usually the result of lacerations, crush injury, or open fractures. Most types of hemorrhage can be controlled with direct pressure over the site of bleeding. Elevation of a lacerated upper extremity may help decrease the rate of hemorrhage. Applying pressure over the supplying arteries at their "pressure points" can be very effective. Blind clamping of bleeding vessels is to be condemned as important tissue may be damaged (i.e., nerves). Tourniquets are used only in truly life-threatening situations where other methods of obtaining hemostasis have failed. They should be as wide as possible, the time of application noted, and an obvious notation made on the athlete that a tourniquet is in place (large red T). The physician should be in charge of tourniquet application and its removal. In the case of open fractures, splinting helps reduce bleeding and prevent further vascular injury. *Occult hemorrhage* is bleeding that goes unrecognized but may significantly decrease the intravascular volume. This may be seen in closed fractures, intraabdominal, or intrathoracic injuries.

Hypovolemic shock is heralded by pallor, thin, rapid pulse, cold clammy skin, hypotension and change in mental status. It should be remembered that 20 percent of the vascular volume can be lost before the blood pressure drops. These findings require restoration of the intravascular volume as quickly as possible. Intravenous crystalloid solutions, such as Ringer's lactate or normal saline, should be administered via several large-bore intravenous catheters at the earliest possible opportunity. Blood pressure should then be obtained and appropriate measures taken to ensure its stabilization.

Cardiac tamponade, a form of hypovolemic shock, is heralded by hypotension, distant heart sounds, tachycardia, respiratory distress, distended neck veins, and pulsus paradoxicus. Subxiphoid pericardiocentesis with 3-inch, No. 18-gauge needle should be attempted under conditions of rapid deterioration. Other conditions that may have dire outcomes are rupture of the aorta, diaphragm, esophagus, or tracheobronchial tree, fractures of the first and second ribs, and pulmonary or myocardial contusion. These are best diagnosed and treated in the emergency room.

REFERENCES

1. Cooper D: This Sporting Life. Emerg Med, 10:24–66, 1978.
2. Rose J, Valtonan S, Jennett B: Avoidable factors contributing to death after head trauma. Br Med J 3:615–618, 1977.
3. Standards and Guidelines for Cardio-Pulmonary Resuscitation (CPR) and Emergency Cardiac Care (ECC). J Am Med Assoc 224:(suppl), 1980.
4. Torg JS, Quedenfeld TC, Newell Wm: When the athlete's life is threatened. Phys Sports Med 3:54–59, 1975.
5. Burman S, Alias D: Emergencies of the respiratory system, in Schneewind (ed): Medical and Surgical Emergencies, ed 3. Chicago, Yearbook Medical Publishers, 1975, p 152.
6. Robin ED: Respiratory medicine, in Rubenstein E (ed): Scientific American Medicine Textbook. New York, Scientific American, 1982, vol I, No. 14, p 10.
7. Hackett PH, Creagh E, Grover R, et al: High altitude pulmonary edema in persons without the right pulmonary artery. N Engl J Med 302:1070–1073, 1980.
8. Hultgren HN: High altitude medical problems. West J Med 131:8–23, 1979.
9. Hackett PH, Drummond R: Rales, peripheral edema, retinal hemorrhage and acute mountain sickness. Am J Med 67:214–218, 1979.
10. Heath D: The morbid anatomy of high altitude. Postgrad Med J 55:502–510, 1979.
11. Krissoff WB: The hazards of exercising at altitude. Phys Sports Med 3(8):26–31, 1975.
12. Spain DM: Coronary atherosclerosis as a cause of unexpected and unexplained death. An autopsy study from 1949–1959. J Am Med Assoc 174:384–388, 1960.
13. Vuori I, Makarainen M, Jass Kelainen A: Sudden death and physical activity. Cardiology 63:284–304, 1978.
14. Gibbon LW, Cooper KH, Meyer CM: The acute cardiac risk of strenuous exercise. J Am Med Assoc 244:1779–1801, 1980.
15. Thompson PD, Stern MP, Paul WS: Deaths during running. J Am Med Assoc 242:1265–1267, 1979.
16. Green LH, Cohen SI, Kurland G: Fatal myocardial infarction in marathon running. Ann Intern Med 84:704–706, 1976.
17. Waller BF, Roberts Wm C: Sudden death while running in conditioned runners aged 40 years or over. Case reports. Am J Cardiol 45:1292–1300, 1980.
18. Kew MC: The heart in heat stroke. Am Heart J 77:324–335, 1969.
19. Noakes TD, Rose AG, Opie LH: Hypertrophic cardiomyopathy associated with sudden death during marathon racing. Br Heart J 41:624–627, 1979.
20. Rose K: Which cardiovascular problems should disqualify athletes? Phys Sports Med 6:63–68, 1975.
21. Barnard JR: The heart needs warm-up time. Phys Sports Med 1:40, 1976.
22. Barnard JR, MacAlpine R, Kattus AA: Ischemic response to sudden strenuous exercise in healthy men. Circulation 48:936–942, 1973.
23. Cushing D: "Cain" death—fibrous coronary artery block. Brief Reports. Phys Sports Med 7:20, 1979.
24. McMillan RL: Sudden death in athletes and Marfan's syndrome. Phys Sports Med 6:105–109, 1978.
25. Standards for CPR and Emergency Cardiac Care. J Am Med Assoc 227(7):(suppl), 1974.

26. Parrish HM: Anaphylaxis of 460 fatalities from venomous animals in the US. Am J Med Sci 245:129–141, 1963.

27. deShazo RD, Evans RE, Ward G: When an insect sting can mean death. Phys Sports Med 6:72–76, 1976.

28. Lamphier TA: Current diagnosis and treatment of acute anaphylaxis. J South Calif Med Assoc 10:449–452, 1979.

29. David J: Immediate hypersensitivity, in Rubenstein E (ed): Scientific American Medicine Textbook, New York, Scientific American, 1982, vol IX, p 6.

30. Siegal AJ: Exercise-induced anaphylaxis. Phys Sports Med 1(8):95–98, 1980.

31. Hendrix SG: Further studies on the safety of polymerized antigens for immunotherapy. J Allergy Clin Immun 67:124, 1981.

14
Common Injuries of the Head and Neck

Richard B. Birrer

HEAD

More fatalities in sports occur as secondary to injuries to the head and neck than injuries to any other part of the body. Though such injuries tend to be most severe in contact sports such as football, rugby, boxing, and the martial arts,[1–6] increasing participation in certain noncontact sporting events (i.e., golf, baseball, skiing, snowmobiling) has produced a corresponding increase in less serious head injuries.[7]

Neurologic Evaluation

Regardless of the extent or type of head injury, the primary care physician must always conduct an evaluation along the same set of priority guidelines:

1. Is the patient breathing and the airway secure?
2. What is the circulatory status of the athlete?
3. Is the patient conscious or unconscious?
4. Is the patient capable of moving all extremities?
5. What is the least stimulus to which the patient will respond?

Once the ABCs of basic life support are secured and all higher priority injuries have been ruled out (abdominal and chest trauma), attention should be directly turned to neurologic status of the patient.

The management of all head injuries begins with a careful neurologic exam. This should be conducted in a serial fashion and the results clearly documented on a flow chart. A more thorough exam of the conscious patient-athlete includes mental status and motor/sensory exams. In the unconscious player, pupillary, respiratory, and reflex changes can accurately predict rostral–caudal deterioration. In addition to basic life support strategies (Chapter 13), the head should be elevated 30° to assist venous drainage of the brain, nasopharyngeal suction should be performed if secretions cannot be cleared, patient's fluid intake should be restricted, and 20 percent mannitol in combination with dexamethasone should be pushed IV. All forms of sedation should be avoided, as level of consciousness is the most sensitive indicator of intracranial pressure. If analgesia must be given, codeine is probably the drug of choice since it does not change pupillary findings.

Remember always to examine the neck and cervical spine in all head injuries since there is a high association between the two. At the hospital, pertinent skull films as well as those of the cervical spine should be obtained in all head injury victims. All concussions lasting more than 5 minutes or those associated with any amount of posttraumatic amnesia should be admitted for observation. Though it is not necessary to admit skull fractures, a linear one—particularly one crossing the venous sinus or middle meningeal artery groove—should be observed in the hospital for 24 to 48 hours for subsequent hemorrhage. All other injuries should prompt immediate neurosurgical consultation. The temporary paralysis of a limb, spontaneous subarachnoid hemorrhage, recurring cerebral concussion, uncontrolled episodes of impaired consciousness, and neurologic deficits from previous injury or other organic brain disease usually disqualifies an athlete from contact sport participation.

It goes without saying that it is much easier to control a conscious cooperative patient than one who is unconscious. For instance, an unconscious, helmeted football player or swimmer who has struck the bottom of a pool must be handled in a very careful but expeditious manner in order to make the diagnosis as soon as possible and effect appropriate treatment. Both athletes require immobilization in order to protect the head and neck, preferably on a spine board. If this is not available, perhaps a team bench will do in the case of a football player; a kickboard could be useful in the case of a swimmer. A helmet should never be forcibly removed but rather used to apply gentle traction to the athlete's neck, with the chin strap serving as a halter and the ear holes as points of attachment for weights or as a means of securing the head in position while the patient is moved on the particular immobilization board. If it is desirable to remove a helmet, the guidelines developed by the American College of Surgeons should be followed. If no rigid object is available, several individuals (preferably five) can be recruited in order to form a human stretcher. Four members should interlock their hands to the elbows of individuals opposite them; the fifth should gently apply traction to the helmet or the head of the injured athlete in order to prevent unnecessary movement until x rays have been taken.

Concussion

With the exception of minor abrasions, lacerations, and contusions of the head and scalp, concussions are the head injury most commonly encountered and of important concern for the practicing sports physician (Chapter 12).

A blow to the head may cause transient impairment of neural function of the reticular activating system, clinically manifested by a variable period of unconsciousness with associated changes in the vital signs (pulse, period of pressure, respiration) and a variable degree of amnesia. By definition, however, a concussion is a temporary and totally reversible event. Concussions can be graded by degree, with first degree representing a "ding" or "bell being rung." Second degree is intermediate, and third degree represents unconsciousness for more than 5 minutes and moderate-to-severe retrograde amnesia.

It is possible for an experienced physician to diagnose a grade I concussion and return the player to game during the same contest. Such action is acceptable if the physician knows the entire history of the particular athlete, witnesses the injury as it occurred, and carefully observes the individual in follow-up. Usually, however, one or more of these items is unknown or unclear. For instance, review of many game films indicates that concussion can be caused from a variety of injuries: obviously by blows to the head, but less obviously by blows to the mid portion of the chest, forcible neck rotation due to face mask grasping, and hyperextension injuries of the neck.

It is recommended that whenever there is any doubt in the examining physician's mind, the player should not be returned to game; rather, a period of observation should be allowed or immediate transport to an emergency facility be arranged for further examination. The possibility of an athlete slowly bleeding into his or her cranial vault from a ruptured surface vessel, while at the same time recovering memory, balance, orientation, and coordination is a distinct reality. The only way a physician can be certain such bleeding is not occurring is with serial examination over a period of observation time or by computerized axial tomogram at an appropriate facility. The Amateur Athletic Union (AAU) boxing and full contact martial arts guidelines clearly state that any amateur athlete who has received a concussion of grade II or III must cease competition at that time.

One of the most difficult areas for a physician to contend with is return to play after a concussion. Because cerebral edema occurs 12 to 24 hours after initial traumatic insult, a period of 24 to 48 hours should be allowed for continued observation of the athlete, particularly during the night following the injury. Parents, close friends, or spouse who remain with the individual that evening should be carefully instructed according to standard "head sheet" guidelines. The athlete should never be left alone during that particular night in case of a sudden deterioration in neurologic status. Occasionally an injured athlete develops the postconcussive syndrome—a throbbing, very painful headache that may or may not be associated with nausea and vomiting.[9,10] Probably secondary to disruption of small pain fibers or small amounts of cerebral edema, the condition usually occurs 3 to 6 days after the injury and lasts for variable periods of up to 1 week. It is imperative that this condition be distinguished from true herniation or more localized forms of cerebral edema secondary to hematoma formation or brain contusion. The neurologic exam is within normal limits. Treatment should involve bed rest, mild analgesics, and removal from light, as it has been found to aggravate the situation.

Occasionally a player will go on to develop migraine headache (footballer's migraine) from a head injury; rarely, continued contact sports participation becomes prohibitive due to incapacitating visual defects.[11] Once again it is important to rule out any expanding mass lesion as the cause for the headache. It is recommended that an athlete, until headache-free at rest, should not resume any form of training. Thereafter, training should be tailored to within the limits of pain; i.e., calisthenics and aerobic exercise can be performed to a degree that does not cause headache, faintness, or dysequilibrium. Return to usual contact sports is appropriate once the athlete can perform regular full training exercises without difficulty. The AAU mandates a 3-month period of competition cessation following a concussion in the ring for amateur boxers and full contact martial arts athletes. The AMA Council on Scientific Affairs for Boxing has also developed a useful set of guidelines. There are, however, no hard and fast guidelines regarding repeated concussions except that, presuming there is no "mental set" of the athlete (secondary gain from external pressures), a specific etiology should be sought for why a particular athlete is receiving such repeated trauma.[12] Perhaps competitive technique or equipment failure is the underlying cause. In general, three concussions, irrespective of degree, are probably enough to prohibit future contact sports participation.

Serious Intracranial Injuries

Cerebral contusions and hemorrhages are discussed in Chapter 13. It should be noted that the most common cause of death in craniocerebral acceleration injuries is acute subdural hematoma, and that intracranial bleeding is the leading cause of death from head injury in sports. The classical presentations of extra- and subdural hematoma may not be present in a young athletic population, and very often if the attending physician waits for the typical findings to evolve, significant morbidity and mortality results. Perhaps the most difficult item following major head injury is the return to play of the athlete. Though the decision should be made in conjunction with the particular athlete, his or her family, the coach, and trainer, the final decision must be that of the team physician. Useful guidelines suggesting return include normal neurologic exam, no headache, no vasomotor symptomatology, and normal EEG, especially if there were posttraumatic neurologic deficits.[13]

Facial Injuries

A variety of contact sports, particularly hockey, football, and lacrosse, produce facial injuries.[14,15] The majority of such injuries are minor and consist mostly of abrasions, lacerations, and contusions. In addition to the basic treatment discussed in Chapter 12, every attempt to care for cosmetic repair should be made, as the area heals rapidly due to rich vasculature. Regardless of the extent of the injury, initial management should always consist of preservation of the airway, establishment of respiration, and maintenance of affected circulation. Because of the rich vascular nature of the facial area, control of hemorrhage is often a problem that is neglected. It is not uncommon for an individual with a nosebleed to lose several hundred milliliters of blood before hemostasis is effected.

Nasal Injuries. The nasal bones are most frequently injured, followed in order by the mandible and the zygoma (Fig. 14-1). The maxilla and frontal bones are the least frequently fractured of the facial bones. The anterior third of the nose is cartilaginous and because of its protuberant nature and its relatively weak structure, is frequently injured in the form of a fracture or contusion. The most common

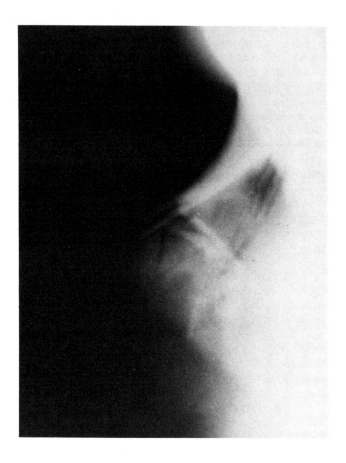

FIGURE 14-1. Nasal fracture.

symptom following trauma to the nose is epistaxis, usually associated with some displacement or a fracture. Presence of a deformity confirms fracture though it is usually most helpful to have the athlete look at the nose in the mirror and state whether it is in any way changed from its previous shape. The diagnosis of more subtle nasoseptal fractures require careful bilateral inspection and palpation of the septum with the thumb and forefinger in an attempt to demonstrate mobility at the inferior suture. A clear fluid discharge may indicate cerebrospinal rhinorrhea and should suggest ethmoid plate fracture. A bulging septum probably represents a septal hematoma which should be drained in order to prevent cartilage necrosis.

The best methodology for controlling bleeding is by external compression of the nose for 10 minutes with the patient's head and neck flexed. Rarely is anterior and/or posterior packing necessary in combination with the application of constrictive medications. Unless the physician is familiar with the technique of posterior packing, the athlete should be handled by an ear–nose–throat surgeon.

Fractures. Fractures of the frontal bone require significant forces (e.g., snowmobiling).[16] The anterior wall can be fractured and, with greater forces, the posterior wall can also be injured with disruption of the dura mater and even the deeper tissue of the brain. Clinical findings include epistaxis, soft tissue swelling, and perhaps an accompanying depression in the area of the fracture. After preservation of the airway and control of hemorrhage, definitive management should be done in conjunction with a skilled surgeon. Maxillary fractures have been classified according to LeFort:

1. Type I fracture consists of separation of the palate from the superior portion of the maxilla, usually secondary to a blow striking the lower portion of the maxillary area. The patient may complain of malocclusion and epistaxis, and physical exam demonstrates mobility of the palate on careful palpation.
2. Type II LeFort fracture consists of separation of the zygoma and frontal bone complex from the nasal bones and middle and lower portions of the maxilla. Symptomatology includes hypesthesia of the cheek, epistaxis, and mobility of both the nose and palate.
3. Type III fracture consists of separation of the zygoma and maxillary ethmoid complex from the frontal bone and craneal bolt. This severe injury is associated with large amounts of edema and the displacement of the middle one-third of the face so that it looks like a dish.

Once again, careful preservation of the airway (as these fracture transverse the nose and paranasal sinus) and control of hemorrhage are the primary factors. With the more severe types of fracture, it is important also to rule our further neurologic damage. Mandibular fractures (discussed in detail in the upcoming section describing dental injuries) should remind the physician that there may be accompanying injury to the teeth. Zygoma fractures are characterized by hypesthesia of the cheek secondary to infraorbital nerve contusion and flattening of the cheek profile due to displacement and depression of the bone.[17] Full extraocular movement should be assessed in order to rule out concomitant "blow out" fracture (see Eye Injuries).

Equipment. The development and regular usage of full facial protective equipment (dental guard, face mask, and helmet) has resulted in a significant decline in facial injury over the past two decades.[18] Continued endorsement by a variety of national organizations in conjunction with individual team physicians can ensure a further decline in the number and severity of such injuries. There has

been some concern that the use of such equipment actually promotes more violent plays, such as face blocking, butt blocking, or spearing in football and facial checking in hockey (see Figs. 14-7 to 14-9). In these particular cases it is important that rules and regulations be supported by major behavioral change in the participating athlete.[6]

Auricular Injuries

The ear is subject to injury not only from such contact sports as wrestling and boxing but also those sports involving differential pressure changes, such as scuba diving and flying.[19] Though recent rule changes have mandated the use of wrestling headgear (in matches as well as practice), auricular hematomas can still be occasionally seen secondary to a direct blow on the ear. The bleeding that occurs between the cartilage of the external ear and its overlying paracondreum, if untreated, produces fibrotic scarring, which over time yields a classic "cauliflower ear." Initial first aid consists of ice and immediate compression of the area to minimize expansion of the hematoma, followed by later aspiration of the hematoma and further compression.

A direct blow that seals the external auricular canal can cause perforation of the tympanic membrane, characterized by pain, a muffled or depressed auditory level, and tinnitus; there may also be associated bleeding. Such an injury has been known to occur in skin and sky diving due to the rapid change in barometric pressure and is termed *barotrauma* (Chapter 10).[20] With a more forceful blow, the ossicular chain can be fractured or dislocated. This has been seen in boxing, full contact martial arts, and water skiing when the side of the head is struck by an object which occludes the auricular canal. Only such injuries from water skiing can be prevented by use of ear plugs; the others require continuous preventive education regarding the appropriate methods of ascent and descent in the case of diving and the proper sparring technique and headgear in martial arts and boxing.

Occasionally the primary care physician may be consulted regarding the loss of hearing due to high noise levels as in shooting sports.[21] The careful fitting of ear plugs or muffs with the appropriate education is required for prevention and protection.

Eye Injuries

Despite the carefully protective design of the skull around the eye, there are approximately 100,000 sports-related eye injuries each year, with 90 percent of these being preventable. Unfortunately, some of these eye injuries lead to blindness—a significant factor being the all too frequent lengthy delay between time of injury and evaluation by the doctor.[22,23] The most important and recurring theme in ocular sports medicine is that accident prevention is paramount and the chief goal is the preservation of sight.

The eye itself is an extremely delicate organ. Well defined lacerations or abrasions can result from blows from sharp objects such as a fingernail or piece of sports equipment (e.g., hockey stick or ski pole) or from field conditions such as a shard of glass or small pebble. On the whole, the prognosis for such injuries is generally good provided that the internal contents are not damaged or expressed through the wound. On the other hand, blows by blunt objects can be far more devastating. Typically such blows are divided into primary global injuries and secondary orbital injuries.

Objects with a diameter smaller than 4 centimeters are usually responsible for primary global injuries: these include golf balls, hockey pucks, squash balls or racquetball balls.[24–26] High-energy forces are transmitted to the delicate internal ocular structures by such items. The usual sequence of injury is deformation of the globe, increase in diameter, increase in intraocular pressure, and globe perforation or a retinal tearing caused by a traction on the vitreous base with rupture of the suspensory of ligaments of the lens with 35 to 50 percent of the eye contents remaining.[27] Such ragged rupture of the globe has the worse prognosis for visual recovery. Of course, the smaller the object the less energy is required since the speeds are higher (e.g., for a bee-bee shot or bullet). The higher the mass (larger diameter) the lower the speed which is required: basketball.

Objects greater than 4 centimeters, such as an elbow, fist, tennis ball, or softball, transmit their forces to the bony margins of the orbit, particularly to the floor [which is thin and functions therefore as a pressure relief valve (blow-out fracture) (Fig. 14-2)]. However, there is a high incidence of occult internal ocular injury in these cases.[23] The usual injury sequence is the following: The object forms a seal at the orbital margin; orbital pressure increases, causing fracture of the floor of the orbit into the maxillary sinus; orbital tissue herniates into the fracture, resulting in diplopia. The normal position of the globe is deformed causing contusion of the resultant angle, a retinal tear of vitreous hemorrhage, submacular hemorrhage, and orbital hemorrhage and edema.

Thus the weakest bony margins of the orbit are inferior and medial, whereas the strongest point of the orbit is the supraorbital rim. An object of 1.4 inches can gain easy access to the eye because half the eye lies anterior to the lateral orbital rim. Not only frontal, but also lateral strikes as from a hockey stick or *shinai* (Kendo) approaching from the side, can strike the globe.[22] Finally it is important that the physician always remember that blows to the cranium can cause indirect injury to eye anatomy and function. The blow could conceivably involve the optic nerve, chiasm, tract, geniculate body, optic radiation, or occipital cortex. For a more detailed discussion, the reader is referred to a standard medical textbook.

Examination. All eye injuries should be considered serious until proven otherwise. The most important exam of eye function is visual acuity and is the most common error of omission on examination of an injured athlete. The injured athlete should be able to read the 20/20 line on a near vision card. Remember to ask whether the victim normally wears glasses or contact lenses. Next, the penlight should be used to observe carefully the pupil and iris region, with particular attention to the pupillary border and the limbus. If either is irregular, this may indicate a laceration of the area with potential prolapse of the iris.

Reactivity of the pupils should then be checked: iritis produces unequal or poorly reactive pupils as does glaucoma. Depth of the anterior chamber can be checked by lateral shining of the light across the anterior chamber. If a shadow is cast along the medial border of the iris, then the anterior chamber is shallow, which indicates elevated intraocular pressure. The cornea and the iris below should be

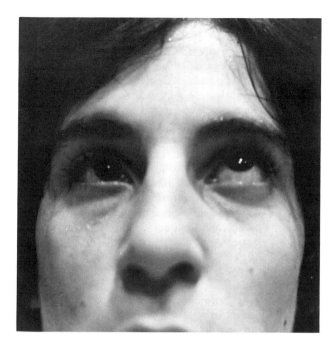

FIGURE 14-2. Blow-out fracture of left orbit following a karate punch.

clear. Any haziness or blood present in the anterior chamber should prompt immediate consultation with an ophthalmologist. If the full curvature of the cornea is carefully observed at an angle with a good light source, foreign bodies and abrasions can be detected without the use of fluorescein, though fluorescein staining should be done in the locker room if necessary.

The conjunctiva, both the bulvar and palpebral portions, should be carefully examined. This includes the areas both under the upper and lower lids. The conjunctiva under the upper lid can be checked by flipping the upper lid over a cotton swab stick. Any observed foreign bodies can be carefully removed with a moist sterile cotton swab without anesthesia. Foreign bodies embedded in the cornea should never be removed. One should pay particular attention to the presence of any black foreign bodies because the interior coats of the eye are black. Such a foreign body may in actuality be a protrusion of the internal contents of the eye through a perforation. Make sure that the extraocular movements are checked in all directions.

Finally, make sure that the globe of the eye itself is intact before proceeding with the evaluation of any lacerations, hematomas, or other problems involving the periorbital tissue or eyelid. For all proven or suspected globe ruptures a hard shield, firmly taped, should be attached to the injured eye. The uninjured eye should also be patched in order to prevent concomitant ocular movements. Before calmly transporting the injured athlete to the hospital for further evaluation, be sure to counsel the player not to squeeze the eyes forcibly.

The primary care physician's ocular examination should thus always proceed in an organized fashion so that entire structure and function of the eye is assessed. If there is any question, the athlete should be removed from competition and referred to a facility for further evaluation (complete slit-lamp examination).

Conditions that prompt an immediate referral are diplopia, suspected or proven globe perforation, shattered or broken contact lenses or eyeglasses, lid marginal lacerations or lid function impairment, irregular poorly reactive asymmetric pupil, decreased vision or visual field loss, blood or haze in the anterior chamber, and embedded corneal foreign bodies. Those conditions treated on site by the physician should be referred at a later date for a complete ocular examination—particularly all blunt trauma to the eye and orbit.

Foreign Bodies/Abrasions. As mentioned, foreign bodies underneath the eyelids or on the conjunctiva should be removed with a moist sterile cotton swab or forceful sterile saline irrigation, antibiotic ointment applied, and play resumed. Superficial corneal foreign bodies should be removed in a similar manner after topical anesthesia (e.g., proparacaine hydrochloride). Play should *not* be resumed after removal of a corneal foreign body; rather, a patch should be applied with antibiotic ointment. The patient should then be seen and followed up by an ophthalmologist or the sports physician on the following day. No attempt should be made to remove an imbedded corneal body with a needle or spud on the athletic field. A fluorescein strip can also be used to diagnose a corneal abrasion after the pupil anterior chamber and globe have been found to be normal and intact. An abrasion shows up as a brightly staining green area under an ultraviolet penlight. The eye should have a topical anesthetic applied, followed by antibiotic ointment and a patch. Play should not be resumed; an ophthalmologic follow-up should be prescribed.

Lacerations. Contact sports, particularly boxing, hockey, and the martial arts often produce brow/lid lacerations due to glancing blows.[28] Lid and brow lacerations which do not impair function or the lid margin can be closed with a sterile closure strip after appropriate cleansing of the area. With the exception of minor superficial lacerations, the player should not be allowed to return to the contest. Full thickness lacerations should be closed in layers with sutures, making sure that the globe itself has not been injured.

Serious Injury: Hyphema. There are several major injuries that occur, though infrequently, during the practice of sports medicine whose diagnosis and initial treatment should be known to the primary care physician. When the major arterial circle of the iris is torn or Schlemm's canal is disrupted there is bleeding into the anterior chamber of the eye;

this is called *hyphema*.[29] This condition can be associated with an inflammation of the iris and the ciliary body (referred to as *traumatic iridocyclitis*). The major pathologic complications of a hyphema is glaucoma, which can result in blindness. The initial inflammatory reaction is usually controlled with topical corticosteroids and cycloplegics. Bed rest is mandatory with both eyes patched. Every hyphema must be examined by the slit lamp for the extent of inflammatory response, possible etiology of the bleeding, and the presence of adhesions. At the time of the slit lamp examination, gonioscopy should also be performed. A useful rule is that opacification of the anterior chamber by more than 50 percent from blood is associated with a very guarded prognosis since there is likely to be a high frequency of serious associated injuries within the eye, especially related to the retina, cornea, and lens.

Perforations. Perforating ocular injuries represent some of the more serious forms of ocular trauma; yet the spectrum of presentation may be from the very subtle to very apparent. Thus even apparently very minor brow/lid lacerations quite removed from the globe itself can be associated with serious perforations. It is important to remember that over 50 percent of all ocular enucleations are performed for trauma, with the greatest proportion being lost due to perforation of the globe. The best prognosis for perforations is related to clean laceration; ragged perforations, especially from blunt objects, have the worse prognosis due to the extent of damage as well as the fact that they often occur at sites distant from the impact and thus are observed at a later time. As mentioned, all diagnosed or suspected perforations should be carefully shielded and immediately referred to the appropriate facility. The eye should not be voluntarily or involuntarily squeezed.

If at all possible, following the acute injury, it is most useful to perform funduscopic examination on the field in order to visualize the retina. In addition to glaucoma, major retinal detachment or small retinal holes are usually responsible for latent posttraumatic blindness. It should be remembered by every practicing sports physician that trauma is the most common, singular cause of retinal detachment between birth and age 16, and that the interval between the diagnosis of the detachment and the actual trauma is often very long. The earlier the diagnosis of a detachment or holes can be made, the better the prognosis. Thus, careful funduscopic examination of the retina should be performed by a qualified person after the injury. The contusion of the choroid secondary to a direct blow can result in fibrotic scarring with loss of vision. Even whiplash types of head and neck injuries can cause macular edema with loss of essential vision. Choroidal tears tend to be concentric and located in lateral portions of the retina. However, peripheral choroidal tears can involve the macular area through the formation of subretinal neovascular membranes. The posterior part of the eye can be involved in a variety of different retinal hemorrhages. Many of these injuries can be successfully treated by laser photocoagulation if diagnosed early. Athletes at high altitudes, mountain climbers, and sport flyers are subject to the development of retinal hemorrhage, probably secondary to hypoxic vasodilatation in combination with rapid rises in the intravascular pressure.[30] Even though these hemorrhages resolve spontaneously when the athlete returns to lower altitudes and normal visual acuity returns, there may be a permanent field defect as well as dark-adaptation problems.

Prevention. The vast majority of eye injuries can be prevented by the regular use of safe eye protectors.[31] It should be noted that there are a variety of such devices on the market that until recently have not undergone rigorous safety performance testing[32]; in fact, it has been suggested that some devices encourage risk taking and a false sense of security.[33] A more thorough discussion of such equipment can be found in Chapter 9.

Dental Injuries

There are two important factors that influence the handling of dental injuries in the sports arena. The first is that the majority of dental injuries are usually not considered serious; the second is that a tooth has one of the lowest potentials for recovery to the normal state following injury. A mild blow to the mandible may not result in any visible injury; however, within a matter of days to weeks the tooth's

vital pulp tissue may be irreversibly damaged, thus resulting in the death of a tooth. Even had the injury been identified in its initial phase, the treatment, which would consist of a root canal procedure, is time consuming, requires precision, and is costly. Thus for a variety of reasons dental injuries are *not* minor in either nature or extent and, for obvious reasons, prevention must be the keynote in sports medicine management of all dental injuries.

Anatomy. It is possible to injure one or more of the structures of the tooth: the crown, periodontal membrane, or supporting bone (Fig. 14-3). The crown consists of an outer portion of *enamel* which cannot repair itself; a dense interior, called *dentine,* which has a very low potential for repair following injury; and an innermost soft portion, called the *pulp,* which consists of the nerve, vein, artery, and lymphatic system of the tooth and also has a low potential for repair. The *root,* consisting mostly of the dentine, contains a hollow canal. The root is covered by a thin layer of connective tissue, called the *cementum,* to which is attached the periodontal membrane which itself connects the tooth to the bone and alveolar socket. Despite the fact that cementum and periodontal membrane have good repair potential, an injured root rarely repairs itself.

Epidemiology. The epidemiology of dental injuries is generally unknown in the majority of sports. The majority of work during the past 30 years has been done in the sports of football, hockey, and occasionally basketball and lacrosse.[34] The incidence of injury is directly related to the presence or absence of mouth guards or facial protection. The injury frequency ranges from 0 percent, where all competitors are required to wear mouth guards, to almost 20 percent, where few individuals wear mouth guards (hockey). On the whole, the rate of injury is lower in football than in hockey; the injury rate in basketball is much lower than that for either hockey or football, but is about equal to football played wearing mouth guards. The majority of dental injuries occurs on the anterior teeth. Such injuries are additionally complicated when they occur in an athlete under the age of 12 years since the roots of the anterior teeth are incompletely formed. Unfortunately, the number of sports-related dental injuries occurring under the age of 10 or 12 is in-

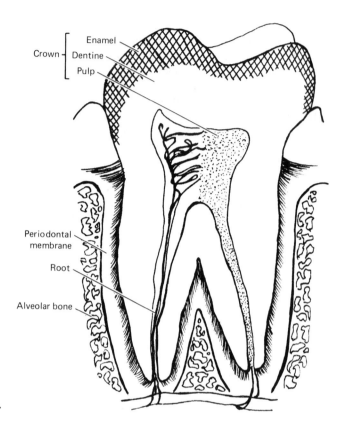

FIGURE 14-3. The anatomy of a tooth.

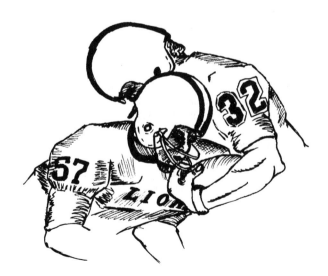

FIGURE 14-4. An example of a traumatic blow to the mandible occurring underneath the face mask during tackle football.

creasing, particularly in youth soccer, boxing, football, and the martial arts (Fig. 14-4).

It should be remembered that not only the teeth are at risk during a direct blow to the chin or jaw, but also the mandible itself and other facial bones as well as the soft tissues—particularly the lip and facial skin. If the blow is strong enough, the force can be transmitted along the mandible to the base of the skull with production of a concussion. In several studies it has been suggested that the wearing of a mouth guard may prevent cranial injuries due to dissipation of the pressure.[8]

Examination. The keynote in treatment of the majority of dental injuries is the speed of the delivery of care. This factor is particularly true in the treatment of partially and completely dislodged teeth. In both cases the tooth must be moved back into good alignment as rapidly as possible. If an athlete receives a sharp blow to the mandible and frontal teeth, the play should be stopped and the athlete examined in the following manner: Visual inspection of the oral cavity should be performed with particular attention paid to the individual teeth, their alignment, their integrity (to rule out fractures), the gingiva, the buccal mucosa, and the lips. Of more importance is the fact that *each individual tooth* should be palpated for integrity, that is, for lateral or anteroposterior motion. Percussion can also be used as a supplementary method to determine whether the tooth has been partially dislodged since it will produce acute pain.

Avulsion and Fracture. If a tooth has been completely dislodged, it should be (1) carefully inspected to make sure there is no compounding root fracture, (2) completely washed, removing all dirt with tap water or sterile saline if available, and then (3) pushed gently back into its individual socket as quickly as possible. Thereafter the athlete, whether with an incompletely or completely dislodged tooth, should be referred for dental follow-up immediately in order to secure the position through splinting with a wire ligature or a fitted orthodontic appliance. It is paramount that dental first aid regarding avulsed teeth be performed on site and that the dislodged tooth not be carried to the dentist or the emergency room. The ability for a dislodged tooth to recover exponentially declines after 30 minutes. Should re-

positioning on the field be impossible due to the degree of injury, then it is best to ask that the player position the loose tooth under his or her tongue until seen by a dentist.

It is not uncommon in certain sports, particularly hockey, that a partial fracture either of the angle or the corner of the tooth occurs. In these particular instances the best advice is to have the injured athlete keep his mouth closed in order to prevent exposure of the sensitive dentine. It is not necessary to discontinue the athlete's continued competition for a fractured tooth, presuming that there is no dislodgement and there is no bleeding from the accompanying lacerations. Thereafter, the athlete can follow-up within 24 hours with dental care. A rare but possible injury is one in which a tooth breaks a portion of the alveolar process of the mandible; in such a case, it may not appear to be loose or broken. It is possible on direct pressure or percussion over that particular tooth to elicit pain and therefore suggest that a more extensive injury may be present. The identification of a fracture of the alveolar process is a most important one in that it must be treated as an open fracture including antibiotics and careful and prompt reduction by a qualified oral surgeon.

Lacerations. Accompanying lacerations of the gingiva, buccal mucosa, and the lips must also be attended to on a first aid basis. There are several useful rules that apply:

1. Lacerations of the mucosa and the face often bleed profusely due to the remarkable vascularization of these areas. The degree of bleeding often does not indicate the necessary extent of severity of the injury.
2. All wounds should be carefully wiped dry by a sterile gauze pad and then observed for their severity and extent once the bleeding is controlled by pressure.
3. Those gingival and buccal lacerations whose sides are closely approximated at rest need not be sutured. Several studies have shown that such wounds tend to heal with minimal scarring and complication whereas sutures tend to produce small scars as well as no decrease in the healing time. Large lacerations which remain open when

the tissues are at rest typically require suturing, though judgment is often required.

Rule 3 is typically applied to through-and-through lower lip lacerations. External facial lacerations usually should be closed with sutures in order to prevent scars and therefore produce the best cosmetic results. Typically, suture material should be very fine, 5-0 nonabsorbable, and placed for 3 or 4 days as healing is rapid. Suturing should not be done on the field but rather in a controlled environment such as the emergency room or doctor's office. The common practice of on-the-field or ringside "butterflying" of facial lacerations with adhesive bandages and topical adrenalin compounds in order to decrease the bleeding is hazardous. Though it is important that the primary care physician render judgment on a case-by-case basis, the general rule should be that temporizing methodologies should

not be employed, as very often the original wound is widened, deepened, or lengthened in further competition.

In terms of the short- and long-term treatment of dental injuries, it is important to bear in mind that the status of the pulp, the lifeline of the tooth, cannot be assessed for at least 5 years after the injury. Therefore, in those situations in which there may be some minimal doubt or in which there is no evident injury other than the history or the observance of a significant blow to the teeth, the athlete should be referred for dental follow-up and perhaps for necessary radiological studies. It is important that the primary care physician become familiar with basic dental first aid and establish a relationship with a community dentist in order to provide continuity of care for all athletes under his or her immediate care. Such continuity becomes very important for those athletes who suffer partial

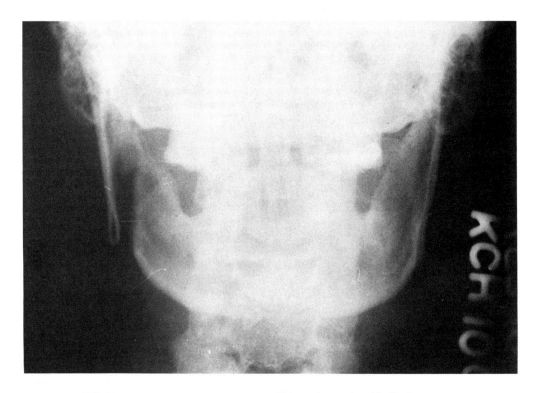

FIGURE 14-5. Fracture of the right mandible at the angle with displacement.

fractures, dislodgment, or injuries which may jeopardize the vitality of the tooth since long-term treatment may very well be mandatory and involve endodontic (root canal) treatment or various orthodontic devices.

Mandibular Injuries. The dental exam should always include a determination of the integrity of the mandible. This includes range of motion and a careful palpation and percussion along the entire condyle and ramus of the jaw. The typical history of a fractured mandible includes a concussive or knock-out blow (Fig. 14-5). Typically it is a contusion that calls first attention to the possibility of a fracture due to a direct blow. As such, any contusion involving the mandible should be carefully examined particularly along the entire inferior border since it is subcutaneous. Careful palpation and percussion determines trigger points, areas of tenderness, local swelling, or irregularities along the margin. This technique is particularly important in hairline or undisplaced fractures of the mandible. Major fractures of the mandible are quite evident: the jaw is usually open, perhaps displaced to the side of the fracture, and the lips may be badly swollen. Often there is an accompanying laceration of the buccal mucosa due to fracture fragments. With respect to less obvious cases, it is imperative to check the range of motion and the opposition of the upper and lower teeth. The best single test of accuracy of reduction of any deformity following a fracture is occlusion without discomfort. The mandible should be carefully observed through its entire range of motion as small amounts of displacement may become obvious.

Anterior fractures, typically involving the tooth-bearing area, are more readily diagnosed whereas posterior fractures often require careful palpation, particularly involving internal oral exam, as well as observing the patient opening, closing, and biting down. Individual condyles should be palpated as they come forward out of the glenoid. Whenever there is one fracture present a careful search should be made for a possible second. Diagnosed mandibular fractures as well as significant mandibular contusions and other dental injuries usually can be treated by the application of a Barton's bandage (Fig. 14-6) which secures the jaw to the maxilla until a more

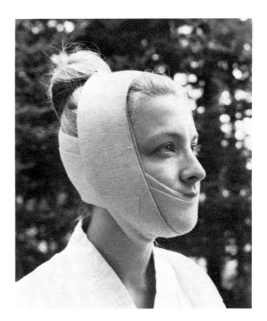

FIGURE 14-6. Barton's bandage.

detailed examination can be made. Once the athlete has been brought to an emergency facility, consultation with an oral surgeon is advisable and radiographic examination involving the anterior, posterior, and lateral plains should be made and carefully interpreted.

Dislocation. A rare but particularly distressing injury is the dislocation of the temporomandibular joint which can occur by a downward, driving blow on an already opened jaw. Occasionally it may be a habitual condition and result from the stretching of the joint capsule by repeated episodes of dislocation. The diagnosis can be easily made by noting that the jaw is locked in an open position, the cotyloid fossae are empty, and the condyle itself has slipped forward in front of the fossa.

If possible, first aid reduction should be performed on the field. The patient should be as relaxed as possible; occasionally the use of intravenous diazepam may be indicated. In a cooperative patient, the physician's gloved thumbs should be placed firmly on the posteroinferior molars or preferably on the retromolar pad while the index fingers are securely locked under the mandibular rami at the junction of the chin. Firm pressure downward should then be gradually applied on the molars until the condyles unlock, followed by superior rotatory pressure forward on the index fingers, thus reducing the anterior dislocation. If the reduction procedure is performed immediately at the time of the injury, operative anesthesia will be rarely required. The athlete should then have a Barton's bandage applied for a week to 10 days with follow-up consultation to an oral surgeon within 48 hours in order to rule out accompanying fracture or other pathology.

Prevention. It is important to bear in mind always that most, if not all, dental and oral injuries could be eliminated if there were mandatory protective rules regarding the use of protective equipment (see Chapter 9). Though the National Collegiate Athletic Association, the Amateur Athletic Union, and the Amateur Hockey Associations in the United States and Canada mandate internal mouthguards for football, hockey, boxing, and martial arts, the rules are not uniformly applied and often not enforced. In addition, there has been little work done on the standardization of protective equipment, particularly by the American Society for Testing and Materials and the Canadian Standards Association.

Types of guard include internal mouth guard and the face guard.[35] The internal mouth guard is further subdivided into its method of formation: custom-made, mouth-forms, and stock-type.[36] Though the custom-made variety is more expensive, it is the most comfortable, producing the least amount of irritation, interfering little with speech and breathing, and is far superior in terms of choice to mouth-forms and stock-type. Most important, it stays in place 90 percent of the time. The mouth-form variety is intermediate with regard to these param-

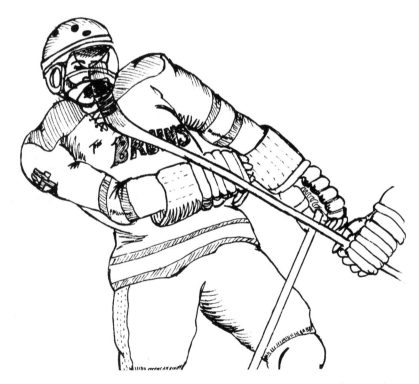

FIGURE 14-7. Facial injury due to a hockey stick sliding under an inadequate face mask.

eters, and the stock-type performs the worst, especially with regard to the fact that it stays in place only 19 percent of the time.

The most commonly chosen type of internal mouthguard is the mouth-form because of its ease of application and its lower cost. If the instructions in the kit are followed carefully, the accuracy of fit is very high. There are a number of these kits on the market but the most successful ones contain a hard plastic molding tray used externally to compress the heated clear plastic material against the teeth and the gums while it sets. It is a good idea for the physician to observe the technique of mouthpiece fitting as done by a trainer and the athlete. If properly formed, the mouth guard remains in place when the athlete opens the mouth wide.

On the whole, face guards, which are invariably attached to a helmet, provide excellent protection against facial injuries, particularly the eyes in the majority of sports (football, lacrosse, boxing). The face guard often does not extend below mid face in order to preserve good downward visibility or prevent fogging or other modes of constriction. This is particularly true in hockey (Fig. 14-7). Thus, despite the fact that the athlete may be wearing a face guard, a stick may be able to strike the unprotected portion of the face or slide up under the guard itself. The same form of injury can occur with a puck or a weapons demonstration and in the martial arts.

NECK

There is no more devastating injury than quadriplegia in a young athlete.[3,9] The likelihood of recovery is extremely small. The research work of White[37] and Reid[38] has shown that it is not possible to protect the neck from the forces to which it is often subjected in most contact sports—this in face of the National Football League (NFL) Management Council statement, which suggests that a professional player's neck can be conditioned to withstand these forces. Thus all cervical injuries should be considered severe until proven otherwise, since the condition of an athlete who has received only a spinal concussion is the same initially as one whose cord has been completely severed. It is not difficult to convert a salvageable case of quadriplegia into a permanent one by improper handling of a fractured or dislocated cervical spine. Furthermore there is absolutely no way clinically to distinguish the stable from unstable spine until x rays have been taken. The physician cannot rely on the mechanism of injury since it is rarely known at the time of occurrence in sports such as football or rugby, though it is easily observed in gymnastics or diving. Thus, under no circumstances should the neck be manipulated on the field without x rays.

Examination

If fortunate enough to have a conscious athlete, it is possible to assess carefully the extent of injury and enlist the player's support during transportation. In examining the conscious athlete, always work within the limits of pain. Initial comfort and reassurance go a long way. The athlete should be then asked to slowly move his or her fingers, hands, and arms, stopping all activity if the player reports any pain or increase in symptomatology. A careful neurologic exam of the sensory, motor, and reflex aspects of the extremity should be made. Once the exam is completed, the player should be placed on a spine board or similar rigid object with helmet in place and traction applied. For the unconscious competitor, the major caveat is to avoid cord damage while establishing an airway and ensuring that breathing and circulation are adequate (Chapter 13). Leaving the helmet in place, bolt cutters or a screwdriver are used to remove the face mask. Traction is applied with sandbags placed on each side of the neck for stabilization. Otherwise, the helmet can be removed by in-line traction being applied above and below.[39,40]

It is always better that the primary care physician err on the conservative side concerning neck injuries. It is not uncommon for the athlete to develop what would appear to be a trivial cervical injury, be allowed to return to play, and then have symptoms insidiously develop at a later time. Any player who complains of neck pain should be removed from the contest and a definitive examination made. Finally, all such neck injuries in the conscious athlete, as minor or mild as they may seem, should be examined with the patient prone and not upright.

Contusions

Blows to the neck can have a serious import especially with regard to the vital underlying structures. Posteriorly, contusions, hematoma underlying the ligamentum nuchae, and cervical fractures may occur. Rarely, cord concussion can result, which is quite alarming, but recovery is the rule. Concussion may be associated with transitory paralysis or paresthesias. Should the deficits persist, a much more thorough search should be made for an intraspinal injury. The contusion can be associated with a cervical strain if the neck is turned in the direction opposite to the direction of the blow. The soft tissue items particularly at risk are the larynx, trachea, and major blood vessels. A not infrequent type of injury in football and rugby is that of "clotheslining." This injury has also been seen in horseback riding and martial arts in which a narrow fixed forceful blow (e.g., of the ridge hand) strikes the player's neck region. Injury to the carotid sheath

can produce thrombosis, a shower of emboli, or symptomatic bradycardia through carotid body stimulation.[41] Laryngotracheal injury has been discussed in Chapter 13. It is not uncommon at ringside to witness a blow to the throat and witness the ensuing extreme dyspnea, discomfort, and speechlessness of the athlete. The usual course is quick recovery of phonation and respiration. Should recovery be incomplete or prolonged, one should consider hematoma formation or more serious injury (fracture of the cartilage).

Mechanisms of Injury

Adequate diagnosis and subsequent treatment regarding cervical injuries is contingent on understanding and elucidating the mechanisms producing the lesions. Generally speaking, cervical injuries are a result of excessive motion caused by stresses forcing the neck beyond its normal range of flexion, extension, rotation, or lateral flexion.[42] Occasionally there may be excessive compressive forces. Often, a combination of forces are present.

Simple marked cervical flexion without an ad-

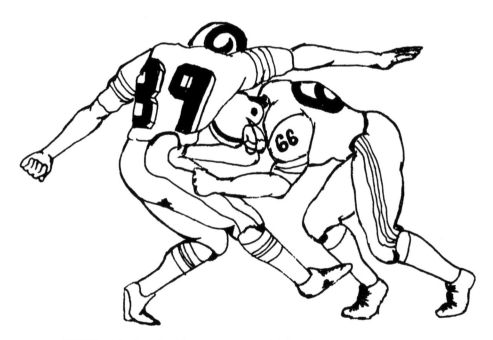

FIGURE 14-8. Butt-blocking can cause neck injury if hyperextension occurs.

ditional passive force rarely produces severe injuries because the chin contacts the anterior chest wall and acts as a check. However, if a passive force is applied, the amount of tissue injury is proportional to the intensity. In mild to moderate circumstances, there is spraining of the supra- and interspinous ligaments; infrequently these may be in avulsion fracture of the spinous process. With larger forces, especially accompanied by some degree of rotation, the above-mentioned ligaments plus the capsular and posterior longitudinal ligament and ligamentum flavum rupture, and there may be subluxation or dislocation of the facets (unilateral or bilateral), facet fracture with or without dislocation, intervertebral disk compression, disruption, or detachment, and possibly cord/nerve root damage.

So-called "whiplash" is caused by hyperextension forces without a passive or compressive force acting. The tissues most frequently injured are the anterior muscles (strains of the scaleni, longus colli, or sternocleidomastoid), anterior longitudinal ligament (sprain), intervertebral disk, esophagus, and trachea (dysphasia and hoarseness), vertebra (subluxation), cord, and vertebral arteries, sympathetic chains, and nerve roots. When hyperextension forces are combined with compressive and rotatory forces, there may be additional injuries such as posterior fracture—dislocation of the apophyseal joints (unilateral or bilateral), bursting fracture of the vertebral centrum, pedicle fracture, spinous process fracture, and serious neurologic damage. This combination of forces often produces an unstable injury. Examples of common athletic hyperextension injuries include diving into shallow waters, "butt blocking" (Fig. 14-8), and "spearing" or face blocking (Fig. 14-9). "Spearing," which involves driving one's face mask into an opponent's numerals can tear the tissues of the anterior neck and compress or tear the vertebral arteries in their bony encasements. In "butt blocking," the top of the helmet is used, but

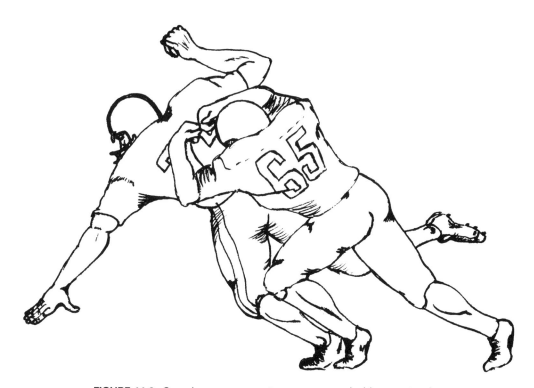

FIGURE 14-9. Spearing an opponent can cause cervical hyperextension.

the injury is the same as for spearing. A knockout blow to the chin of an already dazed fighter whose cervical muscles are relaxed can produce an equivalent injury.

Strains

Because of the size and number of cervical muscles, strains of that area are common and extremely complex. The most commonly strained spinal muscles are of the posterior cervical region and secondary to forcible extension of neck against resistance as would occur in wrestling. *Grade I strains* are treated with rest, reduction of activity, protection from further injury, ice initially, then local heat, and analgesic and anti-inflammatory medication. With careful attention to these parameters, recovery is full and prompt. All too often, however, attention is not paid to protection and rest, and spastic torticollis can develop within 24 to 48 hours following injury.

The wry neck as well as *grade II strains* should be treated with bed rest, light cervical traction of 4 to 8 pounds, local heat, and anti-inflammatory/analgesic agents. Rapid progessive rehabilitation within the limits of pain expedites early return to play. It is possible that a hematoma can be formed secondary to a strain or contusion to certain muscular areas of the cervical region, particularly the sternocleidomastoid. Very often local supportive measures are all that is required, though occasionally aspiration and drainage facilitate drainage.

Sprains

Cervical sprains are common in the athletic population. They are classified according to degree. *Grade I injuries* are the most frequent type. Initially there is little or no discomfort, but over several hours there is worsening pain and limitation of motion, with the athlete unable to move his or her neck from a particular position. X rays should be taken to rule out more significant injury. Treatment consists of rest, ice, analgesics, and anti-inflammatory agents. Progressive resistive exercises should be started after the acute period (48 to 72 hours) and be kept within the limits of pain. A cervical collar is usually helpful in grade I injuries. Recovery can be expected in several weeks.

Grade II injuries are potentially serious and should be treated as such. The athlete complains of moderate to severe pain which may be localized if examined at the time of injury; more often than not, the pain involves the occiput, scapular area, or ipsilateral arm or chest due to generalized muscle spasm. The victim may be noted to hold his or her head vigorously opposing any movement, saying it cannot be kept upright. In the case of a forcible flexion injury, there is interspinous tenderness, whereas forced hyperextension produces tenderness over the posterolateral articulations typically at or above C-5. Associated complaints during the acute phase are vertigo, nausea, headache, diplopia, or blurred vision. A thorough neurologic exam is mandatory. Anteroposterior, lateral, and oblique x rays should be taken in order to rule out more serious injury. Remember to visualize C-6 and C-7, which may require ordering the Swimmer's view. Treatment consists of ice and immobilization of the spine via cervical collar or brace in the direction of injury, bed rest, sedation, analgesics, and anti-inflammatory agents. If the diagnosis is made during the "golden period," an injection of a long-acting anesthetic at the trigger point is diagnostic as well as therapeutic. A minimum of 4 to 6 weeks is required for ligamentous healing. An active physiotherapy program consisting of progressive resistive exercises should not be started until there is full active range of motion without pain. Mismanagement of grade II strains can be responsible for the chronic sprain syndrome or the progression to more serious injury.

Grade III injuries are very serious and should be handled in consultation with an orthopedist and neurosurgeon. Symptoms typical of grade I and II sprains when present are more severe and persistent. The superb conditioning of some athletes may produce only minimal symptoms and signs. Signs include very limited to no motion, extreme tenderness if the rupture site is detected early, and neurologic findings if the cord or nerve roots have been damaged. X rays should be reviewed carefully for concomitant fracture or dislocation. It is possible for the patient to be quadriplegic and the x rays completely normal, particularly in severe hyperextension injuries. If the patient appears stable, serial exams should be performed. The therapeutic goals are (1) protection of the spinal cord and (2) anatomical reduction of dislocations and fractures with fixation. Crutchfield or Gardner–Wells tongs with traction should be applied in the emergency room with all cases of dislocation or fracture dislocations.

Grade III injuries without dislocation can be managed by immobilization with a cervical brace/collar/cast (Minerva jacket), ice, bed rest, sedation, analgesics, and anti-inflammatory agents. Immobilization should be in the direction opposite to the direction of injury. Progressive worsening of the neurologic exam, incomplete lesions not responding to traction, and subarachnoid blocks are indications for immediate surgical intervention. Surgery is also indicated for fracture-dislocations of both the flexion and extension types, intervertebral disk disruption, and disruption of the posterior ligaments.

The chronic cervical sprain syndrome can be frustrating for the physician as well as for the athlete. A careful history should be taken highlighting the original injury, its mechanisms and treatment, subsequent injuries and their management, and an elucidation of the athlete's technique if the syndrome is due to injuries that are similar—e.g., poor blocking technique causing the solid, unyielding posterior helmet rim to impinge on the cervical spine or repeated face mask grabbing so that hyperextension occurs. The prescription of a leather posterior roll or flap would prevent such injuries. X rays are essential in order to rule out a missed fracture-dislocation. Management consists of ice alternating with heat, analgesics, anti-inflammatories, a collar or brace, and a progressive resistive exercise program within the confines of pain. The athlete must be told that return to play is contingent upon the return of normal strength and function. Early return or the failure to prescribe continuing exercises after return are equally harmful.

Nerve Root Injuries

Occasionally neck injuries involve the brachial plexus and nerve roots. Very often the athlete describes what is called a "burner," which is a nerve root injury at the exit point of the C5-6 intervertebral foramen.[43] The natural history of the "burner" is one of progressive damage early on in the player's

experience characterized by short-lived, very intense searing pain. With time the injury, which is usually due to striking with the face mask or head in football, progresses causing neural fibrotic scarring with eventual fixation so that symptomatology includes radiation of pain down the outer aspect of the arm to the thenar eminence. Pain tends to become more frequent after each insult but lasts only 10 to 20 seconds; athletes so affected can often be seen shaking their hands and arms in attempts to relieve the pain. With most advance cases there may be actual weakness of the bicep deltoid and teres major muscle. Eventually movement in any direction causes symptomatology. It is very important to recognize this type of injury early on so that preventive supportive therapy with use of a high collar can be used or the player's position changed in order to prevent further neurologic damage with its prospects of eventual surgical intervention.

It is extremely rare to tear the cervical nerve roots but when such an injury occurs, the physical exam reveals complete loss of function of the particular segment involved. Unfortunately surgical repair of a nerve root tear is impossible though it is very important for the physician to be able to distinguish between a peripheral and nerve root injury of the brachial system because plexus injuries are repairable. A not infrequent plexus injury is "backpack palsy" caused by direct back-strap compression. Symptoms and signs include paresthesias and paresis with possible atrophy of the arm and shoulder girdle muscles. Furthermore, one should be able to differentiate between the "burner" and a herniated cervical nucleus pulposis; a myelogram may be indicated.

Miscellaneous Conditions

Several conditions that can occur in the practicing athlete include the scalenus anticus syndrome which is due to occlusion of the brachial artery or vein and/or pressure on the brachial plexus secondary to anterior scalene muscle spasm. The presence of a cervical rib tends to make the syndrome more frequent and symptoms usually include pain along the ulnar nerve distribution and claudication of the arm musculature when the arm(s) are raised above the shoulders. Furthermore, paresthesias can occur in this position. Although it is not a specific athletic injury it should be considered in a differential of any cervical injury. A classic diagnostic test (Adson's maneuver) is diminution or obliteration of radial pulse if the arm is raised over the head and the neck is turned to the opposite side. Treatment is surgical. This syndrome needs to be distinguished from an extra cervical rib as the symptomatology is very similar. The diagnostic method of choice is radiologic investigation.

Other miscellaneous conditions that should be borne in mind are contusive injuries to the long thoracic and spinal accessory nerves. In the former, winging of the scapula is observed, whereas in the latter, inability or difficulty elevating the shoulder is typical. Both tend to be caused by direct blows and rarely are associated with true nerve rupture. Treatment is usually supportive and surgical intervention is not indicated. Recovery in several weeks is usually complete.

Some athletes are capable of snapping or popping their neck. Very often this becomes a functional or habitual phenomenon and the symptoms tend to be more apprehensive in nature rather than truly functional. It is most important in this case to investigate whether there is any underlying pathology of the cervical vertebra and x rays may be indicated. Typically the etiology is forceful snapping of a tendon over a bony prominence or an articulation irregularity. Once an underlying pathology has been ruled out it is important to educate the athlete to avoid, if possible, getting into a position where such snapping or popping can occur and to establish a fairly extensive physiotherapy regimen emphasizing coordinated movements and strengthening exercises.

Return to Play

It is often unclear when to allow a competitor to return to play after neck injury. Original studies by Albright and colleagues[3] have indicated that a very high percentage of high school and college football players have pre-existing neck injuries many of which carry a high risk of serious damage. Useful guidelines for return to play include absence of muscular spasms which would indicate underlying pathology

and assessment of cervical integrity through the use of a variety of physical therapy equipment. An example of such equipment is that employed by Harvard University, which uses a pulley system attached to a headband in which each direction of motion is tested for maximum strength. The results are recorded and a neck profile is established. Asymmetry of pull or reduction of a pulling force as compared to previous records should prompt further rehabilitation. The athlete should not be allowed to return to play until able to perform up to his or her previous level of recorded neck profile.

REFERENCES

1. Schneider R: Head and Neck Injuries in Football: Mechanisms Treatment, and Prevention. Baltimore, Williams & Wilkins, 1973.
2. Maroon JC: Catastrophic neck injuries from football in western Pennsylvania. Phys Sports Med 9(11):83–86, 1981.
3. Albright J, Moses JM, Feldick HG, et al: Non-fatal cervical spine injuries in interscholastic football. J Am Med Assoc 236:1243–1245, 1976.
4. Silver J: Rugby injuries to the cervical cord. Br Med J 1:192–193, 1979.
5. Lindsay KW, McLatchie G, Jennett B: Serious head injury in sport. Br Med J 281:789–791, 1980.
6. Torg JS, Truax R, Quedenfeld TC, et al: The national football head and neck injury registry, 1978. J Am Med Assoc 241(4):1477–1479, 1979.
7. Mueller FO, Blyth CS: Catastrophic head and neck injuries. Phys Sports Med 7(10):71–77, 1979.
8. Hickey JC, Morris AL, Carlson LD, et al: The relation of mouth protectors to cranial pressure and deformation. J Am Dent Assoc 74:735–740, 1967.
9. Privitera MD, Riggio SP: Post traumatic syndrome. 61:88–96, 1982.
10. Garfinkel D: Headache in athletes. Phys Sports Med 11(1)66–67, 1982.
11. Matthews WB: Footballer's migraine. Br Med J 2:326–327, 1972.
12. Gronwall D, Wrightson P: Cumulative effect of concussion. Lancet 2:995–997, 1975.
13. McLaurin R: Epilepsy and contact sports. J Am Med Assoc 225:285–287, 1973.
14. Wilson KS, Cram B, Rontal M: Facial injuries in hockey players. Minn Med 60:13–19, 1977.

15. Rontal E, Rontal M: Maxillofacial injuries in football players—an evaluation of current facial protection. J Sports Med Phys Fitness 11:241–245, 1971.
16. Rigg BM: Facial fractures and snowmobile accidents. Can J Surg 20:275–277, 1977.
17. Bertz JE: Maxillofacial injuries. Clin Symp 33(4):19–25, 1981.
18. Vinger PF: Too great a risk spurred hockey mask development. Phys Sports Med 5:70–73, 1977.
19. Lee S: Athletic hazards related to otolaryngology. In The Medical Aspects of Sports. Proceedings of the 15th National Conference. Chicago, American Medical Association, 1974.
20. Strauss M, Cantrell R: Ear and sinus barotrauma in diving. Phys Sports Med 2:39–43, 1974.
21. Odess J: The hearing hazard of fire arms. Phys Sports Med 2:65–68, 1974.
22. Horns RC: Blinding hockey injuries. Minn Med 59(4):255–258, 1976.
23. Cullen GC, Luce CM, Shannon GM: Blindness following blow-out orbital fractures. Ophthalmic Surg 8:60–62, 1977.
24. Vinger PF, Tolpin DW: Racket sports: An ocular hazard. J Am Med Assoc 239:2575–2577, 1978.
25. Rose CP, Morse JO: Racquetball injuries. Phys Sports Med 7:88–92, 1979.
26. Easterbrook M: Eye injuries in squash and racquetball players: An update. Phys Sports Med 10(3):47–56, 1982.
27. Delori F, Pomerantzeff O, Cox MS: Deformation of the globe under high speed impact: Its relation to contusion injuries. Invest Ophthalmol 8:290–301, 1969.
28. Pashby TJ, Pashby RC, Chishom LD, et al: Eye injuries in Canadian hockey. Can Med Assoc J 113:633–666, 1975.
29. Beale H, Wood TO: Observations on traumatic hyphema. Am Ophthalmol 5:1101–1104, 1973.
30. Schults WT, Swan KC: High altitude retinopathy in mountain climbers. Arch Ophthalmol 93:404–408, 1975.
31. Garner AT: An overlooked problem: Athlete's visual needs. Phys Sports Med 5:75–82, 1977.
32. Wigglesworth EC: A comparative assessment of eye protective devices and system of acceptance testing and grading. Am J Optom 49:287–304, 1972.
33. Bishop PJ, Kozey J, Caldwell G: Performance of eye protectors for squash and racquetball. Phys Sports Med 10(3):62–69, 1982.
34. Park RD, Castaldi CR: Injuries in junior ice hockey. Phys Sports Med 8:81–84, 1980.
35. Castaldi CR: Mouthguards in contact sports. J Conn State Dent Assoc 48:233, 1974.
36. Stevens OO: Mouthprotectors: Evaluation of twelve types—second year. J Dent Child 32:137–145, 1965.
37. White AA, Johnson RM, Panjabi MM, et al: Biochemical analysis of clinical instability of the cervical spine. Clin Orthop 109:85–96, 1975.
38. Reid SE, Tarkington JA, Epstein HM, et al: Brain tolerance to impact in football. Surg Gynecol Obstet 133:929–936, 1971.
39. Long SE, Reid SE, Sweeney HJ, et al: Removing football helmets safely. Phys Sports Med 8:119, 1980.
40. American College of Surgeons Committee on Trauma: Techniques of Helmet Removal from Injured Patients. Chicago, 1980.
41. Lyness SS, Simeone FA: Vascular complications of upper cervical spine injuries. Orthop Clin N Am 9(4):1029–1038, 1970.
42. Fink F, Wells RE: Injuries of the cervical spine in football. Clin Orthop 109:50–58, 1975.
43. Rockett FX: Observations on the "burner": Traumatic cervical radiculopathy. Clin Orthop 164:18–19, 1982.

15
Common Injuries of the Back

Richard B. Birrer

THORACIC SPINE

Contusions

The most stable section of the vertebral column is the dorsal or thoracic spine. Contusions of the thoracic area are relatively common although rarely severe. Such muscular contusions should be treated the same as contusions elsewhere on the body. However, because there is a variety of thoracic muscles, muscular strain is frequent and often debilitating. Treatment is usually supportive and conservative followed by rapid progressive rehabilitation within the limits of pain. If a particular trigger point can be located, anesthetic injection with or without hyaluronidase may be of value should hematoma formation be present also.

Sprains

Mention should also be made of dorsal sprains which are frequently indistinguishable from and occur simultaneously with contusions. Treated in the same fashion as sprains elsewhere, bed rest, protection from further injury, and muscle relaxants followed by rapid progressive rehabilitation are the keynotes. Occasionally a fitted corset or adhesive strapping should be considered as supplementary treatment for strains or sprains of the thoracic spine. Interlocking basketweave, heavy 3 inch adhesive strips should be used, with the first strip being placed low enough to protect the inguinal canal. Each vertical and horizontal strip should overlap the previous by one half. The strapping should be extended 4 to 6 inches on each side of the spine. Chronic back strains are usually the result of an inadequately treated acute strain or sprain and require prolonged consultation, physical therapy, and protection from further injury. Very often psychological factors need to be elucidated by the attending physician. Diathermy, ultrasound, and a variety of physical therapy techniques are useful in rehabilitating such an athlete. If a trigger point can be localized, an injection of a corticosteroid/anesthetic combination is often useful.

Dislocations/Fractures

Dislocations of the thoracic spine are rare, though compression or bursting fractures, particularly at T-11 and T-12 are common particularly in such sports as baseball, basketball, football, track, and more violent sports such as polo and automobile racing. The usual history is sharp forward flexion motion which compacts the cancellous bone on itself while preserving the posterior ligaments. Examination may reveal point tenderness over the involved vertebra which can be confirmed by having the player flex his or her neck or bend at the upper back, though more often than not such maneuvers tend to produce generalized pain in any direction. A neurologic exam should be performed in order to rule out cord injury especially from posterior displaced fragments. Radiologic examination is imperative coupled with accurate measurement of the vertebrae. Unfortunately this may be misleading since one or more of the dorsal vertebrae may be of smaller size than others normally.

Careful examination of the bone appearance itself may reveal a fracture line or an increased density due to compaction. Treatment should be performed in conjunction with a competent orthopedic surgeon. For dislocations, reduction is imperative and local hyperextension according to the "jack method" is by far the best. Once reduction has been performed, a suitable plaster jacket should be applied in order to preserve local extension without generalized hyperextension. It should be noted that not all compression fractures need be immobilized. The majority of compression fractures can be managed conservatively: the application of a well padded cast extending from below the clavicle to the symphysis pubis while the patient is in traction with the spine neutral, and bed rest for 6 weeks followed by another 6 weeks of weight bearing; the cast is removed after a total of 12 to 14 weeks. Hyperextension exercises are begun immediately but flexion exercises start after the cast is removed. Though bed rest probably offers the best chance for maintenance of the correction, it is difficult to keep an athlete at bed rest. Careful cast application in order to place the entire weight of the injured spine on the articular processes and careful follow-up is in order; bed rest may then be curtailed.

Scoliosis

Although cases of lateral deviation of the spine or *scoliosis* are rarely disfiguring or functionally compromising, the condition produces undue anxiety for the athlete and family. Seventy percent of cases are idiopathic and are eight times more frequent in adolescent girls than boys.[1] Risk factors appear to be rapid precocious growth and positive family history (autosomal dominant with incomplete penetrance). It can appear in one of three forms:

1. Infantile type (birth to 3 years), more common in males with left thoracic curvature and a good prognosis (85 percent of cases)
2. Juvenile type (age 3 to 10), with predominant right thoracic curvature, which is usually progressive, and equal gender preference

3. Adolescent type (age 10 to skeletal maturity), characterized by mostly right thoracic and thoracolumbar curvature.

The evaluation of the patient should include a history directed toward the chronological age of the patient, age of recognition of the deformity, family history, developmental history (Tanner staging, rate of growth), and associated symptoms (fatigue, pain, cardiopulmonary difficulties, range of motion). The exam should be directed at trunk alignment, shoulder girdle symmetry, assessment of the specific curve (degree of flexibility/rigidity/range of motion), and a careful neurologic and cardiopulmonary inventory. Finally a maturity index should be calculated. Radiologic studies should include an anteroposterior (AP) and lateral of the spine, as well as a left hand and wrist in the adolescent. Whether one chooses the Cobb (more accepted) or Risser-Ferguson method, the curvature should be measured, graded, and recorded. The examination should be repeated every 3 months or sooner if one suspects a rapidly evolving scoliosis.

Prognostic indicators of major import are the following:

1. Age—the younger at the onset, the greater the tendency to deformity
2. Pattern—the degree of thoracic component is main determinate of overall deformity
3. Apex curvature alteration on x ray—more rapid progression seen with osteoporotic vertebrae, irregularly narrowed disk spaces, and marked wedging adjacent to the apex.

Treatment rests on the presupposition that each deformity has its own natural history including the potential for progression and interference with visceral function. Even after maturity has been reached the curve can increase another 15° over the next 20 years.[2] Thus, early identification of a scoliosis is critical; management should be aggressive with a carefully prescribed physiotherapy exercise and stretching regimen. Symmetric (develop general body musculature and tone) and asymmetric (reduce convexity and strengthen ipsilateral muscles) exercises should be performed. For nonrigid curvatures of less than 40°, a Milwaukee brace can hold a variable degree of the condition until maturity is reached. Surgery is indicated for rapidly progressive cases, pain especially in adults, curves greater than 45° in adolescents, truncal deformity regardless of whether spinal growth has ceased, and decreasing cardiopulmonary function. Recently nocturnal muscle stimulation has been used with some success.

LUMBAR SPINE

The lumbar area is the most commonly injured area of the spine. The National Center for Health Statistics considers chronic back complaints the single most common medical ailment. At least 70 million Americans have experienced one severe prolonged episode secondary to a low back injury, according to the U.S. Public Health Service report. The athletic population is not immune to lower back problems. Several Olympic studies have shown that it is a common problem area in highly trained athletes.[3] Fortunately, the majority of such injuries involve a contusion, sprain, or strain and rarely involve herniation of the nucleus pulposus or spinal fracture. Greater mobility and inherent stability of the lumbar spine due to its massive vertebrae and large muscle supporting masses is offset by weak abdominal muscles and hip flexors in combination with inflexibility and tightness, especially of the hamstring hip extensor muscles.[4] Such a fact may seem to be incongruous with the highly trained capacities of most athletes. However, in several studies it has been clearly shown that many world class athletes have markedly underdeveloped abdominal muscles, many being unable to complete one or two bent-knee sit-ups. The sports population tends to have strong back and hip extensor muscles but much weaker anterior flexor muscles. Individuals particularly at risk include gymnasts who hyperextend while dismounting, runners who compete in forced extension, divers who extend while entering the water, and finally weight lifters, shot-putters, and discus throwers who extend their back while hoisting heavy weights.

Examinations/Common Conditions

As with cervical and thoracic injuries, the acute lumbar injury should be treated with care. Examination should be initially performed on the field and movement should not be attempted until a careful neurologic exam has ruled out any form of impairment. Because of the structure of the lumbar spine, it is most uncommon to fracture or dislocate the vertebra. Bowel and bladder function should be checked as part of the neurologic exam. Each of the spinous processes should be carefully palpated for the detection of a trigger point which might indicate possible fracture or sprain of the interspinous ligaments. Compression fractures typically involve the first two lumbar vertebrae and, like spinous or transverse process fractures, are usually stable, though it is essential that the athlete be transported on a spine-board until x rays are taken and clearly establish the underlying problem. Palpation should also include the large paraspinal muscles as well as the side, flexor, and rotator muscles. Mild swellings often create a diagnostic dilemma in that a contusion, strain, sprain, or a combination of these may be present. Larger swellings may indicate hematoma formation. The primary care physician should be familiar with diagnosis of herniated nucleus pulposus (slipped disk), which may present with pain along the involved nerve root and may be accompanied by motor signs such as paresis and diminished reflexes. Typically any form of strain such as coughing, sneezing, laughing, or passage of a bowel movement or urine tends to make the pain worse. The initial treatment for a herniated disk as well as the majority of strains, sprains, and contusions is conservative and involves bed rest, protection from further injury, muscle relaxants, and anti-inflammatory and analgesic agents followed by rapid progressive rehabilitation within the limits of pain. A very small percentage of more serious injuries and persistent neurologic deficits (e.g., absence of a particular reflex or muscular atrophy along a root distribution) should prompt neurosurgical consultation, myelography, and possibly surgery.

Miscellaneous Conditions

A variety of miscellaneous lumbar conditions may present themselves to the physician. Lumbarization of the first sacral vertebra and sacralization of the fifth lumbar vertebra are usually of no significance from an activity viewpoint. There may be mild pain or slight lower back imbalance if the fusion is incomplete, but usually reassurance is all that is necessary.

Spina bifida occulta represents failure of arch fusion of one or more vertebrae posterior. Although it is a common finding, it is of no significance and the player should not be alarmed by the reporting of the condition; rarely, back support with a corset may be recommended during particularly strenuous sports activity.

Lastly, *spondylolysis,* which is defect in the pars intra-articularis and *spondylolisthesis,* which is spondylosis and displacement of superior vertebrae forward on the one below, may occur with some frequency but are often asymptomatic and therefore rarely diagnosed. There are four grades of spondylolisthesis and, if there are incapacitating symptoms (particularly in the younger population) associated with grades III or IV, definitive treatment of the condition should be considered rather than interdiction of sports activity. If the symptoms are minimal, then perhaps a change in the exercise prescription is warranted. It should be kept in mind, however, that degenerative changes do occur over time; this factor must be carefully weighed against encouragement of persistent and increased activity. On the other hand, prescribing less activity for the active, eager athlete or endorsing indolence in the already sedentary individual should warrant consideration for a possible surgical correction.

Rehabilitation

The treatment program of back injuries should be threefold: management of acute pain and spasm, progressive rehabilitation, and preventive educa-

tion.[5] Treatment of the acute stage is best made with the use of ice and anti-inflammatory/analgesic agents, muscle relaxants, rest, and protection from further injury. The majority of lower back strains usually respond within 24 to 48 hours. The second phase of the program should begin as soon as possible after the injury before muscle weakness and stiffness sets in. Rapid progressive rehabilitation within the limits of pain should be established in conjunction with ultrasound, diathermy, and transcutaneous electric nerve stimulation. It is a wise idea for the physician to become familiar with back strain and flexibility testing. A pillow or similar form of padding should be placed under the upper hips while the patient is prone upon the examining table. While fixating the buttocks and legs to the examining table, the back extensor muscles can be tested by asking the patient to raise the head, chin, elbows and back off the examining table. In a similar fashion, lower back muscle integrity can be tested by fixation of the head and trunk and asking the athlete to raise the knees and legs from the table. For both tests, 10 seconds of lift indicates weak musculature whereas 20 seconds or more indicates strong muscles.

A variety of stretching methods can be used to assay the flexibility of the athlete as well as counsel for rehabilitative exercises. A useful test for the patient lying supine includes the straight-leg raise and a nose-to-toe touch with one leg on a waist-high table for the hamstrings; a single-knee raise and double-knee hug assess the hip extensors, hamstrings, and lower back. While standing with locked knees, the athlete should attempt to place both hands on the floor, thus testing lower back/hip extensors and hamstrings. In the early phase of rehabilitation it is wisest to apply ultrasound dia-

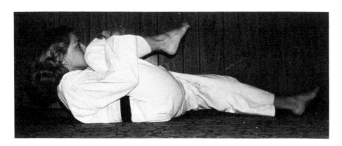

FIGURE 15-1. Single-knee hug.

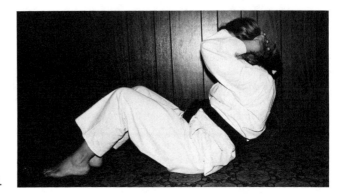

FIGURE 15-2. Abdominal curl.

thermy or other forms of heat treatment to the lower back before and after the exercise interval, which should be ideally done twice daily. It is imperative that all exercises be done within the limitations of pain and that they be done slowly and progressively. As far as strengthening the lower back muscles, the standard Williams flexion exercises are usually recommended. It is wisest to begin with the simplest exercises such as the back flattener, in which the supine patient attempts to flatten the back against a surface by tilting the pelvis (which requires tensing of the gluteal and abdominal muscles) and the single-knee raise and hug, which is also done in the supine position and is used to stretch the lower back, hip flexor, and hamstrings (Fig. 15-1); through the intermediate exercises such as the double-knee hug and the single-leg raise, which stretch the lower back and hamstrings and strengthen the abdominal and hip-flexing muscles; to the most difficult, which include the partial and advanced sit-up or abdominal curl (Fig. 15-2). Regular sit-ups and double-leg raises should not be done under any circumstance as they will aggravate back injuries.

The athlete's progress should be kept continually monitored by the physician and each stage should be completed before advancement to the next step. As part of the third phase of preventive education, the athlete should be taught the posture check (Fig. 15-3), which involves assessing the amount of lordosis when the head, upper and lower back, and buttocks are placed firmly against a wall and the heels are 4 inches from the same wall. If there is a space between the lower back and the

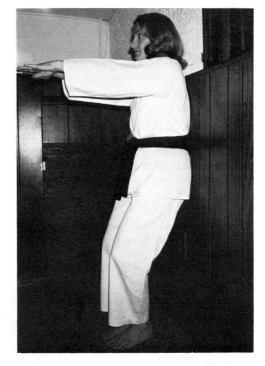

FIGURE 15-3. Posture check. Note: heels 4 inches from wall, back flat against wall, head and cervical spine upright.

wall, posture is poor. The individual should be taught to keep his or her knees slightly flexed 10° to 15° and abdominal muscles tightened up in order to tilt the pelvis and rotate it superiorly and posteriorly. This flattens out any lordotic curve.

The most important aspect of preventing further back injury is the teaching and maintenance of proper posture, which requires tensing the gluteal and abdominal muscles, slightly flexing the knees, and walking, standing, and sitting as tall as possible. Leaning or standing for long periods of time in high-heel shoes should be avoided. When leaning, it is important to bend the knees, and when bending over to lift an object, it is important to squat first and then lift the item with a straight lower back.

Regarding the sitting position, it is best to avoid chairs on rollers, swivel chairs, soft or overstuffed chairs, ottomans or footstools, or sitting in the same position for a prolonged period. When sitting it is best to allow the lower back to be flat or slightly rounded outward but never with a forward curve. The most desirable type of seat is one with a hard back that begins contact with the lumbar area in a flat manner approximately 4 to 6 inches above the seat. Sleep or rest should be only on a very flat, firm mattress which it is often wise to supplement with a ¾-inch piece of plywood.

Finally, some effort should be made to retrain an athlete in a given sport if it has been aggravating

the problem. For instance, in power lifters, in order to avoid forced anterior flexion of the spine ("good morning sing"), it is important to teach the athlete to keep the head and chin always extended with the eyes looking up as the weight is lifted. The runner, gymnast, equestrian, and diver should be reminded that their sport tends to hyperextend the spine and that every effort should be made to maintain good abdominal and gluteal muscletone. Baseball, volleyball, softball, handball, and tennis players should be reminded to keep their knees bent rather than their backs while playing. In order to avoid hypertension while serving in a racquet sport, it is best to keep the ball slightly forward of the body. There is no question that the majority of athletic back injuries can be prevented if the sports physician continually educates and the athlete is responsible.

REFERENCES

1. Keim HA: Scoliosis. CIBA Clin Symp 24(1):2, 1972.
2. Collis DK, Ponseti IV: Long term follow-up of patients with idiopathic scoliosis not treated surgically. J Bone Jt Surg (Am) 51A:425–445, 1969.
3. Harris WD: Low back pain in sports medicine. J Arkansas Med Svc 74:377–379, 1978.
4. Ferguson RJ: Low back pain in college football linemen. J Sports Med 2:63–80, 1974.
5. Smith CF: Physical management of muscular low back pain in the athlete. Can Med Assoc J 177:632–635, 1977.

16
Common Injuries of the Chest and Abdomen

Richard B. Birrer

CHEST

Contusions

Contusions to the chest are common due to its size as well as its central location. Very often a direct blow will cause the "wind to be knocked out" of the athlete followed by immediate muscle spasm and later localized tenderness. The diagnosis of chest wall contusion is usually not a difficult one. By sliding the skin upward or downward over a rib one can distinguish between a superficial contusion and one involving the rib itself. In the latter, there is direct rib tenderness whereas in the former the pain is constant in the skin.

It is possible with a major direct blow to fracture a rib. This can be readily diagnosed by point tenderness as well as positive "bucket handling"— i.e., pain in a specific area of a rib replicated by compressing the chest with one hand placed adjacent to the thoracic spine and the other over the ipsilateral parasternal area. Occasionally a complicating hematoma may form which, if large, should be aspirated and then compressed to prevent reformation. Breast contusions, particularly in the female, can be most distressing as the loose subcutaneous tissue is conducive to hematoma formation. One may note on clinical examination a hard indurated area underlying the areola which is exquisitely tender, and there may be some serious

exudation from the nipple. Very often diagnosis and treatment is delayed because of the embarrassment to the athlete. The usual treatment for contusion and hematoma is indicated and return to play should be rapid. Rarely there may be subcutaneous fat necrosis, which can be an alarming cosmetic problem. Reassurance and careful follow-up are important. It is advisable to prescribe protective contact pads over the contused area.

Abrasions

Simple frictional stress over the nipple region produces erythema and edema with repeated insult (jogger's nipples). The condition occurs in women who do not wear brassieres, as well as in men. Treatment is a well fitted bra in the female and petrolatum or tape over the nipples in males. Shirts should be made from a hard silk or polyester fabric.

Strains

Because of the large number of muscles on the chest wall strain can occur secondary to overstretching on violent exertion. Typically, the strain is more likely to involve an area connecting to the chest rather than within the chest itself. This is particularly true of the trapezius, serratus, scapular, and abdominal muscles. Treatment of such strains is in the usual fashion and return to competition is expected. It is important that the athlete not be reintroduced to full play too soon because reinjury can result. Interim measures such as the application of rib belt or elastic bandage wrapping may be expedient.

Sprains

Ligamentous injury to the rib more often occurs at its anterior attachment, though its posterior or vertebral site can also be damaged. It should be noted that a direct blow to the rib usually causes a fracture rather than a sprain or dislocation. With progressive lateral compression of the chest or direct driving force to the sternum there is a forward thrust of the ribs with subluxation and eventual dislocation if the pressure is great enough. First- and second-degree sprains respond well to conservative management: local anesthetic injection, ice, rest, and chest strapping. More serious injuries should be handled in conjunction with a specialist. Occasionally a severe rib sprain or fracture may be associated with a costochondral injury such as subluxation or dislocation. X-ray diagnosis is usually not possible as the cartilage is radiolucent. Unfortunately, most of these injuries require surgical intervention due to delay in diagnosis or presentation. A more common condition is *costochondritis* or Tietze's syndrome, an idiopathic inflammation of the costochondral junctions, classically of the second and third ribs, though other sites can be involved. Reassurance, rest, analgesics, and anti-inflammatory agents produce good results.

Fractures

Most physicians are familiar with rib fractures as they are a common injury in a variety of settings. It is important to keep in mind the fact that radiologic evaluation may be negative due to the oblique course of the rib, the overlying soft tissue, the frequent lack of displacement, and the depth of the thorax. In the uncomplicated fracture local therapy is all that is required. This consists of local anesthetic, analgesics, and some form of immobilization. A rib belt is very useful as it produces support for the local area which has been injured rather than for entire hemi- or bilateral thorax. Adhesive strapping of the area can also be applied but is often

irritative and difficult to apply in the region of the breast. One should allow 3 or 4 weeks for healing and it is wise to have the athlete wear a binder in any contact sport for at least 6 weeks in combination with an incorporated local protective pad. Complicated rib fractures consist of fragmentation and comminution of the bone in association with internal mammary artery damage, injury to the intercostal nerves and vessels, with hematoma pneumothorax or hemopericardium.

From a clinical viewpoint, one should suspect a more serious injury when the athlete does not recover from the initial period of breathlessness following the blow. Furthermore, the dyspnea may be progressive and cyanosis may intervene. Rarely there may be clinical evidence of subcutaneous emphysema. As in all emergency situations, the ABCs of basic life support are imperative, followed by subsequent treatment of the underlying pathology; these have been discussed in detail in Chapter 13. Fractures of the first three ribs, in particular, should raise the suspicion that more serious underlying injury may be present.

Injuries to Sternum

Forces applied directly to the sternum can produce contusions, sprains, subluxation, dislocations, and fractures. Usually the athlete experiences some degree of shock reaction in association with variable amounts of dyspnea if the blow was severe. Invariably the athlete recovers within a short period of time and perhaps complains only of mild pain on forced expansion or extremes of chest movement. There may be some point tenderness on examination, though fingertip ballotment often identifies the trigger point. Nondisplaced fractures, subluxations, and reduced dislocation can be treated conservatively with the elimination of all contact sports for the interim period of 5 to 6 weeks and the instillation of local anesthetic, analgesics, rest, and an active physical therapy program. Once the athlete begins sports participation it is wisest to prescribe a tailored contact pad or similar device for protection against reinjury (e.g., custom plastic molding). Finally, it is always important to remember that the forces needed to fracture-dislocate a sternum often produce damage to the underlying tissue and organs.

ABDOMEN

The abdominal area extends from the diaphragm superiorly to the pelvis inferiorly and consists of massive bones and heavy muscle forming the posterior wall, several crisscrossing layers of synergistic muscles anterior which together provide motion in any direction (flexion extension, lateral bending, rotation, or any combination of these), and a variety of internal abdominal viscera responsible for important bodily functions. Thus, athletic injuries to the abdominal area can be divided into two distinct categories: (1) injury to the abdominal wall and (2) injury to the abdominal contents.

Though the abdominal area is large and well padded, the nature and localization of an athletic injury may not always be apparent due to the indirect accessibility of diagnostic maneuvers. It is important for every primary care physician to bear in mind the fact that many abdominal injuries are occult in nature and may present over several hours to several days. The assessment for such injury, however, is not different from that of the head, chest, or similar orthopedic injuries. Furthermore, the diagnostic inventory must be organized, reproducible and complete in order to identify the most serious potential injuries.[1] Finally, it is paramount that injury prioritization be kept foremost in the physician's mind. Thus, airway, breathing, and circulation should be guaranteed before further evaluation of possible internal abdominal injury is made.

Injury to the anterior abdominal wall is common, though serious injury is uncommon in most major sports. The reasons for this are threefold:

1. Muscles of the anterior abdominal wall are extremely pliable and resilient.
2. The area is less exposed to injury since it is on the flexion side of the trunk.
3. The abdominal wall is usually protected in most sports by well designed pads of individual equipment.

Abrasions/Hematomas

Skin abrasions are infrequent and are treated in the usual manner with particular attention being paid to thorough cleansing, scrubbing of the area, and updating of tetanus immunization. Dressings on lacerations and abrasions should be sterile and kept to the minimum. Antibiotic ointments and topical anesthetics should be avoided. Blunt trauma to the subcutaneous tissue can cause an arteriolar or venous hematoma. The typical story is that of an athlete coming in to see the team physician the day after a contact game complaining of an egg-shaped discolored mass in the rectus sheet. A careful abdominal exam, particularly with the abdominal musculature tense (straight-leg raise), demonstrates that the mass is anterior to the abdominal wall muscles. Treatment is the same as for any hematoma—RICE (Rest, Ice for 48 to 72 hours, Compression, Elevation and avoidance of reinjury). Rarely does a subcutaneous hematoma require additional treatment in the form of aspiration. Aspirin and the nonsteroidal anti-inflammatories may be useful supplemental forms of treatment. If an athlete continually develops repeated subcutaneous hematomas, an investigation for an underlying blood dyscrasia should be made (leukemia or idiopathic thrombocytopenic purpura).

Contusions

The most frequent abdominal wall injury is contusion of the musculature—recti, external and internal oblique muscles, and the transversus abdominis muscle. The injury is typically due to blunt trauma (a batted ball or blow from a weapon or fist), although it can also be due to a sharp-pointed object causing penetration (skate point or ski pole). Most penetrating injuries should be surgically explored and observed for appropriate hemostasis or further complication. Complete abdominal exploration is indicated if the peritoneal membrane has been pierced. Abdominal wall contusions should be treated in the usual fashion. Rarely, the deep epigastric arteries or veins can be ruptured due to blunt trauma; this results in an expanding deep hematoma which eventually becomes self-tamponading. Such injuries require surgical exploration, vessel ligation, and evacuation of the expanding hematoma.

Contusions of the abdominal wall may also involve the bony iliac crest or the lower tenth, eleventh, and twelfth ribs. These contusions, like those involving other bones, can be at times extremely distressing and debilitating due to subperiosteal hematoma formation and concomitant pain. It is extremely unusual to dislocate or fracture lower ribs as they are mobile and are well protected by large muscle groups.

Strains

Muscle strains of the abdominal wall periodically occur to the active athlete. Strains can occur at the musculotendinous insertions at the iliac crest, rib, or pubic attachment or occur within the body of the muscle itself due to vigorous overstretching, especially when the trunk is twisted or hyperextended secondary to contact or particular motion. Most of these strains are mild, though it is possible to tear the aponeurotic sheath from its site of attachment to the muscle. Such injuries tend to occur in gymnasts, high jumpers, or pole vaulters. Most of these injuries are mild to moderate in nature and are characterized by local tenderness, perhaps accompanied by a small nodular swelling which develops over a matter of hours: rarely is the onset acute and incapacitating; in such cases it is indicative of more serious underlying injury. Treatment consists of ice for prolonged periods, rest, protection from further injury, and slow but progressive rehabilitation performed within the limits of pain. Local injections of steroids and anesthetic solutions are contraindicated. The efficacy of ultrasound and deep diathermy remains to be established. Abdominal corsets and similar support devices provide some abdominal support and restrict motion so that passive tension on the injured area can be eliminated, but do little to prevent vigorous abdominal muscle contraction. They are recommended for acute or short-term injuries.

It is essential to bear in mind that any abdominal wall injury can be associated with and should suggest the possibility of more serious internal abdominal injury. Occasionally a unilateral rectus abdominus strain on the right side must differentiate from a case of acute appendicitis or, on the left side, from a possible splenic rupture.

Hernia

Though a more thorough discussion of hernias is well beyond the scope of this book, it is essential that the primary care physician bear in mind that active athletics and hernias do not mix. The majority of sports increase abdominal pressure and tend to aggravate hernias which were formerly asymptomatic. Hernias should always be considered an important portion of differential diagnosis of all abdominal wall and inguinal masses. All symptomatic and the majority of asymptomatic hernias should be repaired if an individual is contemplating or is involved in various athletic endeavors.

Intra-Abdominal Injuries

Examination. All intra-abdominal injuries are acute surgical emergencies. Though extremely infrequent in sports competition, such abdominal injuries carry a high degree of morbidity and mortality. Very often (30 percent) intra-abdominal injuries are associated with significant trauma to other anatomic areas (head, chest, or extremities).[2] The abdominal area is often quite difficult to evaluate clinically and, in many instances, significant intra-abdominal injuries are not initially apparent, becoming so only after a significant period has elapsed.[3] Therefore, a careful and thorough history of the mechanism of injury together with a complete physical examination should be a benchmark for every physician with regard to abdominal injuries.[1] It is important to get as accurate a description of the incident as possible: details as to the type of object (blunt or sharp, helmet, elbow, knee), position of body at time of impact, location of the particular injury, tone at the time of impact, elapsed time since the injury, the athlete's perception of the degree of injury, history of previous abdominal injury, time of the last meal, whether the athlete's bladder was full or empty at the time of impact, and time of last bowel movement. Vital signs should be taken and carefully noted and compared to any previous vital signs taken at the field.

The abdomen should be carefully inspected for any obvious swellings, discolorations (Cullen's or Grey-Turner's signs) or lacerations. Furthermore, the general contour should be noted (scaphoid vs distended). The most informative method in examining the abdomen for injury is careful palpation, which should be undertaken after reassurance and hand warming by the physician. The most reliable physical sign indicating peritoneal irritation is the presence of involuntary spasm, which tends to make the wall tense and boardlike. Voluntary spasm can be diagnosed by noting the decrease in muscular spasm under the examining hand as the patient is asked to breathe deeply. Involuntary rigidity, secondary to peritoneal irritation, remains constant. Localized rigidity (that is, tenderness underneath one or two fingers) is suggestive of a walled-off lesion with local bleeding or leakage from a particular viscus. This diagnostic finding can be confirmed by noting rebound tenderness to the primary site under consideration.

The lower portion of the chest, the flanks, the inguinal areas, and all four quadrants of the abdomen should be carefully examined. In the nonrigid, nontender abdomen, the liver, spleen, bowel, and kidneys should be palpated for carefully. The most tender area always should be examined last. As a technique, percussion has the lowest sensitivity and moderate specificity. Auscultation is not terribly useful although the absence of bowel sounds is a frequent sign of early hemorrhage or significant abdominal injury. Finally, rectal and pelvic exams should always be performed.

Laboratory Evaluation. A CBC and urinalysis should be performed as well as a flat and upper right abdominal x ray. In those athletes whose course is unstable and progressively downhill, a diagnostic paracentesis or lavage should be performed.[4] This involves an infrapubic incision following the application of a local anesthetic, the insertion of a peritoneal dialysis catheter or trocar, or use of a simple angiocatheter. The aspiration of nonclotting blood essentially confirms the diagnosis of hemoperitoneum. If no blood or other material is aspirated, 1 liter of Ringer's lactate should be rapidly instilled into the peritoneal cavity, the patient rotated from side to side (presuming the absence of any major bony fractures), and the fluid siphoned out. Depending on the protocol in use in one's particular institution, the removal of 20 to 100 thousand red cells per cubic millimeter, 300 to 700 white blood cells per cubic millimeter, an elevated amylase, and the presence of bile or bacteria within the material are indications for immediate laparotomy. The sensitivity and specificity of this procedure approach 95 to 97 percent. Complications include the puncturing of intra-abdominal viscera, particularly the small and large bowel, the mesenteric vessels, and the production of a retroperitoneal or abdominal wall hematoma.

In conjunction with a surgeon, all penetrating injuries should be explored thoroughly in order to determine the presence and/or depth of a foreign body. As already mentioned, if the peritoneum has been penetrated, the abdomen should be explored. If the patient's condition has been stable or improving since the injury, a period of observation in the hospital may be indicated. This should be at the discretion of the physician in conjunction with an abdominal surgeon.

Splenic Injury. The spleen is the abdominal organ most frequently injured secondary to blunt trauma. It can be ruptured during mononucleosis due to its friability (Chapter 12). The history of trauma to the left lower chest or the left upper abdomen should suggest splenic injury. Fractures of the overlying rib often cause accompanying injury to the spleen. Symptomatology ranges from negligible to distressing incapacitation and usually involves abdominal pain or, in certain cases, left shoulder discomfort secondary to phrenic nerve irritation. Spectrum of physical findings also ranges from unremarkable to left upper abdominal, left flank, or left lower chest exquisite tenderness and hypovolemic shock. X-ray examination of the abdomen occasionally demonstrates obliteration of the splenic shadow of the colon, depression of the colonic flexure, elevation of the left hemidiaphragm, and perhaps prominence of the gastric rugae. Though the diagnosis of splenic rupture is predominantly a clinical one, radionuclide scanning and angiography may be required for confirmation.

If these techniques are unavailable, it is wise to observe an athlete with potential flank injury over a period of 24 to 48 hours inside the hospital providing he or she is stable. It is possible that occasionally a subcapsular splenic hematoma can rupture several days to weeks after the initial trauma. Once the diagnosis has been made or the patient's course is downhill, treatment is surgical removal of the spleen or its direct repair (splenography) in order to preserve the organ.

Liver Injury. The liver is the second most commonly injured organ in blunt trauma. Right flank, lower chest, or upper abdominal strikes can cause liver contusion or laceration. The typical course of liver injury consists of a rapid progressive downhill course secondary to hypovolemic shock. Since mortality is very high with liver injuries, it is imperative that the physician make the diagnosis as quickly as possible and take the injured athlete to surgery.

Pancreatic Injury. Pancreatic injuries are extremely uncommon in the sports arena but, when they occur, usually involve the junction of the head and the body of the pancreas. Though serum amylase is usually elevated, physical findings tend to be scanty and evolve over a prolonged period. Thus consideration for abdominal laparotomy should be made when the condition is strongly suspected even though there may be few peritoneal signs. Ultrasound may be useful especially if a pseudocyst is suspected.

Bowel Injury. The majority of bowel disruptions occur distal to the duodenum and usually involve the proximal half of the jejunum or distal ileum. The mechanism of injury involves blunt trauma directed at the bowel overlying the vertebral column or a sheering/tangential force against a relatively fixed bowel or mesentery, i.e., at the ligament of Treitz or the iliocecal valve. Because the symptomatology and clinical findings evolve slowly over time, it is wisest to perform serial abdominal examinations in order to detect progression of the intra-abdominal injury. Radiologic investigation may not reveal free air within the abdominal cavity as there is very little gas present in the small bowel in the resting state. Though tearing of the mesentery is usually associated with massive hemorrhage and hypovolemic shock, it is possible that a small tear could become clinically manifest hours or days after the original injury secondary to progressive ischemia and the necrosis of the bowel.

Stomach and large bowel injury are most uncommon although it is possible that a forceful direct blow could cause injury; both are typically associated with free air in the abdominal cavity. Clinical signs and symptoms of peritoneal irritation develop early in stomach injury due to high acid content, whereas they are delayed in large bowel injury until an infection is well established.

Duodenal Injury. Duodenal injury, though rare, is often insidious and overlooked due to association with other abdominal organ injury. The duodenum is susceptible to blast rupture, laceration, or perforation from direct anterior blows as well as a possible fall upon the back because: (1) Gas can be trapped between the closed pylorus and the sharply angulated duodenal jejunal junction; (2) It is located retroperitoneally; and (3) It lies immediately anterior to the vertebral column. Once other intra-abdominal organ injury has been ruled out, the athlete must be carefully observed for worsening of abdominal symptomatology and clinical findings. As a result of serial examinations, a barium swallow or endoscopy may be indicated as serum amylase studies, lavage, and roentgenograms of the abdomen are often reliable. Milder forms of duodenal injury include intramural hematomas, which often present as small bowel obstructions.

Kidney Injury. Despite their well protected location in the upper retroperitoneum, the kidneys are subject to direct as well as contrecoup injuries. The most common injury to the kidney is contusion, which may be secondary to an elbow, helmet, or similar strike to the flank region. The majority of renal contusions are minor and involve the extravasation of a small amount of blood underneath the renal capsule. There may be mild flank pain existing for several days and perhaps micro- or macroscopic hematuria. The majority of these injuries have no long-term side-effects though the mechanism of injury is distinctly different from the microscopic hematuria associated with vigorous exercise. It is wise for the physician to follow up with the patient who has a renal contusion, ordering urinalysis within a month to make sure that there is no long-term sequela. More forceful strikes or blows to the flank area can produce capsular rupture and laceration or rupture of the renal parenchyma or tear of the renal pedicle. The symptoms and signs are related to the type of injury. With more serious injury, flank pain and tenderness tend to be severe. Renal colic may be present if a thrombus obstructs the collecting system or ureter. Expanding flank mass hypovolemic shock may be present if there is severe hemorrhage, usually extrinsic to the kidney. Flank and lumbar muscles are noted to be in painful spasm and occasionally the differential diagnosis for muscular hematoma or contusion may be difficult; in fact, the entities may coexist. Hematuria may be gross or microscopic. Abdominal plain films may show a loss of the renal outline, associated rib or vertebral fractures, blurring of the psoas margin, and/or elevation of the ipsilateral hemidiaphragm or pulmonary atelectasis. An emergency intravenous pyelogram should be ordered and consultation with a urologist should be placed. Typically there is no surgical intervention indicated for contusions, cortical lacerations without urinary extravasation, or intrarenal lacerations without disruption of the renal capsule. Renal pedicle injuries, transcortical or transcapsular lacerations with evidence of extravasation, and all injuries associated with massive hemorrhage are indicative of immediate surgical intervention. Finally, it is important to bear in mind that other organs within the abdominal cavity, as well as other genital and urinary organs, may be involved in the renal injury.

Though rare, the ureters may be injured in a concomitant, severe renal injury, or in fracture of the pelvis or vertebrae. Unfortunately, such injury is not suspected until a complication or significant urinary extravasation occurs. Bladder injury is most uncommon because the competitive athlete tends to maintain an empty bladder. However, direct strikes or a blow to the suprapubic area, as in the martial arts, has been known to cause bladder contusion and, rarely, a rupture. A patient may or may not complain of lower abdominal suprapubic pain and/or blood in the urine. If the patient is unable to void, a catheter should be placed and a urinalysis done immediately. An emergency urethrogram and cystogram should be performed and it is important to bear in mind that the upper tracts should also be evaluated by an intravenous pyelogram. Most bladder contusions can be managed with conservative treatment but bladder rupture requires early surgical intervention and repair.

Urethral/Genital Injuries. Urethral injuries in males and females are not common in the sports world.[5] Gymnastics, cycling, and the martial arts have been associated with lacerations and contusion of the distal urethra in the female and the membranous urethra in the male. It is most rare to injure the anterior urethra in the male as it is very mobile. Urethral injuries in females have also been noted with the use of tampon inserters. Diagnosis is made by urethrography and panendoscopy which is best handled by a competent urologic surgeon.

The external genital area in both sexes can be injured in a variety of sports. The most common cause for vulvar and scrotal injuries is a direct blow to the area when unprotected by an athletic cup. In the female the highly vascular and loose subcutaneous tissue of the labia predisposes to hematoma formation. In the male, scrotal hematomas are common sequelae to direct blows. In either case the treatment is ice for 48 to 72 hours, elevation, and rest. In the male, testicular contusion, epididymitis, and torsion can also occur. It is particularly important that the physician be able to differentiate testicular torsion from epididymitis. The most reliable sign in distinguishing the two is that the testicle, when torsed, tends to be elevated and extremely painful even when lifted by the palpating hand, whereas in epididymitis the epididymis tends to be swollen and tender, but pain is relieved when the testicle is elevated. Diagnosis must be made as rapidly as possible as the viability decreases after 2 to 3 hours. If diagnosis is uncertain, a urologic surgeon should be consulted and a radionuclide scan made if available. The scan is "hot" in the case of epididymitis but "cold" in torsion due to the absence of perfusion.

REFERENCES

1. McSwain NE: Systematic evaluation of the abdomen. Curr Concepts Trauma Care 4(2):5–8, 1981.
2. Davis JJ, Colin I, Nance FC: Diagnosis and management of blunt abdominal trauma. Ann Surg 183:672–677, 1976.
3. Nance FC: The early management of abdominal trauma. Curr Concepts Trauma Care 2(2):9–14, 1979.
4. McSwain NE: Tips and techniques—peritoneal lavage. Curr Concepts Trauma Care 4(2):21–22, 1981.
5. Presky L, Hoch WH: Genitourinary tract trauma monograph, Curr Probe Surg 9:1–64, 1972.

17
Common Injuries of the Upper Extremity

Richard B. Birrer

There are two important ingredients to the understanding of any injury to the upper or lower extremity. The first is normal biomechanics of the entire process involved. (For example, the complex sequence for throwing is as follows: push-off rotational thrust, contralateral leg kick, trunk thrust, and forward acceleration and derotation of the upper extremity. For running, the sequence is: support phase of the foot strike, midsupport phase of the take-off, and recovery phase of the follow-through, forward swing, and foot descent.) The second important feature is the mechanism of injury. How did the injury occur and during which phase of the particular motion was the injury sustained? Knowledge of either the mechanism of injury or the biomechanical factors of the particular motion alone results in inappropriate treatment and subsequent dysfunction. Finally, a comprehensive synthesis of the athlete's injury should include a more than superficial understanding of the demands of the individual's sport or performance requirements, because often treatment and expectations after recovery are directly related to the demands of the individual competitive sport.

SHOULDER

The complexity of shoulder girdle anatomy is surpassed only by its impressive array of function. The shoulder is able to move forward, backward, upward, downward, and in a rotational manner. It is constructed from the humerus, scapula with its important features of the acromion and coracoid processes, the clavicle, an impressive assortment of ligaments (acromioclavicular, coracoclavicular, and sternoclavicular) and a variety of supporting muscles. Thus, in a very important anatomical sense, shoulder stability is sacrificed for controlled mobility in which very smooth, coordinated, synchronous movement of the upper extremity is enabled. One of the earliest signs of a shoulder girdle lesion is a disturbance of this coordinated movement.

Examination

In addition to shoulder anatomy and the biomechanics of throwing, a careful orderly examination must be coupled with a good history and mechanism of injury.[1] Inspection of the athlete's posture, station, and gait should be made before more detailed shoulder evaluation in order to assess overall symmetry and freedom of coordinated arm swing. The sternoclavicular, acromioclavicular, scapulothoracic, costernal, costovertebral, and costotransverse joints should then be in turn inspected and palpated for deformity, discoloration, edema, crepitus, and tenderness. Each joint should be assessed through its full range of motion, first actively then passively. Because *active movements* consist of contractile as well as noncontractile components, they tend to be nonspecific in identifying particular anatomical pathology. *Passive movements* stress the noncontractile component and are, therefore, very useful in eliciting pathology in a variety of tissues: ligaments, joint capsule, fascia, nerves, vessels, or bone. Specifically, the following motions should be tested:

- sternoclavicular joint (rotation, superior and posterior glide)
- glenohumeral and acromioclavicular joints (traction, anterior and posterior glide)
- scapulothoracic joints (circumduction, rotation, protraction, retraction, elevation, and depression)
- costosternal and costovertebral joints (anterior and posterior glide)

Supplemental tests can then be chosen, based on the suspected pathology:

- Yergason test—bicipital tendinitis/strain
- apprehension test—glenohumeral subluxation/dislocation
- drop arm test—supraspinatus strain
- impingement syndrome test—biceps and supraspinatus tendons
- Gilcrest, Lippman, or Ludington tests—biceps tendon
- Booth and Marvel transverse humeral ligament test—transverse humeral ligament

A neurovascular examination should conclude the shoulder exam. Pulses (radial, ulnar, and brachial), deep tendon reflexes, motor strength, and sensation should be evaluated and recorded.

Contusions

The top of the shoulder is the most commonly contused area although the clavicle, the spinal portion of the scapula, and the deltoid muscle are also frequently contused. Contusions of the bony area, particularly that of the clavicle, can produce a subperiosteal hemorrhage. There is nothing unusual about contusions in the shoulder area, and standard therapy including ice, rest, immobilization, protection from further injury, and rapid progressive rehabilitation are in order.

Strains

Strains, unlike contusions, can often be a debilitating problem about the shoulder area and are classed from mild or minor (grade I) through severe, complete rupture of the musculotendinous unit (grade III). Strains of the deltoid can occur anywhere within the muscle belly, but most commonly at the site of its attachment to the shaft of the humerus. Scapular strains are also common and may be quite debilitating due to the number and variety of muscular insertions on the body: inferiorly the latissimus dorsi, superiorly the levatur scapulae and rhomboideus minor, medially rhomboideus major, and laterally the teres minor and triceps. Extension with external rotation of the humerus can cause injury to the rotators, such as the subscapularis, the latissimus dorsi, teres major, and pectoralis major. The infraspinatus supraspinatus and teres minor composing the rotator cuff can be damaged on forced internal rotation (swimmer's shoulder).[2] Finally, the biceps tendon passing through the intertubercular groove of the humerus can frequently be strained or subluxated for a variety of reasons and a wide range of sports (e.g., weight lifting, rowing, slot machine tendinitis). Subluxation (snapping shoulder) of the biceps tendon occurs following tearing of the fibrous bicipital groove covering in combination with a shallow congenital groove. The tendon can be strained at the glenoid attachment but more commonly tends to become irritated and inflamed particularly in the bicipital groove, producing a tenosynovitis. From a functional viewpoint either of these injuries is particularly debilitating since most shoulder/joint motion becomes quite painful and limited, particularly abduction in external rotation. Diagnosis is made by noting tenderness along the bicipital groove and accentuation of pain by active bicipital contraction against an extended elbow.

Very often chronic bicipital synovitis can produce calcification of the tendon and sheath. Rarely, adhesive tenosynovitis may result and the tendon altogether ceases to slide through the bicipital groove. Grade III strain on the bicipital tendon (acute rupture) rarely occurs and is usually due to a forceful contraction of the biceps or a forced extension while the biceps is contracted. The rupture, which may occur anywhere from the glenoid attachment to the muscle belly, is characterized by acute, sharp pain, followed by tenderness along the tendon's course, when the elbow is flexed to 90° and the arm abducted and externally rotated. The muscle belly moves away from the rupture when the patient contracts the biceps. All acute ruptures, except perhaps in the older age group, should be surgically repaired. A biceps strain or tenosynovitis must be distinguished from a subluxating tendon due to a congenitally shallow bicipital groove. Symptoms are often undistinguishable, though a snap or pop may be reported and the clinical exam elicits a painful snap as the tendon slips out of and into the groove on arm rotation. Treatment is surgical repair.

The treatment of a majority of shoulder strains and acute tenosynovitis is supportive and includes ice, rest, immobilization, protection from further injury, analgesics, and anti-inflammatories where indicated. Thereafter, rapid progressive rehabilitation within the limits of pain is important for early reintroduction to sports competition while at the same time protecting the athlete from reinjury. Most cases of chronic tenosynovitis can be treated with aggressive physiotherapy (diathermy, ultrasound, hot packs for stretching, and ice for cool-down), analgesics, anti-inflammatories, and (in certain select players) careful steroid injections. Rarely does tenosynovitis require surgery, although it is indicated in the adhesive case in which more conservative forms of treatment are not successful.

Sprains, Subluxations, and Dislocations

These constitute the spectrum of a single injury with increasing forces. *Class I or mild sprains,* representing less than 25 percent ligamentous rupture, are common throughout the shoulder joint. There is no major displacement between the two sides of the joint. Usually only minimal sensitivity can be palpated over the injured area. Rest, protection from further injury, ice, appropriate strapping, and progressive reconditioning over a 1- to 3-week period is usually necessary for full return to sports activity. *Second-degree (class II) sprains* or subluxation can be thought of as resulting from disruption of 25 to 75 percent of the ligamentous support of a particular joint. Swelling and tenderness is more marked over

the injured area and there may be some joint instability. Though the treatment is generally conservative, the period of healing is usually prolonged to 4 to 6 weeks. Finally, *class III sprains or ruptures,* which represent essentially tearing of the ligamentous structures of a joint and are associated with dislocation, are accompanied by severe pain and tenderness as well as abnormal joint function or position. Surgical intervention is often necessary in such injuries in order to achieve the best anatomical and functional result.

Sprains of the shoulder mechanism usually involve three sites: sternoclavicular, acromioclavicular, and glenohumeral joints.

General Treatment Guidelines

Because laboratory evidence of healing (histochemical, cytological, and strength criteria), correlates poorly with athletic performance, it is often wisest to err on the conservative side as long as progressive resistance rehabilitation is in progress. In the case of class III injuries, 4 to 6 months of rehabilitation are often required. However, the determination of reintroduction into play is often most difficult in class II injuries.

Very often the primary care physician is faced with a young athlete (e.g., a competitive gymnast) who has suffered a class II injury with resultant moderate joint laxity and who is eager to return to competition as early as possible. If the player is allowed to return to activity too early, conversion to a class III injury is a distinct possibility. On the other hand, prolongation of the rehabilitation and reconditioning progress can produce a variety of psychological frustrations and disappointments on the part of the young athlete. As competition is an all-or-nothing event, it is important that both the counseling physician and athlete come to an understanding regarding the distinctions between conditioning and full-scale competition. Usually the involved player has difficulty accepting anything less than competition when feeling generally healthy. It is wisest for the physician to perform serial clinical examinations with careful assessment of the injury in terms of anatomical and functional healing. The results of this examination, in conjunction with good knowledgeability of the healing process and rate, the demands of the particular sport, and associated factors such as adequate protective gear and the utilization of carefully prescribed physical therapy, should promote early return to the game and preserve the greatest amount of tissue anatomy and function.

Sternoclavicular Injuries. Direct forces, such as from a pile-on, can tear the sternoclavicular ligaments. Indirect forces, which thrust the shoulder girdle forward and backward, drive the clavicle posteriorly or anteriorly, respectively. Anterior sprains are much more common than posterior ones. Conservative treatment is recommended for grades I and II sprains of the joint and includes ice acutely followed by sling and swathe or figure-of-eight wrap for 3 to 4 days in grade I injuries and 4 to 6 weeks in grade II sprains. Extensive disruption of the ligament or malposition of the fibrocartilaginous disk (grade III) should prompt early surgical open reduction, though there is considerable controversy as to whether anterior dislocations require repair at all; reduction with the application of a figure-of-eight dressing is often sufficient.

On the field, initial concern should be given to the underlying vascular structures. The athlete may complain of dyspnea and there may be plethora of the ipsilateral extremity, face, and neck as well as diminution of pulses on the affected side. If there is compromise, an attempt should be made on the field to reduce the dislocation, always a posterior one, by simple traction being applied to the shoulder in a backward and outward direction with simultaneous outward pressure on the inner end of the clavicle, usually with a towel clamp. Major disruptions require at least 4 to 6 months for functional and anatomical repair. Although strapping and taping of this joint is particularly ineffective, a specially designed piece of protective gear should be considered.

Acromioclavicular Injuries. Sprains of the acromioclavicular (AC) joint are common in a variety of sports, particularly football and wrestling.[3] The mechanism of injury can be direct—as would occur from a sharp blow to the acromium or from a fall with the arm adducted to the side—or indirect, in which a force is transmitted to the acromioclavicular joint along an outstretched arm (polo or missed

judo fall). The extent of injury often parallels the tenderness produced on joint palpation as well as observed deformity.

Grade I sprains are characterized by tenderness of the AC joint and minimal edema. X rays, including stress films, are negative. Treatment is a simple sling and swathe for 1 to 3 weeks; strapping is not well tolerated by the athlete and usually produces maceration. The athlete should be counseled that occasionally AC arthritis may be a late complication requiring arthroplasty.

Grade II sprains or AC subluxation consist of disruption of the acromioclavicular ligament with the coracoclavicular ligament remaining intact. There are moderate amounts of pain and swelling. Routine films are normal, though bilateral stress films (5 to 10 pounds suspended from each arm) reveal subluxation with the pathognomonic finding being separation of the distal clavicle by not more than one-half its diameter from the acromion. There is no increase in the distance between the coracoid and clavicle. A sling and swathe for 2 to 3 weeks is the recommended treatment, although some physicians prefer to use a compressive dressing which pushes the clavicle down and the arm upward (e.g., Kenney Howard sling).

There is complete dislocation at the AC joint with upward displacement of the clavicle and disruption of both the acromioclavicular and coracoclavicular ligaments in third-degree injuries (Fig. 17-1). The treatment of an AC dislocation is somewhat controversial though some surgeons recommend surgical fixation of all third-degree sprains. Others prefer immobilization for 6 to 8 weeks. Overall, the literature tends to support AC immobilization for 6 weeks (Kenney Howard sling) as the results are the same as for surgical repair. Regardless of management choice, these injuries should be handled in conjunction with an orthopedic surgeon in order to obtain the best anatomical and functional result.

The impingement syndrome represents an entity causing a decrease in shoulder arc motion due to a narrowing of the coracoacromial interspace.[4] Sports requiring overhead movement of the upper extremity, such as tennis or swimming, can lead to inflammation of the rotator cuff or subacromial bursa.

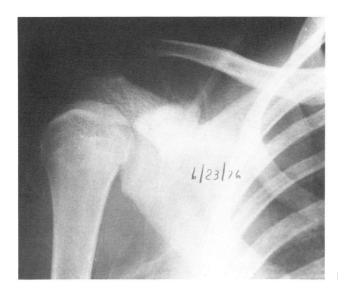

FIGURE 17-1. AC separation, grade III.

The resulting bursitis or tendinitis reduces shoulder motion. Chronic inflammation or trauma to the acromion can lead to osteophyte formation and so mechanically reduce full range of motion. Once the underlying condition is diagnosed treatment is tailored appropriately. Surgical excision of a bony spur may occasionally be necessary. Progressive resistance exercises are essential for good function and strength.

Glenohumeral Injuries. Ninety-eight or 99 percent of glenohumeral injuries are to the anterior portion, with the remainder being posterior.[5] The reasons for this distribution include the flattened anatomical lip of the glenoid labrum and the usual mechanism of injury—abduction and external rotation of the arm. Internal rotation in moderate forward flexion and adduction can result in the posterior dislocation of the joint. The two must be carefully distinguished clinically and radiologically as their treatments are distinctly different. The mechanism of injury is usually a trapped ski pole in combination with a moving skiier or a football player performing an arm tackle (Fig. 17-2). Glenohumeral injuries are classified in the same manner as all sprains. A grade I (mild) sprain is treated with a sling preferably placed under the shirt so that the

arm is supported at the side and external rotation and adduction are prevented. It is not necessary to immobilize the shoulder completely. Early range of motion and aggressive physical therapy within the limits of pain are indicated. Usually healing is complete in 2 to 4 weeks, although grade II sprains often require 4 to 6 weeks for the initial phase of healing to be complete. Early reintroduction to sports participation or overmanipulation during rehabilitation injures the healing ligamentous fibers possibly causing fibrotic scarring with eventual formation of the impingement syndrome (swimmer's shoulder).

Grade III sprains or dislocations represent the end point of continually applied force to the shoulder girdle. Minimum forces are actually required if there is inherent capsular laxity, attenuation of the glenoid labrum, or previous dislocations. If the player complains of a forward pop and a snapping back, a subluxation can probably be diagnosed. In the case of true dislocation, the athlete often complains of a severely painful, immobile arm which he or she holds away from the side and externally rotated. Clinical examination reveals that the acromion is very prominent and there is a palpable defect below it rather than the usual fullness of the deltoid mus-

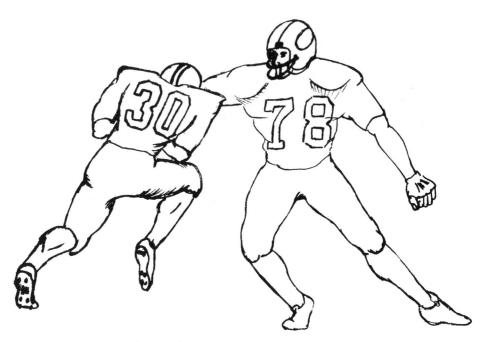

FIGURE 17-2. An example of an arm tackle, which commonly leads to shoulder dislocation or rotator cuff tear.

cle. The flattening can be detected by sliding the examining hand under the shoulder pads. The humeral head can be palpated as it lies firmly against the coracoid anteriorly.

In the well muscled or heavy individual the clinical diagnosis of dislocated shoulder by examination alone may be difficult. Any attempt to manipulate the arm or elbow, especially abduction, causes severe pain. The complete examination includes evaluation of the neurovascular status since the brachial plexus can be damaged, particularly during an anterior dislocation. Because dislocation of the shoulder joint is an acute emergency, reduction should be made as fast as possible before muscle spasm and severe pain develop. Very often such reduction may be done on the field or in transport before the hospital facility is reached. It is desirable that prereduction radiographs be made in order to assess whether there are other skeletal injuries present. However, reduction should be accomplished as soon as possible and in certain circumstances

(ringside or the playing field) before x rays can be made. Of course, a postreduction film must be made in order to ensure complete reduction as well as the absence of other skeletal tissue injury.

A thorough discussion of the numerous methods for shoulder relocation are beyond the scope of this book, although the practicing sports physician should be familiar with at least one of them. Examples include the simple elevation of the ipsilateral hand above the head, the Hippocratic method, the weight pendulant method, the Kocher maneuver, and the traction–countertraction method. Provided that they are instituted early and done properly, all of these methods work well without anesthesia. It is important to remember that serious damage to the brachial plexus can be produced by an improper Hippocratic technique in which the foot is placed directly on the thorax while the arm is levered over the foot (as opposed to the foot being placed against the axillary wall while traction is made at a 45° angle). Perhaps the most physiologic, least painful, and least time-consuming method for the physician is the pendulant technique, in which a weight is applied to the suspected wrist while the patient is either prone or seated.

A certain proportion of anterior dislocations are in actuality inferior dislocations due to the forcing of the arm into straight abduction. This particular form of dislocation tends to be resistant to any type of reduction method other than straight traction. A clinical examination cannot determine whether the head has gone primarily anteriorly or inferiorly and careful radiographs are indicated to determine the exact position. Rarely, the abduction force is so great that the humeral head locks under the glenoid with the shaft of the humerus pointing directly superiorly (luxatio erecta) so that the capsule is completely detached and the rotator cuff is torn. This is a very serious injury requiring immediate intervention as brachial plexus damage is common and, even after closed reduction is obtained, surgical intervention may be necessary to repair the rotator cuff and shoulder capsule.

The rarer posterior dislocation, typically in alcoholics, tends to be diagnosed late because initial presentation is unclear and the diagnosis is often missed. Acutely there may be increased prominence of the coracoid and decreased fullness of the humeral head anteriorly. There is usually no gross deformity of the shoulder evident because in a short period of time there is rapid swelling and disability, motion of the shoulder is sharply restricted, and radiologic examination difficult to interpret. Radiographic views should be taken bilaterally and overlapping of the humeral head and the glenoid noted—displacement is usually absent. Special views in the case of a possible posterior dislocation should be ordered, particularly on axillary view. Reduction by forward traction or pressure on the humeral head is usually sufficient though very often anesthesia must be given. Post reduction films are also critical as fracture of the posterior portion of the glenoid rim is a frequent complication of this dislocation.

Recurrent dislocations are most commonly anterior and may be due to repeated acute traumatic injuries or congenital glenohumeral joint deviation, which is usually bilateral and requires surgical intervention. The younger the athlete with a first dis-

location, the greater the chance of recurrent dislocation developing. The recurrence rate (75 to 80 percent) is particularly high, especially in individuals with lax ligaments and with reduced amounts of muscle mass. With each successive dislocation, less force need be applied and reduction is accomplished more easily. Eventually it is possible that simple abduction and external rotation by the player cause a dislocation with actual trauma.

In summary, the physician should be aware that there is considerable debate regarding proper management of dislocations following postreduction. It appears that the majority of physicians prescribe 3 to 4 weeks of shoulder immobilization for the young athlete (1 week for those over age 50) followed by progressive rehabilitation programs prior to returning to full competition. Surgical reconstruction is recommended for subsequent dislocation or where there is history of subluxations or shoulder joint instability so that the individual is not capable of participating in the chosen sport. Some physicians feel that considerably less time (2 to 3 weeks) is all that is necessary, whereas others feel that prolonged periods (6 to 8 weeks) are important in order to reduce the incidence of redislocation. In the highly competitive athlete it may be of merit to consider early interventive surgical correction—perhaps even after the first dislocation.

Fractures

Fracture of the clavicle is a common athletic injury particularly in the preadolescent or adolescent competitor, although clavicular injuries tend also to involve ligamentous support structures. Clavicular fractures are common and initial x rays confirmatory (Fig. 17-3). These fractures should not be disregarded as unimportant as they may progress into significant angulation, perhaps with complete displacement. The standard AP view should be ordered as well as a vertical view. In the case of a diagnosed clavicular fracture, or if there is doubt, a standard figure-of-eight splint or similar clavicular yoke (Fig. 17-4) for a period of 4 to 5 weeks is all that is usually necessary. Repeat x rays in 10 to 14 days can determine that a fracture occurred by demonstrating initial callus formation. A visible or palpable callus in the young athlete eventually under-

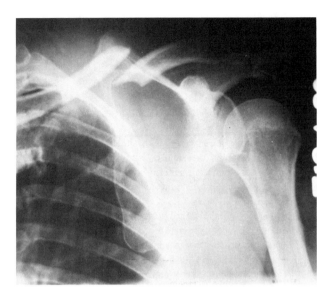

FIGURE 17-3. Severe displacement with mid shaft clavicular fracture.

goes resolution during the remodeling process; however, the callus remains in the adult athlete. Fractures in the outer portion of the clavicle should be treated as an AC separation.

Bursitis

Bursitis is commonly a source of agonizing distress to an active athletic population. Although there are at least ten bursae associated with the shoulder girdle, subacromial (subdeltoid bursitis) is the most frequent. The condition may be caused by direct trauma over the shoulder at the acromion process, though this is uncommon. Usually, bursitis is secondary to rotator cuff injury; therefore careful search for a primary lesion should be made with every case of subacromial bursitis. Symptoms include shoulder motion pain (particularly on abduction), point tenderness inferior to the acromial process, and pain on rotation of the shoulder (particularly internal rotation). Usually rest, protection from further injury, local heat, diathermy, or ultrasound, analgesic and anti-inflammatory agents produce complete recovery. With repeated trauma or inappropriate treatment during acute episodes, chronic adhesive subacromial bursitis can result. Calcification may be noted in the supraspinatus region on x ray. Very

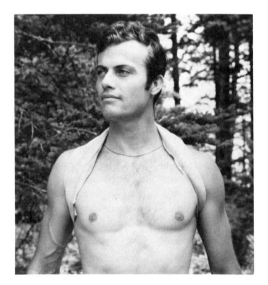

FIGURE 17-4. Makeshift clavicular figure-of-eight from an elastic bandage.

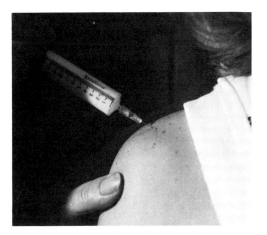

FIGURE 17-5. Proper injection site for subacromial bursitis.

often there is crepitation and occasional snapping of the shoulder on extremes of motion, particularly abduction. In such cases a careful, accurate corticosteroid injection is indicated (Fig. 17-5). Rarely is surgical excision of the bursae necessary. Less common locations for shoulder bursitis include the bursae surrounding the subscapularus tendon, which produces pain and tenderness in the area of the coracoid process that is aggravated by external and internal rotation of the arm. There are numerous bursae associated with the scapula, where symptoms tend to be diffused and usually involve motion of the scapula against the chest wall. Diagnosis can be confirmed in this case by the production of pain and crepitation when the patient is asked to tense his or her crossed arms anteriorly.

Miscellaneous Conditions

Miscellaneous shoulder girdle injuries include the scapula fracture, a rare injury in athletics due to the large amounts of muscle encasing the scapula. Such a fracture usually occurs only on a violent direct blow. Symptoms are usually those of a severe contusion; the clinical finding is typically swelling of the entire scapula so that its outline is visible. It should be noted that scapular fractures are often associated with underlying pulmonary contusion.

Treatment is usually conservative, employing the use of a sling or a swathe for 7 to 14 days, and rapid progressive rehabilitation thereafter. A direct blow over the deltoid may not only produce contusion of that muscle and possible hematoma, but also a contusion of the axillary nerve. Such damage is associated with severe parethesia and weakness of that shoulder. Recovery is rapid, usually within a few hours, and complete. Occasionally there is an associated, delayed paralysis of the deltoid. Thus, initial and serial neurologic examinations of that area should be performed and, if there are questions, early consultation with a competent surgeon should be made.

UPPER ARM

Contusions

Upper-arm injuries include contusions of the large muscle groups of the biceps and triceps. Ice, compression, rest, and protection from further injury are the keynotes. Repeated contusive blows to the subcutaneous area of the distal deltoid attachment produce chronic fibrositis and periostitis, a condition termed *exostosis* or "blocker's node" due to use of a rising arm bar to check the impetus of the charging opponent. Early on, local measures including injection therapy and protection from further injury are useful. With further blows, the irritative exostosis extends anterolaterally and inferiorly with a rather sharp leading edge. Surgical excision of the exostosis is usually recommended.

Blows to the arm can also contuse the radial nerve as it courses in a spiral fashion superomedially to inferolaterally. Symptoms and signs include variable amount of paresthesias in the lateral posterior portion of the hand and motor weakness (wrist drop). Conservative management including a volar splint is the best course initially with surgical intervention being reserved for worsening symptoms/signs over several months.

Strains

Strains of the arm muscles are common especially in those sports requiring violent forces—pitching, weight lifting, rugby, and football. Very often strains accompany contusions and it may be difficult to distinguish the two. The biceps muscle is most often strained due to location and the fact that it is often contracted at the time of trauma. Rupture can be ruled out by careful palpation and inspection of the muscle during contraction and relaxation. Strains are treated in the usual fashion with surgery being reserved for complete rupture.

ELBOW

While the elbow primarily functions as a hinge point via the articulation of the coronoid and olecranon process of the ulna with the humeral trochlea, it is capable of secondary rotation through the radial head and capitellum. Both joints are very stable. The annular (orbicular) ligament fastens the radial head to the ulna and, in conjunction with the lateral collateral ligament, reinforces radiohumeral articulation. The interosseus membrane also unites the radius and ulna, whereas the medial collateral joins the distal humerus to the olecranon.

Contusions and Related Conditions

The subcutaneous nature of the elbow joint makes it prone to easy contusion. A forceful blow can cause simple contusion, laceration, abrasion, periosteal hematoma (especially on the lateral side), triceps tenosynovitis, olecranon bursitis (student's or dart thrower's elbow), or ulnar neuritis. A direct blow to the ulnar nerve as it passes through its shallow medial groove produces severe, often incapacitating tingling and shock sensations along the ulnar distribution (fourth and fifth fingers); these transient paresthesias led the point of impact to be termed the "funny bone." Repeated blows can lead to chronic fibrosis with resultant ulnar palsy and intrinsic wastage (ulnar compression syndrome). Treatment of these conditions is, on the whole, conservative in nature. Ice, rest, protection, compression, elevation, and analgesic/anti-inflammatory drugs go a long way. Installation with a corticosteroid/analgesic preparation following aspiration may be required for cases of bursitis. Rarely, the bursitis may become suppurative due to its sub-

cutaneous location. Obviously, antibiotics with surgical drainage are necessary in such cases.

Strains

Elbow strains are common as the joint is critical to many sports, especially baseball. Strains are more frequent over the medial aspect of the joint involving the flexor–pronator musculotendinous unit. Less frequently, the lateral extensor–supinator muscle group is involved. As these strains often involve their respective epicondyle, it is useful to discuss the problem at this juncture.

Tennis Elbow. *Tennis elbow* is a general term that does not signify either the type of injury or its location.[6] It includes radiohumeral bursitis, radio-ulnar bursitis, and strain of the extensor–supinator aponeurosis, either at its attachment to the lateral epicondyle (true epicondylitis) or directly over the radial head. The history of each is usually similar (i.e., any forceful, new activity requiring lateral wrist movement in conjunction with vigorous gripping). The poorly conditioned weekend athlete is at risk for the development of "tennis elbow." Originally described in tennis, it has been seen in players of other racquet sports, carpenters (hammer use), electricians (screwdrivers), ice fishermen (hooker's elbow), or from the simple shaking of hands.

Examination usually differentiates the various forms of "tennis elbow." All conditions produce pain on gripping, but bursitis pain can be localized at its respective anatomical sites; in epicondylitis, however, there is point tenderness over the lateral epicondyle which may extend along the supracondylar ridge. Medial epicondylitis (golfer's/Little League elbow) is similar in history and clinical presentation except that the medial flexor–pronator muscle group is involved. Treatment for epicondylitis requires rest, analgesics, anti-inflammatory agents, and, in severe cases, a volar splint which produces slight wrist dorsiflexion and flexes the elbow to 90°.[7,8] Supplementary physiotherapy (diathermy, hot packs) in conjunction with a steroid/anesthetic instillation are most useful (Fig. 17-6). Finally, as prevention is the keynote, the athlete should be reeducated concerning throwing or volley style. Very often a slight change in technique or a

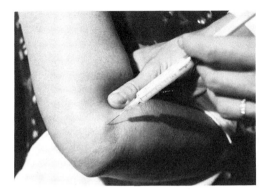

FIGURE 17-6. Lateral epicondyle injection site.

modification of the hand grip or racket tension is all that is required. In addition, progressive resistance exercises should be initiated once inflammation has subsided and range of motion is pain free.

Sprains, Subluxations, Dislocations

The inherent stability of the elbow joint makes it fairly resistant to sprains and dislocations; however, severe hyperextension forces in either abduction or adduction can rupture the collateral ligaments and anterior capsule and push the olecranon posteriorly (Fig. 17-7). Such dislocations are emergencies due

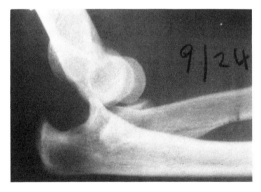

FIGURE 17-7. Posterior dislocation following fall on outstretched arm in football game.

to the possibility of irreversible circulatory damage. All pulses should be palpated and neural function (especially that of the median nerve) assessed. Because such an injury is initially numb and soon becomes markedly painful and edematous, reduction should be attempted on the field or en route to the treatment facility. Very gentle traction should be applied along the long axis of the forearm at the wrist in extension and the extremity slowly moved into flexion. The neurovascular status should be monitored and, if the reduction is unsuccessful, the athlete should be taken to the operating room. Post-reduction films and plaster splints are mandatory. In all actuality, most radial head dislocations probably occur with olecranon subluxation/dislocation–relocation or ulna fracture (Monteggia's fracture). Careful x rays of the radial head should be taken and reviewed in conjunction with an orthopedist.

Fractures

Fractures of the elbow are uncommon. They may occur in association with dislocations or secondary to strong traumatic forces such as pitching (pitcher's elbow). Fractures of the epicondyles are best handled with surgical fixation although this is not always necessary. Remember to obtain comparative views with the "normal" side in order to distinguish avulsion fracture from normal epiphysis. Osteochondral fractures, particularly of the capitellum, are overlooked—for the most part being dismissed, after falls on outstretched arms, as epicondylitis or contusion. Repeated or severe contusive blows to the joint can lead to osteochondritis dessicans (Panner disease). There is often transient aching pain especially in forced extension; x rays reveal lucent defects over time.

Supracondylar fractures are true emergencies particularly in children as there may be irreversible vascular damage with forearm ischemia as a complication. Brachial artery spasm causes rapid hand swelling, pallor, numbness, and coolness. Pulses are absent. On-field management includes splinting and transport to the emergency facility as soon as possible. A vascular and orthopedic surgeon should be consulted at the earliest opportunity.

FOREARM

Contusions/Hematoma

The large subcutaneous area of bone in the forearm makes it very vulnerable to contusions. Very often subperiosteal hematoma or traumatic tenosynovitis can result. Standard therapy is warranted, with aspiration and injection of an anesthetic indicated for hematoma. Rest with elimination of painful motion and protection from further injury are essential for the earliest return to play. Repeated injury fosters the formation of myositis ossificans, a discussion of which is reserved for a section dealing with thigh injuries (see Chapter 18).

Fractures

Occasionally, a forearm blow is severe enough to fracture one or both of the forearm bones. The typical mechanism is a fall on an outstretched arm, as in a missed wrestling or judo throw. Careful radiological evaluation must be made and it is wisest to consult an orthopedist: even nondisplaced forearm fractures can become markedly angulated due to rotational forces along the axis of the forearm.

True Colles fracture does not occur in the younger population since there is radial epiphyseal separation or more proximal radial fracture which occasionally is misdiagnosed as a wrist sprain. Careful examination reveals point tenderness and x rays often demonstrate the fracture site. Epiphyseal separations should be managed in conjunction with a specialist. Falls on the outstretched hand can also cause greenstick or torus fractures of the radius. Careful radiologic evaluation with a good clinical exam secures the diagnosis. Usually a long arm cast for 2 to 3 weeks followed by a short arm cast for another 2 to 3 weeks produces good results. Greenstick fractures angulated more than 15° should be referred to an orthopedic surgeon for fracture completion and reduction.

Other less common forearm injuries are avulsion fracture of the radial styloid, reverse Colles (Smith's fracture), and Barton's fracture (distal radius fracture with carpus subluxation). These fractures and their management should be familiar to all sports physicians. Their accurate reduction is ideally achieved by local anesthesia though, occa-sionally, regional block must be performed with casting in the functional position.

Strains

Any of the musculotendinous units of the forearm can be strained so that there may be painful flexion, extension, pronation, or supination. Treatment is conservative in most instances unless a complete rupture is present. Complicating tenosynovitis suggested by "snow-pack crepitation" must be vigorously managed in order to prevent a chronic adhesive inflammatory response. Immobilization, protection from further trauma, and local instillation of a long-acting corticosteroid/anesthestic combination is indicated.

WRIST

The functional integrity of the hand is predicated on the normal anatomy and physiology of the wrist, which includes the distal radius and ulna and proximal metacarpals as well as the intervening eight carpal bones. The volar carpal ligament and radial and ulnar collateral ligaments bind these bones into a functional unit, with the volar carpal ligament forming the carpal tunnel.

Contusions

Contusions of the wrist proper are due most frequently to direct blows, as from a helmet or cleat. Although fractures are the usual worry, it is more common to damage the delicate adventitial structures such as tendons, nerves, and vessels. X rays in the AP and lateral direction should be supplemented with oblique views. Range of motion should be carefully assessed as chronic tenosynovitis is a potential outcome. The usual treatment is in order and should include a volar splint, which should be extended above the elbow if there is pain on pronation or supination.

Strains

Muscular strains of the wrist are not common, as there are no muscles within the anatomical wrist. A direct tendon blow or repeated overuse is the most common cause of wrist strain (e.g., Space

Invader's or Pac Man wrist).[9,10] The usual injury involves one or more of the numerous tendons. Immobilization in the position in which there is relaxation of the involved tendon is central to treatment. Thus extensor injuries should be splinted in extension and flexor trauma in flexion. Rehabilitation should begin only after there is no discomfort, and then kept strictly within the limits of pain. Complications such as chronic adhesive tenosynovitis require instillation therapy and a vigorous physiotherapy program, while being sure to prevent reinjury.

Similar chronic compressive forces to the wrist can produce an ulnar neuropathy termed "cyclist's palsy" or "handle bar neuropathy."[11] The history usually involves cycling over several days and the athlete complains of hand weakness and paresthesias of the fourth and fifth fingers. Rest and change of hand grip are curative.

Tenosynovitis

Constrictive tenosynovitis of the long abductor and short extensor of the thumb secondary to overuse of the thumb and wrist (de Quervain's disease) causes increasing pain and swelling with a palpable click acutely. Eventually, all movement ceases due to

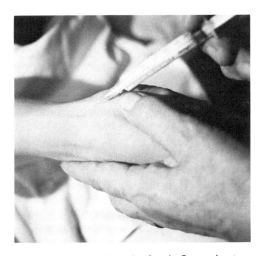

FIGURE 17-8. Injection site for de Quervains tenosynovitis.

fibrotic thickening of the retinacular roof over the radial styloid. Diagnosis is made by grasping the flexed thumb and deviating the wrist to the ulnar side; severe pain in the area of constriction results. Local aggressive treatment is initially indicated (corticosteroid injection and rest) (Fig. 17-8), but refractory or severe cases should be handled by an orthopedic surgeon.

Carpal Tunnel Syndrome

The carpal tunnel syndrome is more frequent in the athletic population than one would think. In this syndrome, the impenetrable and rigid transverse carpal ligament does not allow expansion from internal swelling, due to a direct blow, fall on an outstretched hand, tenosynovitis of the flexor tendons, fracture of a carpal or distal forearm bone, or even an intrinsic mass (ganglion or exostosis). Initially, there are tingling paresthesias of the index and long fingers with deep pressure pain over the transverse carpal ligament. Thenar atrophy is a late finding. Bilateral x rays are very valuable, especially of the carpal tunnel. Early on, rest and immobilization in a volar splint goes a long way. Chronic cases can be treated additionally with instillation of a long-acting anesthetic/steroid preparation, administered medial to the palmaris longus tendon so that the median nerve is avoided. Surgery is often required for the refractory case or one in which muscular atrophy is present.

Ganglion

A brief mention should be made of ganglia, which are most common on the wrist dorsum (Fig. 17-9). Whether the pathology is one of synovial degeneration or herniation, it is relatively unimportant to the athlete complaining of a painful mass on the back of the wrist that causes excruciating pain in forceful throwing or gripping. There may be a history of trauma, although chronic overuse and strain are significant contributing factors. It is important to distinguish the mass from other tumors and effusions. A ganglion may be soft or hard, usually mobile when the involved tendon is moved, and may be erythematous and warm if inflamed. Treatment is fraught with problems. Multiple sterile injections of a corticosteroid following local anes-

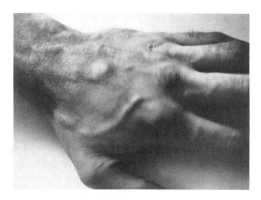

FIGURE 17-9. An example of a ganglion over the dorsum of the hand.

thesia and aspiration can be useful. Surgery should be reserved for painful or refractory ganglia. Both modalities of treatment are associated with recurrences.

Sprains, Subluxations, Dislocations

The sprain–subluxation–dislocation complex of the wrist is probably responsible for more undue physician anxiety than similar injury elsewhere in the body.[12] Much of the worry is due to unfamiliarity with the anatomy as well as diagnosis of these sports injuries. There are several useful rules that the primary care physician should follow. The diagnosis of wrist sprain should be viewed with suspicion; more often than not, such injuries are actually tendinous strains or carpal fractures, as the ligaments are very strong and tend to cause carpal subluxation before actually tearing. Thus, all negative x-ray wrist studies should be treated with splint immobilization and careful follow-up, including serial clinical and radiological evaluations. A linear fracture, particularly of the navicular, may be picked up 2 to 3 weeks after the initial trauma.

The most common wrist dislocation involves the lunate bone and results from forced dorsiflexion and compression, as in a fall on an outstretched hand. The dorsal carpal ligament is usually torn even in a subluxation. Dorsal tenderness and edema just distal to the radius, in combination with a painful, limited range of motion, should prompt careful

x-ray study including bilateral views. A palpable mass under the flexor tendons and median nerve dysfunction secondary to carpal tunnel compression clinches the diagnosis. If diagnosed early, closed manipulation is usually successful. Unfortunately, this injury is overlooked all too frequently so that delayed open reduction becomes necessary with its attended complications of avascular necrosis and poor function.

Perilunate dislocation is rarely pure, more often than not involving dislocation or fracture of the navicular, intercarpal dislocation, or any combination thereof. Early accurate reduction of this serious fracture–dislocation is mandatory as functional outcome progressively declines with the passage of time. Even near perfect, immediate reductions are associated with arthritic changes. Since slowly healing wrist sprains can be masquerading perilunate dislocations, no wrist injury should be treated for a long period without reevaluation.

Fractures

The most common carpal fracture involves the navicular or scaphoid bone. Predisposing factors include its narrow waist, its bridging function between the carpal bones, and the fact that radial deviation and dorsiflexion forces compress it. Hyperextension forces similar to those causing a lunate dislocation or Colles fracture and present in a variety of sports (particularly roller skating[13]) can fracture the navicular. Complaints may include wrist pain at the base of the thumb and anatomical snuffbox tenderness. X rays are usually negative. The diagnosis of sprain is acceptable only if the wrist is immobilized adequately for 2 to 3 weeks, followed by reevaluation. X rays may then reveal faint callus formation or a fracture line. A negative exam in the face of a positive clinical picture should prompt another 2-week period of immobilization followed again by an exam and x rays. Recently, radionuclide scans have been useful in detecting occult navicular fractures.

Undisplaced fractures should be immobilized in a thumb spica cast—mid arm to the interphalangeal (IP) joint of the thumb with the wrist in 25° of extension and forearm in midposition. Often, it is weeks to months until healing is complete. Displaced fractures should be seen in conjunction with a specialist as nonunion is common.

The triquetrum, pisiform or hamate (tennis wrist), can also be dislocated or fractured by hyperextension forces. The athlete may complain of wrist weakness or wrist clicking, though hamate fractures produce pain at the top of the hand due to associated neuritis and tendinitis. Bilateral radiologic exams are usually diagnostic. Treatment is usually conservative though specialty consultation is wise. Posterior driving blows against the neutral thumb can fracture the greater multangular. Functional disability and pain is often worse than navicular fractures. Open reduction is recommended.

Miscellaneous Conditions

Those athletes who complain of chronic discomfort following repetitive stresses to the wrist, as would occur in baseball, tennis, golf, or hockey, should be investigated for the possibility of focal avascular necrosis, particularly of the carpal lunate (Kienboch's syndrome).

HAND

Contusions

Because the hand is so critical to the majority of human activity it should not be surprising that a high number and variety of injuries occur during sports competition.[12] Contusions, abrasions, and lacerations are extremely common and, with the exception of the following caveats, are treated in the usual fashion. Injuries to the dorsum of the hand should prompt careful evaluation since the extensor tendons lie subcutaneously and are easily injured. Palmar trauma can be particularly distressing due to the tight arrangements of the palmar muscles which effectively produce a closed space; any swelling, particularly that due to a hematoma, can therefore be very painful and debilitating. Contusion of the proximal hypothenar and thenar eminences, as would occur by falling on an outstretched hand, can damage the intrinsic muscles of the thumb and fifth finger. "Cuber's thumb" results from repeated compressive forces against the volar aspect of the thumb base while working Rubik's cube. Ice, immobilization, rest, and progressive rehabilitation within the confines of pain are indicated. Large or recurring hematoma, particularly of the dorsum of the hand, should suggest a defect in the clotting mechanism.

Lacerations. Laceration, puncture wounds, and bites of the hand should be carefully inspected and debrided. Careful attention must be paid to transection of local tendons and nerves which are often not visible on superficial examination. Puncture wounds, and in particular bites as would occur in the accidental striking of a human tooth, require careful wound care including debridement, antibiotics, and tetanus prophylaxis.

Infections. It is not uncommon for a simple abrasion or minor laceration or puncture wound to lead to a significant hand infection. A minor nail contusion can result in debilitating, paronychial infection or felon.[14] Such infections require careful and immediate incision and drainage. In particular, a felon must be drained adequately as a complicating osteomyelitis of the phalanx can result. Because the pus is contained in compartments deep within the fat pad of the fingertip, an adequate fishmouth or through-and-through incision of the terminal pulp involving all compartments must be made in order to provide drainage. Thereafter, the wound should be kept open either with a petrolatum gauze or iodoform wick and allowed to close after 48 to 72 hours. Antibiotics are not usually indicated. More serious infections include tendon sheath and palmar space abscesses. The primary care physician should be familiar with the diagnosis of such infections (Kanaval's signs) because they are often minor appearing but become rapidly extensive throughout the hand and up into the forearm. The physician may often mistake a small palmar abscess for a collar-button abscess—a small visible abscess superficial to the palmar fascia secondary to a large, deep abscess of one of the palmar spaces.

Fingertip Injuries. Fingertip injuries are usually made light of by both competitor and physician; however, a simple nail contusion followed by a subungual hematoma can lead to incapacitating throbbing pain that often is prohibitive to further competition. An immediate application of ice, elevation of the injured finger, and then drainage of the hematoma at the playing field allows continued play. Though there are a variety of means of draining a subungual hematoma including the application of a red-hot paper clip or battery operated electrocautery unit, the easiest and least painful method is the careful drilling of the affected nail with a No. 18 gauge needle. Very often it is the athlete who performs the procedure. Ethylchloride refrigerant can also be applied during the drilling though it is not very helpful. Thereafter it is wisest to provide a protective splint and to make sure that the drainage site remains open. Nail lacerations and avulsions should be treated conservatively and usually include removal of the torn nail. The athlete can then be allowed to return to play as long as the fingertip is protected.

Strains

The overstretching of a digit or its overuse against resistance can cause a strain of the long flexors and extensors or the extrinsic muscles of the hand. Repetitive excessive use is the etiology for intrinsic muscle strains. It is typical in those sports requiring constant gripping, such as rowing, golfing, tennis, or gymnastics, and is characterized by fatigue and cramping of the muscles and pain on resistive function. Strain of the long musculotendinous units usually is manifested as pain in the area of the injury (musculotendinous junction or at the attachment of the tendon to the bone). "Tennis thumb" is tenosynovitis of the flexor pollicis longus secondary to repeated overuse and friction. Stenosing tenosynovitis of the abductor pollicis longus and extensor pollicis brevis (de Quervain's disease) is characterized by pain over the radial aspect of the wrist and a positive Finkelstein's test. Painful blocking of flexion and extension of the middle and ring fingers at the proximal interphalangeal joint is referred to as "trigger finger." Trigger finger represents a chronic form of stenosing tenosynovitis due to repeated strains or blows to the flexor or extension tendon/sheath unit of the metacarpal–phalangeal joint. Treatment of these conditions can be conservative with periodic steroid injections (Fig. 17-10). Surgical excision of the fibrous thickening can also be successful. Strain of the short flexors is most often within the muscle belly itself. Third-degree strains

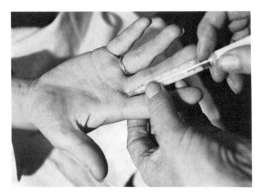

FIGURE 17-10. Injection site instillation of a corticosteroid for trigger finger.

or tendon rupture mandate surgical correction. The flexor tendon can be ruptured when there is forced extension during flexion (e.g., a football player grabs an opponent's jersey and cannot hold on). Rarely, the flexor digitorum profundus tendon can be avulsed as would occur with a forceful blow to the dorsum of the digit which is flexed. There is inability to flex the distal interphalangeal joint which represents detachment from the base to distal phalanx. Early surgical repair is indicated.

Sprains, Subluxations, and Dislocations

The sprain–subluxation–dislocation complex in the hand probably causes the most worry for the sport physician. Forced motion in any direction beyond the strength of the ligamentous support of the carpal–metacarpal joint causes a sprain.

Thumb. The carpal–metacarpal thumb joint, in order to allow the motion of opposition, is extremely mobile and hence predisposed to easy sprain. Overvigorous Aikido grasping, improper bowling technique, or an inadvertent wall collision in racquetball or squash can cause grade II sprains or even frank dislocation with rupture of the joint capsule (Fig. 17-11). Six to 8 weeks or more may be necessary for healing of the grade II or III injury, and, if the joint is initially unstable, serious consideration for internal fixation should be made. It

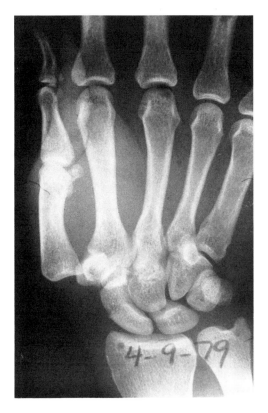

FIGURE 17-11. Dislocation of the carpal–metacarpal joint of the thumb following a collision with the wall during a squash tournament.

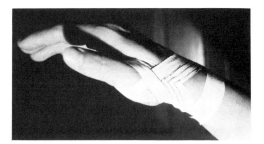

FIGURE 17-12. Interlocking basket weave from $\frac{1}{2}$-inch, adhesive tape.

is wisest that the athlete wear some form of supportive strapping (e.g., basket weave) for the remainder of the season (Fig. 17-12).

The metacarpal–phalangeal (MP) joint of the thumb is very vulnerable to sprain because forced abduction and rotation of the thumb due to hyperextension forces fix the metacarpal, and the force then becomes directed against the joint capsule itself or the ulnar collateral ligament (gamekeeper's or skier's thumb). Inadequate treatment of the acute injury is usually responsible for chronic instability.

Such instability often is the case in catchers who suffer repetitive hyperextension forces when catching high-speed pitches. As discussed previ-

ously, the treatment of such mild sprains is conservative with the degree of immobilization, duration of protection, and application of rehabilitation proportional to the healing response. Continued protection for the remainder of the season is imperative.

Because there is usually only moderate local discomfort and rarely any major deformity, the diagnosis of a major sprain is often not made. With appropriate nerve block and stress films, more than 15° to 20° of angulation between the noninjured and injured metacarpal–phalangeal joint suggests a major sprain. Surgical repair is indicated since subsequent functional disability in the form of compromised pinch strength and early degenerative arthritis results (Fig. 17-13). The sprain can be associated with an avulsion fracture of the proximal phalanx of the thumb. The radial collateral ligament is sprained and there is an avulsion fracture of the radial portion of the proximal phalanx as in mechanical bull riding—"bull rider's thumb."[15]

Fingers. Hyperextension forces on the metacarpal areas of the finger rays can produce sprains and even open dislocation (Figs. 17-14 and 17-15). In such instances there is tearing of the volar plate and perhaps of the transverse metacarpal ligament. This is a serious finger injury and requires careful and early repair by a qualified specialist. Often the athlete or a friend attempts to reduce this dislocation and the proximal phalanx is dorsally displaced but parallel to the metacarpal. Unless the primary care physician is versed in the reduction of this dislo-

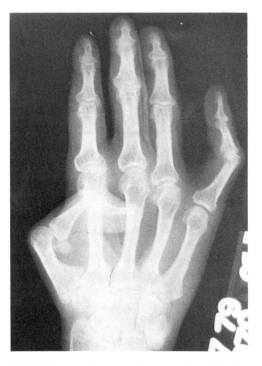

FIGURE 17-13. Degenerative arthritis following ulnar collateral strain of the MP joint of the thumb in bowling.

cation, which is difficult due to entrapment of the volar plate and collateral ligaments, it is best to refer as soon as possible. Continued inappropriate manipulation only aggravates the edema, producing pain as well as further damage.

General rules regarding the reduction of dislocations are the following. First, an initial range of motion and neurovascular status check should be made. If swelling is not severe, then progressive traction should be applied along the long axis of the dislocated bone. Once traction has been instituted, pressure should then be applied to the proximal base of the dislocated unit in the direction opposite to the dislocating force. A click will be heard or palpated upon relocation. Usually a prereduction film cannot be attained at the time of acute injury but a postreduction film is mandatory as there is a high incidence of avulsion or splinter fractures. If a reduced dislocation spontaneously subluxes or dislocates, the injury is more complex and consultation is warranted. Presuming that the diagnosis is simple dislocation without fracture, the usual course is 2 to 3 weeks in a supportive splint followed by rapid progressive rehabilitation, with the understanding that it takes at least 6 weeks for good ligamentous healing to be achieved. Finally, it is important to bear in mind that dislocations can be

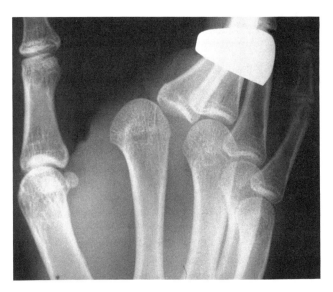

FIGURE 17-14. Dislocation of the index MP joint following a "jam" injury during a rugby meet.

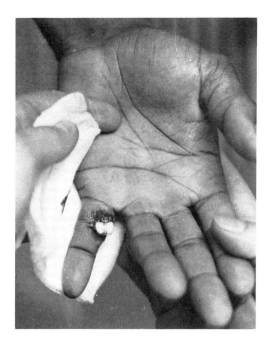

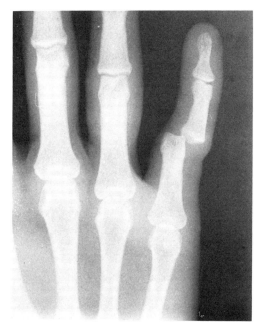

FIGURE 17-15. Open dislocation of the fifth inter-phalangeal joint. *(Courtesy of William Towey.)*

FIGURE 17-16. Missed judo grasp causing dislo-cation of the interphalangeal joint.

associated with major ligamentous and tendon in-jury; full functional recovery thus not only depends on reduction and fracture healing but also on treat-ment of the associated conditions.

Injury to the interphalangeal joints usually leads to sprains of the anterior capsule, though continued force produces a dislocation (Fig. 17-16). Sublux-ations and dislocations are serious injuries and should be high on the suspicion list when the athlete pre-sents with a history of interphalangeal trauma as it is usually reduced by the time the visit is made. Nonreduced injuries usually indicate that the pha-langeal head is caught either in the flexor tendon or joint capsule. As mentioned relocation should be performed at the time of injury since with delay edema and pain require procaine block for adequate manipulation. Occasionally the dislocation is open and, after thorough surgical scrubbing and reduc-tion, the tissue including the capsule should be pri-marily closed. Immobilization is best achieved in the position of function or the "blade of the hoe"

position (Figs. 17-17 and 17-18) with a suitable aluminum splint, though first aid treatment is per-formed by taping to an adjacent ray. Once again it is important to get a postreduction film and carefully assess for accompanying fracture. Concomitant fracture fragments can usually be molded into the

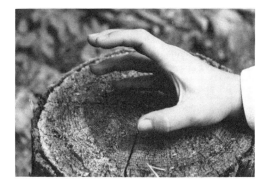

FIGURE 17-17. Position of hand function.

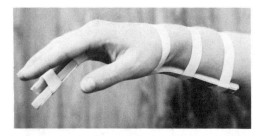

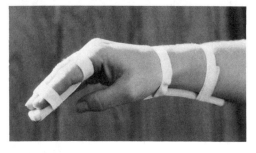

FIGURE 17-18. "Blade of the hoe" position.

proper position; however, significant displacement and inability to reduce a small splinter fragment should prompt surgical consideration. Furthermore, it is always important to check range of motion after reduction including lateral deviation, which occasionally requires the use of stress films to assess collateral integrity. There is a large number of athletes who never see a doctor following digital dislocation or who visit one several days or weeks after the injury, at which time there may be fusiform swelling of the joint with instability and stiffness. Early reconstruction of the collateral interphalangeal ligaments appears to be the treatment of choice but once the injury is delayed and chronic, good functional and anatomic results significantly decline.

Fractures

Thumb Fractures. Because fracture of each of the individual bones of the hands presents its own problems, there are no hard and fast rules other than the single goal of satisfactory hand function. A careful therapeutic balance must be struck between perfect anatomic reduction with joint stiffness

and possible adhesive tendonitis versus good intrinsic and extrinsic muscle function with bony malposition. Fractures can occur from direct trauma or indirectly in association with ligament or tendon injuries. A good example is the Bennett fracture, which is a fracture–dislocation of the carpal–metacarpal joint of the thumb. The typical mechanism of injury is an inexperienced boxer closing his fist around the thumb which is tucked into the palm. Direct force down the intercarpal shaft also drives the metacarpal base dorsally and proximally so that there is tearing of the dorsal ligaments and capsule as well as bone fracture. There is foreshortening of the thumb with increased base width. Traction and abduction reduce the deformity but, upon relaxation, the deformity promptly recurs. Regardless of the method of treatment, nearly perfect reduction is critical. External elastic traction through an outrigger with pull directed along the metacarpal shaft for several weeks produces good union. A cast can then be applied with the thumb held in abduction. Alternatively, Kirschner wire fixation can be performed.

Metacarpal Fractures. Fractures of the metacarpals of the finger rays are usually due to transmitted forces of a direct blow because the bones are in close approximation particularly at the bases. Displacement may not be evident and, in fact, no fracture line may be visible on the initial x ray. There may be extreme tenderness at the site of the break from direct pressure or tapping at the end of the bone. For obvious undisplaced fractures, careful splinting with the wrist in slight dorsiflexion is usually sufficient (Fig. 17-19). The splint should include the fingers of the involved metacarpals. Cases of slight angulation can often be reduced providing that traction is placed on the involved finger and direct pressure is applied over the metacarpals adjacent to the fracture site so as not to entrap the extension tendons while plaster is being applied. Unstable and markedly angulated fractures are best treated in consultation because open fixation is often necessary.

The boxer's or karate practitioner's fracture of the neck of the fifth metacarpal is very common due to poor punching technique (Fig. 17-20). Typically there is marked flexion deformity and on ex-

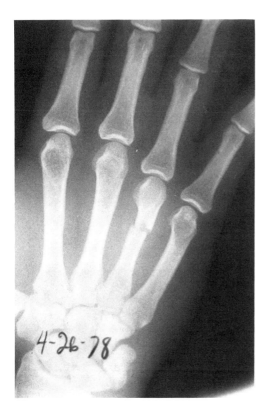

FIGURE 17-19. Minimally displaced fourth metacarpal fracture following a "pile-up."

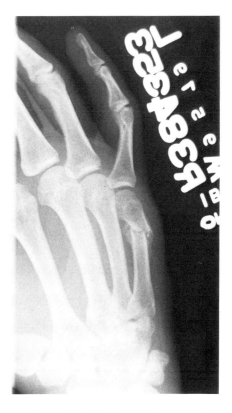

FIGURE 17-20. Missed boxer's fracture demonstrating callus formation.

amination the defect is readily palpable. A complicating impaction usually occurs and reduction with disimpaction must be performed before a cast is applied. If a good reduction is achieved, simple splinting with maintenance of the fingers in the position of function while preventing rotation is all that is necessary; otherwise, definitive surgical correction may be required.

Phalangeal Fractures. The most common fracture of the hand involves the common phalanx. Very often an improper boxing technique or indiscreet karate blow can fracture the base of the proximal phalanx and even be associated with dislocation. Because the head does not lock out of position, the dislocation spontaneously reduces. Very often the athlete presents with an exquisitely tender, swollen metacarpal–phalangeal joint without obvious deformity. If the fragment is anterior, the finger should be placed in flexion; if it is posterior, the joint should be splinted in slight extension in order to achieve good apposition. If there is any question as to whether the fragment is correctly positioned, consultation should be made and perhaps consideration given to open reduction. If the fracture involves the lateral margins, the physician should think of compounding capsular or ligamentous injuries. Less severe blows over the metacarpal–phalangeal joint can cause "boxer's knuckle" or traumatic bursitis.

The midshaft is the portion of the proximal phalanx which is most commonly fractured, and it is usually transverse or oblique with the distal fragment angulated dorsally. Simple splint fixation with the digit in moderate flexion is indicated for stable fractures. Dorsally angulated fragments should be held in position by a well-padded dorsal splint for about 3 weeks and then gradually mobilized. Any fracture which is comminuted, oblique, or spiral typically requires traction via an outrigger mechanism; this is best handled in consultation with an orthopedic surgeon. It is unusual that open reduction of such a fracture requires surgery. Fractures of the distal end of the proximal phalanx are due to forceful flexion and are readily treatable by immobilization in slight extension for 10 to 14 days.

Longer periods of splinting result in undue stiffness and longer periods of rehabilitation. More complex fractures, such as a T fracture of the distal end of the proximal phalanx and fractures causing marked comminution and rotation should be handled by consultation. It is mandatory after reduction of any metacarpal fracture to check for normal rotatory alignment. In the normal state each finger ray when individually flexed points toward the base of the thumb. In addition, lines drawn down the axis of each of the middle phalanges converge at the navicular tubercle. Thus, traction and reduction should be along this line. Improper alignment results in finger overlap. Fractures of the middle phalanx are handled in the same manner as those of the proximal phalanx. For simple nondisplaced fractures, immobilization should be for 3 to 4 weeks since longer splinting causes joint stiffness and adhesive tendinitis. Because of the various tendon insertions on the middle phalanx, angulation and rotation is often a problem. A fracture between the flexor sublimis and the extensor tendon causes the distal fragment to glide forward whereas the proximal fragment tends to be pulled backward. A rigid splint with the finger in mild extension (relative to the position of function) is usually sufficient in order to maintain alignment without direct pressure over the fracture site. If the fracture is distal to the sublimis attachment, there is forward angulation of the proximal fragment; the treatment is then the same as that for a proximal phalangeal fracture (i.e., flexion of the finger in all joints). Unstable spiral or comminuted fractures require traction and possible fixation.

Combination Injuries

There are certain combined bone and ligamentous injuries that should be familiar to the primary care physician. Avulsion of the central extensor tendon slip at the proximal interphalangeal joint produces the classic Boutonniere's deformity. The diagnosis is often missed initially as the finger appears normal and range of motion can be achieved through other supporting ligaments. Later on, flexion-contracture of the joint occurs with inability to extend the proximal interphalangeal joint actively. A large paper clip or clothespin splint applied to the dorsum for 4 to 5 weeks produces an excellent functional result. Delay in diagnosis is synonymous with reconstructive surgery. Forcible flexion on an actively ex-

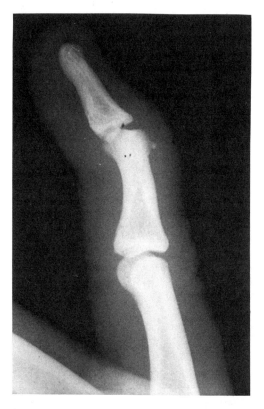

FIGURE 17-21. Mallet finger with splinter fracture pulled proximally due to rupture of extensor tendon.

tended finger causes an avulsion fracture of the distal phalanx in association with rupture of the extensor tendon (Fig. 17-21). The so-called "baseball" or "mallet" finger can be treated definitely by a posterior paper clip splint or similar device in which the finger is held in extension for 6 to 8 weeks. The results are generally good, although O'Donoghue reports that open reduction and internal fixation produce better results, as complications (arthritis, recurrent dislocation, and joint instability) are reduced.[16] Avulsion of the flexor tendon on the distal phalanx (jersey finger) must be surgically repaired. Distal phalangeal fractures are almost always due to crush injuries and usually involve the tuft of the digit—that is, the distal portion of the distal phalanx. Treatment consists of immobilization with a metal splint or its equivalent, protection against further trauma, and appropriate care of the concomitant soft tissue injury. Fractures which involve the articular surface in the nature of a T or Y fracture require consultation.

Miscellaneous Injuries

A less common but distinctly possible sports injury in any activity requiring repetitive contact with a hard object, such as baseball, hockey, bowling (bowler's thumb), and kendo, is pressure on a specific digital nerve leading to neuroma formation. Preferential treatment is prolonged rest although selective cases may respond favorably to appropriate steroid instillation. Surgery may rarely be necessary. Osteoarthritis can complicate the picture chronically.

REFERENCES

1. Davies GJ, Gould JA, Larson RL: Functional examination of the shoulder girdle. Phys Sports Med 9(6):82–104, 1981.
2. Bateman JE: Cuff tears in athletes. Orthop Clin N Am 4:721–745, 1973.
3. Behling F: Treatment of acromioclavicular separations. Orthop Clin N Am 4:747–757, 1973.
4. Hawkins RJ, Kennedy JC: Impingement syndrome in athletes. Am J Sports Med 8:151–158, 1980.
5. Neer CS, Welsh RP: The shoulder in sports. Orthop Clin N Am 8:583–591, 1977.
6. Nirschl RP: Tennis elbow. Orthop Clin N Am 4:787–800, 1973.
7. Froimson AI: Treatment of tennis elbow with forearm band. J Bone Joint Surg 53A:183–184, 1971.
8. Nirschl RP, Sobel J: Conservative treatment of tennis elbow. Phys Sports Med 9(6):43–54, 1981.
9. McCowan TC: Space-Invaders wrist. N Engl J Med 304(22):1365, 1981.
10. Neiman R, Ushiroda S: Slot machine tendinitis. N Engl J Med 304(22):1368, 1981.
11. Burke ER: Ulnar neuropathy in bicyclists. Phys Sports Med 9(4): 52–56, 1981.
12. Posner MA: Injuries to the hand and wrist in athletes. Orthop Clin N Am 8:593–618, 1977.
13. Perlik PC, Kalvoda DD, Wellman AS, et al: Roller skating injuries. Phys Sports Med 10(4):76–80, 1982.
14. Walker FW, Lillemore KD, Farguarson RR: Disco felon. N Engl J Med 301(3):166–167, 1979.
15. McConnell RY, Rush GA: Mechanical bull syndrome. South Med J 75(6):681–686, 1982.
16. O'Donoghue DH: Treatment of Injuries to Athletes. Philadelphia, WB Saunders, 1976, pp 377–379.

18
Common Injuries of the Lower Extremity

Richard B. Birrer

This chapter deals with sports injuries related to the pelvis, thigh, leg, foot, and the intervening joints. Because the lower extremity is responsible for weight bearing and ambulation, it is injured with some frequency and its dysfunction often produces marked disability in the majority of sports. Before launching into a discussion of the many varieties of lower extremity injury, it is useful at this juncture to review general stretching and rehabilitative exercises for that area.[1]

REHABILITATION

Ballet stretches with alternating legs being raised to shoulder height and then the trunk flexed forward on the leg, holding the position for 20 seconds, stretch the hamstrings (Fig. 18-1). By leaning against the wall with hands and forearms and straightening the back and lower extremity in a continuous line, the calf muscles and Achilles tendon on each side are stretched for a count of 15 to 20 seconds (Fig. 18-2). With the legs spread as far as possible, the hamstrings can be stretched by slowly bending forward from the hips to the ipsilateral foot in the sitting position for a count of 20 seconds. The feet can then be brought together and the entire trunk pressed downward toward the knees as far as possible also stretching the hamstrings (Fig. 18-3). A hurdler's or dancer's stretch is best for the leg adductors and should be done in a slow, progressive

fashion (Figs. 18-4 and 18-5). Finally, the hip adductors and joint ligaments can be stretched by placing the foot soles together and pulling them as close as possible to the groin. Thereafter, the knees are slowly pressed toward the floor while the yoga position is assumed. Added stretch of the lower back is achieved by pulling the chest and trunk to the feet. All of these exercises should be done pre- and postathletics in a very slow progressive and dynamic fashion. Bouncing should be discouraged as it can produce spasms and strains.

There is a wide variety of protocols and methods for strengthening the muscles in and about the knee. Whether one chooses the West Point protocol or that used at a local rehabilitation center, the exercises should involve all direction of motion and be tailored to the prospective activity of the athlete. There should be some methodology available for progress measurement. The physician should be able to prescribe his or her own set of exercises incorporating the use of a weight boot, Velcro snap weights, prefabricated home weights or even by using makeshift weights of sand bags, stones, bricks, lead shot, or coins placed in a small travel bag, handbag, or even nylon hose or knee socks. Whether one chooses to prescribe isometric, isotonic, or isokinetic exercises, the keynote is that they be progressive resistance exercises (PRE). The goal is equal strength in both extremities as the weaker limb is usually injured. A single maximum effort (SME) should be determined for each muscle group. This

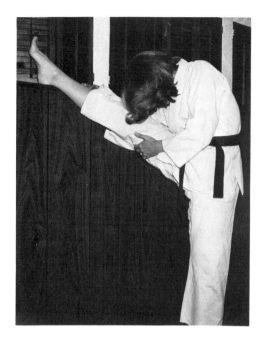

FIGURE 18-1. Ballet type of stretch for the hamstring muscle.

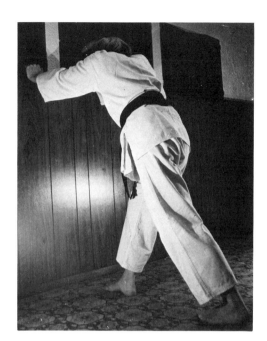

FIGURE 18-2. Achilles tendon stretch.

can be done with a dynamometer in the case of isometrics and taken as the single largest weight being lifted in isotonic exercises, or the highest reading from the pressure gage of an isokinetic device. The unaffected side of the body is then used as a comparator for the rehabilitation of the injured limb. Seventy percent of the SME is used as the amount of weight or effort to be regularly incorporated in the PRE program. Six to eight repetitions holding at the extremes for five to ten counts should ideally be done twice a day. Weight should be incrementally increased when ten repetitions can be easily performed. Examples of commonly prescribed exercises include knee extensions (quadri-

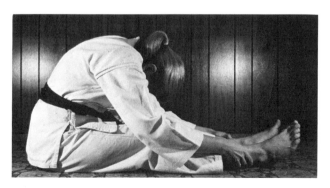

FIGURE 18-3. Hamstring stretch.

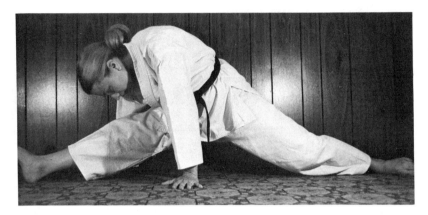

FIGURE 18-4. Hurdler's stretch.

ceps), hip flexion and side leg lifts (hip abductors), cross-overs (adductors), and straight leg raises (quadriceps and hip flexors).

PELVIS

The pelvis has as its primary function the mechanical transfer of weight through its various bones, joints, ligaments, and muscles; its secondary role is to cradle and protect the abdominal viscera.

Contusions

The location and construction of the pelvis predisposes it to a variety of characteristic injuries. The subcutaneous nature of iliac crests and spines and the pubic bone predispose them to contusive forces. In particular, a blow in the region of the anterior iliac crest can produce extremely painful nodular swelling referred to as a "hip pointer." Running and ambulation are extremely distressing. Although typically a periostitis, it is possible to strain or avulse the muscles attaching along the crest and produce

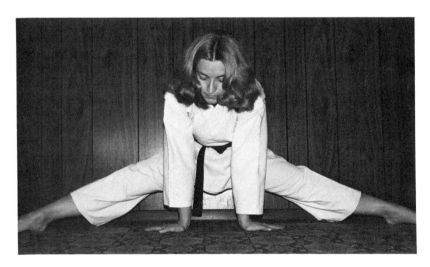

FIGURE 18-5. Dancer's stretch.

similar symptoms. The treatment of contusions and strains is discussed in detail in Chapter 12.

Injuries in the region of the sacrum are typically contusions secondary to direct blows due to the subcutaneous nature of its posterior surface and are rarely sprains due to the very strong sacroiliac ligament. In fact, one should be wary of the diagnosis of sacroiliac "sprain" since typical forces applied usually result in lumbosacral ligamentous tears. Contusions of the sacrum and coccyx, while uncommon due to the requirement for sacral pads in contact sports, often produce pain in excess of true disability. While it is important to rule out the possibility of the subluxation of one of the sacroiliac joints or fracture, simple supportive therapy is usually all that is necessary.

The most common injury to the buttock is from a direct blow and can cause sciatic nerve contusion, ischial bursitis with calcification and spur formation, and hematomata of the muscles or periosteum. In cases of sciatic nerve contusion (e.g., cycling), the athlete complains of nonradicular pain and paresthesias along the entire distribution of the nerve.[2] Straight-leg raising (Laseque's or Gaenslen's maneuver) replicates the pain in the area of the contusion. Usually, conservative therapy in association with a good rehabilitation program provides complete functional recovery. Bruising of the ascending ramus of the ischium or the descending pubic ramus frequently occurs in the form of a straddle injury, as would occur in cycling or gymnastics (balance beam). Subperiosteal hematomas can be quite painful and debilitating though they rarely lead to such a complication as osteomyelitis. The physician should remember that a localized collection of blood can at a later time lead to infection and calcification; with repeated trauma, myositis ossificans may be made. Finally, all major buttock and perineal blows should remind one of possible injury to the genitourinary system.

Strains and Avulsion Fractures[*]

Because tremendous forces are often exerted at the site of pelvic attachments, it is not uncommon to encounter strains and avulsion fractures. Examples of such injuries include avulsion of the iliac crest aponeurosis; avulsion fracture of the anterior superior iliac spine secondary to tensor fasciae lata

and sartorius strains in association with unusual muscle violence (as in running or jumping, particularly from a height); and avulsion of the ischial tuberosity (hurdler's injury) secondary to forced flexion of the hip with the knee extended requiring contraction of the biceps, femoris, and semitendinosus muscles as in the case of high kicks (football, martial arts) or the leading outstretched leg of a hurdler. In each instance, the athlete usually complains of localized pain and variable forms of disability when walking or running. The clinical exam often detects localized tenderness and pain on direct palpation and aggravation of these findings when passive motion is performed in the direction of the original injury. Rest, protection from reinjury, and simple immobilization are often curative for the majority of these injuries providing that there is good approximation. However, separations that are complete or wide should merit consideration for surgical repair. With the exception of simple contusion, it is most uncommon to injure the posterior iliac spine since the ligamentous attachments in this region are not conducive to acute avulsive forces.

Forced abduction, which occurs in such sports as gymnastics, horseback riding, dancing, and the martial arts, can produce a straddle injury—a strain with possible rupture of the adductor longus muscle. The athlete limps and resists forceful passive abduction of the thigh or active adduction against resistance when examined. The usual site of the tear is at the site of its attachment to the ramus and, presuming that the injury is only mild to moderate, conservative therapy with a rehabilitative program is indicated. Complete avulsion, if diagnosed early, should be treated with surgical repair. In the young female, forced abduction in straddling can also cause a pubic symphyseal strain. Differential diagnosis includes contusion as the treatments are distinctly different. Usually a lumbosacral corset or circumferential pelvic adhesive strapping, in combination with rest, analgesics, and anti-inflammatories, produces a good result.

Strains of the gluteus medius muscle are caused by overactivity of the muscle (e.g., mechanical bull syndrome) and are mostly chronic in nature.[3] A good functional test for this strain consists in asking the patient to elevate the involved leg against resistance while lying on his or her thigh, thus putting stress on the abductors. Grade III strains are associated with avulsion fractures of the trochanteric epiphysis, particularly in the adolescent. These are best repaired surgically if there is displacement or if the fracture is complete; otherwise, immobilization of the thigh in abduction and slight external rotation for at least 6 weeks with rehabilitation thereafter is suitable. The differential diagnosis should include trochanteric bursitis.

Injuries in the vicinity of the groin or inguinal region are common (e.g., mechanical bull syndrome) due to the complex arrangement of tendons, ligaments, and muscles; most are minor in nature and extent.[3] Perhaps the most common is strain of the iliopsoas tendon which can occur in the musculotendinous junction or at its attachment to the lesser femoral trochanter. The usual mechanism of injury is a flexed thigh being forced into extension. The player is noted to be in severe pain and holds his or her thigh in adduction flexion and external rotation. There is direct tenderness on clinical palpation and internal rotation, and active contraction of the muscle produces severe pain. It is important especially in the adolescent to perform radiologic evaluation in order to rule out avulsion fracture. Conservative therapy with bed rest, immobilization with the thigh flexed and externally rotated, ice, analgesia, and anti-inflammatory agents produces good healing in several weeks. Rarely is surgical repair necessary though it is important to bear in mind that, regardless of the degree of strain, iliopsoas injury can be very disabling as the muscle is critical for running and jumping. Thus complete recovery is absolutely imperative before unrestricted activity can be permitted. Strapping is usually not effective as it does not prevent overactivity.

Other injuries that can occur in the inguinal area include strain of the abdominal muscles which attach along Poupart's ligament, a conjoined tendon strain and injuries to the other underlying neurovascular bundle, in particular, traumatic phlebitis and phlebothrombosis secondary to a direct blow.

Other Fractures

Although it is possible to fracture the larger bones of the pelvis, such as the ilium and ischial and pubic rami, these injuries are uncommon due to the large

forces required. They have been occasionally seen in such sports as parachuting, football, rugby, and judo. With the exception of underlying pathologic conditions or very severe direct blows, it is most uncommon to fracture or dislocate the hip in athletics. The athlete is immediately and completely disabled and no attempt should be made to reduce such a major injury on the field. Because the incidence of aseptic necrosis of the femoral head varies directly with the duration of dislocation, it is important that this injury be reduced at the earliest possible moment under anesthesia.

THIGH

Trochanteric Bursitis
The superficial position of the greater trochanter predisposes it to easy injury from direct blows. Very often such injury is manifested by the development of an acute bursitis, although infection or friction are other etiologies. Flexion, extension, or rotation of the hip and thigh causes the tensor fasciae femoris to irritate the bursa. In addition to local tenderness detected by direct palpation, pain can be elicited by adduction of the thigh with the knee extended, followed by internal or external rotation. The differential diagnosis should include gluteus medius strain. With repeated injury or recurrent inflammation an audible and palpable snap occurs secondary to chronic bursitis. Chapter 17 details treatment of bursitis (section on shoulder bursitis).

Contusions
Strains and contusions are the most common injuries of the thigh, with contact sports being the leading etiology in the latter. The anterior anterolateral region of the thigh most commonly receives a direct blow which is invariably mild to moderate in extent and does not produce significant disability (charley horse). With more severe blows there is hematoma formation, and repeated blows or repeated irritation following a single blow can cause myositis ossificans. Regardless of the force of the blow, the athlete is usually able to complete the contest before the onset of aching soreness or pain on motion significant enough to prompt complaint. Contusions in

this region are handled in the usual fashion. Unfortunately many such contusions are slighted by the coaching staff, other athletes, and even physicians. The standard philosophy of "working it out," as well as early locker room treatments such as massage and kneading, can lead to enlargement of underlying hematomas and set the necessary conditions for the development of myositis ossificans. The extremity should be stretched in order to allow some compression around the hematoma.

It is most important that an injury, even a mild or minor one, be given the appropriate time to heal and that rehabilitation progress within the confines of pain; muscle activity beyond the injury limit results in chronic irritation and the reparative response of calcification and ossification. Minor forms of ossification are probably very frequent following muscle contusions of the thigh. However, with repeated irritation in the form of overenthusiastic massage or early reintroduction to play, massive amounts of bone formation may result. Misdiagnosis, early surgical biopsy, or attempts at removal can lead to the diagnosis of tumor as well as invite recurrence of the lesion. The common differential diagnostic error is confusion with osteogenic sarcoma. It is wisest to allow the lesion to mature before any decision is made regarding surgical removal or biopsy, which should be done by a specialist.

Strains
Strains of the thigh are common in the running activities of track and field events. The rectus femoris on the anterior portion of the thigh and the hamstring muscles can be torn. Conservative therapy in combination with an aggressive rehabilitation program within the limits of pain produces good functional and anatomic healing. More serious grade II or III strains with complete muscle rupture particularly of the hamstrings can follow very vigorous sprinting or stretching. It is important to examine these injuries as early as possible before edema occurs because it can be difficult to differentiate contusion, hematoma, and rupture several hours after the initial injury. A direct blow, as from a helmet over the rectus femoris while it is in fixed contraction, can produce a rupture. Conservative management often suffices in the case of a hamstring tear

due to its multiple components, although early surgical repair is indicated for larger ruptures for the best functional results. Appropriate conditioning including pre-exercise warm-up and cool-down are essential ingredients in the prevention of such strains. This fact is especially true when one considers the 10:6 strength ratio between the quadriceps and hamstring synergy and the fact that the hamstrings, being antigravity muscles, are in a constant state of functional tension. Thus, it becomes necessary to stretch these muscles on a daily basis.

Occasionally the strong circumferential vaginal fascia of the thigh is torn in an athletic injury particularly along its anterolateral aspect where it is in close relationship to the iliotibial band. A fascial hernia may then present itself as a palpable tumor-like mass when the muscle is relaxed and disappearing when the muscle is contracted. Large tears are mostly asymptomatic whereas smaller tears tend to produce some amount of pain by actual ischemic pinching and compression of connective and adipose tissue. Treatment, therefore, is usually conservative.

Fractures
A final brief mention should be made of femoral shaft fractures which, though rare, are very serious. Their emergency management has been outlined in Chapter 12 and more definitive management should be carried out in consultation with an orthopedist.

KNEE

Anatomy
In discussing sports injuries of the knee it is wisest to remember that the knee is the most vulnerable joint in the body from a sports medicine viewpoint. Furthermore trauma to the knee constitutes the most frequent seriously disabling injury in sports. The knee is functionally a hinge joint but physiologically a gliding joint—in particular, the patellofemoral joint. Knee joint stability is primarily the result of a series of strong check ligaments *(static stabilizers)* that, together with muscles *(dynamic stabilizers),* tendons, meniscal cartilage, and bones, provide the unique functioning of this joint.

The static stabilizers consist of the medial, lateral, and posterior compartments. The *medial* compartment (collateral) is further subdivided into the tibial collateral ligament, which has a primary superficial portion (superficial medial collateral) inserting on the tibial and femoral condyles, and a less important deep component (medial capsular ligament), which inserts on the medial meniscus and the condyles. The tibial collateral ligament is the primary medial stabilizer against external rotatory and valgus stress, and it is the most commonly injured knee ligament. Normally it limits rotation, abduction, and the forward glide of the tibia on the femur, but it is taut only in extension.

The *lateral* compartment is extracapsular, does not attach to the lateral meniscus, and extends from the lateral femoral condyle to the fibular head. There is no primary lateral stabilization; rather, the lateral collateral, popliteus tendon, and posterior cruciate share in the functional integrity of the lateral compartment. In general the lateral compartment is injured infrequently but when trauma occurs, combined injuries are the rule. Varus forces tend to be resisted by the lateral collateral, popliteus, and posterior cruciate. The cruciate functions as the primary check at 90° of knee flexion whereas the lateral collateral is primary in midrange flexion. In some instances the popliteus tendon and lateral collateral may provide stability during internal and external rotatory forces.

The *posterior* compartment, consisting of the posterior capsule, becomes taut only in extension and is paramount in preventing valgus stress, external rotatory instability, and hyperextension.

The cruciates are extracapsular static stabilizers and extend from the femoral intercondylar fossa to the tibial eminence. The ligaments (anterior and posterior) are named according to their insertion site on the tibia. The prime check on hyperextension, anterior tibial displacement, and internal and external rotation in extension is the anterior cruciate, which also prevents valgus stress in flexion and extension, valgus stress in extension, and external (secondary) rotation in flexion. It is also important to knee extension (screwing home mechanism).[5] The cruciate primarily prevents posterior tibial displacement and internal tibial rotation in flexion and,

secondarily, hyperextension varus stress in extension and valgus stress in flexion and extension.

The dynamic stabilizers consist of the semimembranosus, pes anserinus, quadriceps tendon, the iliotibial tract, biceps femoris, and the popliteus muscle. Stability via the semimembranosus is achieved through the popliteal ligament, which attaches to the posterior capsule and tightens it when stressed; its attachment to the medial tibial condyle, which serves to flex and internally rotate the knee; and its insertion on the posterior horn of the medial meniscus, which causes the meniscus to be pulled posteriorly during flexion. Excessive knee rotation and valgus motion is inhibited by the pes anserinus formed from the confluence of the graciles, sartorius, and semitendinosus tendons. The quadriceps tendon, formed by the conjoined tendons of the vastus lateralis, medialus, and intermedius, is the primary dynamic stabilizer of the knee. Lateral knee joint stability is aided by the iliotibial tract or band which passes distally from the tensor fasciae lata as the vaginal fascia of the thigh to the distal femur through the intermuscular septum, thence crossing the knee to the upper tibial plateau to the tubercle of Gerdy. The popliteus tendon provides secondary and tertiary support in resisting internal tibial rotation in flexion and extension. Finally the biceps femoris assists knee flexion and rotation through its lateral stabilization with its fibular head insertion.

The weight-bearing cartilage of the knee consist of the medial C-shaped and the lateral O-shaped menisci. The medial meniscus is less mobile than the lateral due to its attachment to the medial compartment. With flexion, the menisci move posteriorly secondary to their attachment to the semimembranosus and popliteus tendons; with extension, they move anteriorly.

Examination

Nowhere can the case be made more strongly than in the knee joint for a careful and accurate review of the mechanism of injury (Tables 18-1 to 18-4).[4,5] In the acute situation, if the trauma was not directly observed, then an accurate account from either the player, coach, trainer, or other team members must be obtained. It is important to determine when the injury occurred and whether the player was im-

TABLE 18-1. VALGUS STRAIN[a]

Flexion with external rotation	Extension
↓	↓
Medial collateral ligament injury	Medial collateral ligament injury
↓	↓
Anterior cruciate injury	Anterior cruciate and medial portion posterior capsule injury
↓	↓
Medial meniscus and/or posterior cruciate injury	Deep medial capsular ligament injury
	↓
	Posterior cruciate injury

[a]When a valgus stress is applied to the knee in flexion and extension, a different sequence of events is initiated. Serious flexion injuries are often referred to as the *unhappy triad*. *(Reprinted from Simon RR, Koenigsknecht SJ: Orthopedics in Emergency Medicine. New York, Appleton-Century-Crofts, 1982, p 380, with permission.)*

TABLE 18-2. VARUS STRAIN[a]

Extension with internal rotation	Extension or flexion	Flexion with internal rotation
↓	↓	↓
Anterior cruciate and/or lateral collateral and/or popliteus tendon injury	Lateral collateral injury	Lateral collateral injury
	↓	↓
	Iliotibial band and/or biceps femoris injury	Lateral posterior capsule and/or lateral meniscus injury
↓	↓	
Posterior cruciate and lateral posterior capsule injury		Posterior cruciate injury

[a]When a varus stress is applied to the knee in flexion or extension with or without internal rotation, a different sequence of events is initiated. *(Reprinted from Simon RR, Koenigsknecht SJ: Orthopedics in Emergency Medicine. New York, Appleton-Century-Crofts, 1982, p 380, with permission.)*

mediately disabled, was able to leave the playing area unassisted, or continued to play. Was there a sensation of snapping or popping present? What were the degree, location, and quality of pain and swelling? What course was followed since the original injury? If a chronic injury is present, a careful assessment of the knee "giving way" must be made in addition to a detailed history of all previous traumata. Remember that hip, lumbosacral, and cord pathology can also cause knee joint pain via obturator nerve referral.

Acute Injuries. If at all possible, it is best to carry out the clinical exam as soon as possible following the injury, particularly during the "golden period"—the first 20 minutes after an injury. The

athlete should be carried from the field (rather than bear weight on the injured joint) and placed in an area where a thorough comfortable exam can be carried out. It is always wisest to examine the opposite normal knee first; this provides useful comparison and reduces the player's apprehension. Before proceeding with any manipulative tests, much information can be gleaned from careful inspection and observation made as the extremity lies still and then throughout the full range of knee motion. Valgus and varus deformity should be noted as well as patellar alignment.

It is wisest to ask the patient to move the knee through its full range of motion if possible, noting any abnormalities, in particular the last 15° to 20°

TABLE 18-3. HYPEREXTENSION STRAIN[a]

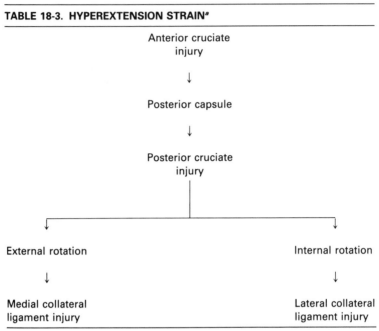

Anterior cruciate
injury

↓

Posterior capsule

↓

Posterior cruciate
injury

External rotation   Internal rotation

↓   ↓

Medial collateral   Lateral collateral
ligament injury   ligament injury

[a]When a hyperextension strain is applied to the knee the sequence of structures injured is as above. *(Reprinted from Simon RR, Koenigsknecht SJ: Orthopedics in Emergency Medicine. New York, Appleton-Century-Crofts, 1982, p 381, with permission.)*

of extension, which are in locking rotation (screwing home phenomenon). Erythema and edema should be recorded in location and extent. Swelling after acute trauma most often represents a serious injury (hemarthrosis is common with an anterior cruciate tear). Gentle palpation should then be applied in order to assess degree of swelling and presence of fluid, and to search for painful trigger points. Very often, simple palpation of the medial joint line as the knee is internally rotated and extended can identify medial meniscus injury. Joint line tenderness also occurs in lateral meniscus damage though the cartilage itself is not palpable. Do not overlook the popliteal fossa in terms of masses and pulsations. The neurovascular status of the knee as well as distal leg (dorsales pedis and posterior tibialis) pulses should be noted and recorded.

No attempt at manipulation should be made until careful palpation and inspection have been performed. Furthermore, passive range of motion should be performed only after the patient has been asked to move the extremity actively. It is a good idea during the active range of motion test to apply the hands during that period of time and feel for crepitation, snaps, clicks, pops, or shifting fluid. A history or clinical finding of a pop or snap is highly suggestive of an anterior cruciate tear. True mechanical locking caused by a torn meniscus or cruciate ligament or a loose body must be distinguished from false or pseudolocking secondary to muscle spasm and effusion and inflammation characteristic of grade I and II ligament sprains.

Chronic Injuries. In addition to the historical and clinical factors pertaining to acute injuries the sensation of "giving way" must be thoroughly evaluated in chronic knee injuries. The athlete may com-

TABLE 18-4. ROTATIONAL STRAIN[a]

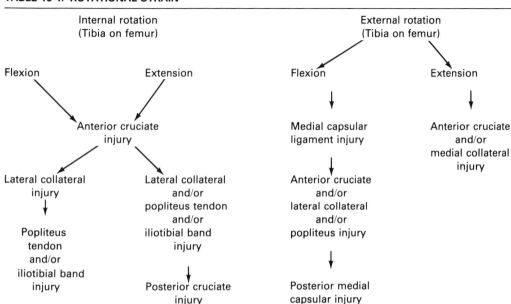

[a]When a rotational stress is applied to the knee the above sequence of events may occur. *(Reprinted from Simon RR, Koenigsknecht SJ: Orthopedics in Emergency Medicine. New York, Appleton-Century-Crofts, 1982, p 381, with permission.)*

plain of a knee that "collapses," often unpredictably and painlessly. The differential diagnosis should include quadriceps dysplasia, anterior cruciate sprains, patellar pathology, or true mechanical locking.

The patella is often involved in chronic knee pain, which is frequently anterior and diffuse though it can radiate medially and to the popliteal area. With patellar pathology, prolonged sitting with the knee flexed aggravates the pain (movie sign); "giving way" is usually preceded by pain. If an effusion is present, patellar ballottement is useful in assessing its quality and quantity. The patella should be checked for tenderness, crepitation, and instability on medial and lateral glissement. The latter can be graded according to the amount of displacement (grade I, normal, to grade IV, subluxation/dislocation).

Measurements. Several important anthropomorphic measurements particularly in the chronic situation should be made. Circumferential measurements should be taken at the joint line, the level of the tibial tubercle 8 to 10 centimeters above the tibial plateau, at the belly of the gastrocnemius muscle, measured at a reproducible distance from the tibial tubercle, and the suprapatellar region 2 centimeters above the superior border of the patella with a comparable reproducible recording in centimeters of this site above the tibial tubercle. While performing these tests it is wise to assess the tone, volume, shape, mass, and strength of such important muscles as the quadriceps, especially the vastus medialis, and gastrocnemius. For instance, weakness of the vastus medialis often constitutes a major factor in the lateral subluxation of the patella and later knee pathology. Quadriceps weakness can lead to anterior knee instability as well as difficulty in fully extending the leg. Goniometric measurements (degrees of flexion and extension) are useful for baseline reference information.

Stress Tests. The successful performance of stress tests is highly dependent on a relaxed cooperative patient ("golden period" in the acute situation). Once swelling and pain has occurred, an adequate examination may not be possible, although a systemic analgesic in conjunction with knee aspiration and the injection of 5 to 10 cc of 1 percent lidocaine may facilitate the assessment. Otherwise examination under anesthesia usually is indicated. The quality of the endpoint as well as the nature and degree of pain associated with the stress test are key interpretive elements to an accurate diagnosis. Moderate to severe pain usually accompanies sprains. A "mushy" endpoint is characteristic of a complete ligament tear whereas a firm endpoint is more typical of a mild to moderate sprain. For simplicity the test can be conceptualized in two planes: anterior–posterior (drawer tests) and medial–lateral (valgus and varus stress).

Rapid assessment of knee stability is done in 0° and 30° of flexion with valgus and varus stress. Valgus and varus stresses alternatively applied are positive in cases of medial and lateral sprains, respectively. With the knee in 90° of flexion the drawer test, which assesses cruciate integrity, can be performed with the foot immobilized in the neutral position. The upper posterior leg is grasped with the fingers; the thumbs are placed along the edges of the inferior patellar tendon with the hamstrings and gastrocnemius muscles relaxed. Gentle traction is applied in an anterior and posterior direction. Increased amounts of motion in either direction by comparison with the uninjured side indicates possible anterior or posterior cruciate sprains, respectively. The posterior cruciate can also be assessed during valgus stress particularly in full extension. The knee should be flexed to 30° so that the collaterals can be tested; in full extension the posterior capsule prevents medial and lateral instability. The physician should also be familiar with one or more of the more complex knee joint examination maneuvers that assess rotatory instability and multiple structures. Though such tests are helpful in con-

firming a diagnostic impression, they are not essential; the "simple" tests are the bulwark of diagnosis.

Flexion–rotation tests are useful in determining instability on rotation and also the possibility of concomitant meniscal tear. In the *McMurray test* the examiner forces the foot into alternating external and internal rotation while the knee is flexed. The other hand is placed over the medial and lateral patellar groove and the underlying collateral and meniscus cartilage, respectively. The joint is then slowly extended completely, and pain, tenderness, the palpation of an audible click, or the sensation of sponginess is noted. Underlying abnormalities suggest a collateral strain or possible meniscus tear especially of the medial portion. It should be noted that this manipulation is often difficult following an injury due to pain and swelling. Anterior cruciate integrity can be accurately assessed by the sensitive Lachman and pivot shift tests. The *Lachman test* is essentially an anterior drawer maneuver done in 30° flexion. With one hand behind the tibia and the other under the thigh, the tibia is then pulled forward while the thigh is pushed posteriorly. The amount of excursion and quality and sensation of endpoint is noted. The test is very sensitive in the acute as well as chronic situation because biomechanical studies have shown maximal tibial displacement at 30° flexion when the anterior cruciate is torn. A false-negative result may occur if the anterior displacement is blocked by a bucket-handle meniscus tear. The *pivot shift test* or "jerk test" is anterior subluxation of the tibia at 20° to 40° of flexion marked by visible, palpable, and audible changes ("clunk or thud") when the examiner produces 10° to 15° of internal rotation of the involved leg on the femur, lateral compartment compression by gentle valgus stress, and flexion of the knee. The test is normally graded 1 to 3, with grades 2 and 3 indicating anterior cruciate tear. Grade 1 may occur in the athlete with ligamentous laxity. The test may be often negative in the acute situation due to guarding; in such cases it is almost always positive under anesthesia. The *Apley grind test* is performed in two parts. The first part consists of lateral foot rotation and fixed leg flexion with the patient prone. Pain at the lateral knee suggests tibial collateral strain.

The second part is then performed by applying tibial condylar pressure via the examiner leaning on the foot. Pain indicates a medial meniscus tear.

The *Childress duck waddle* is done by asking the patient to waddle on the balls of his or her feet. Inability to complete the maneuver, in association with pain and clicking, suggests a tear of the posterior meniscal horn. The duck waddle can be supplemented by jumping, squatting, jogging in place, figures-of-eight (clockwise–counterclockwise), hops, and cuts (sudden turns), all of which should be performed in a large space adjacent to the examining room.

Radiologic studies should be ordered on the basis of the clinical findings. An initial film "as the joint lies" is often most revealing. Thereafter, routine AP and lateral views may often demonstrate osteochrondral defects or degenerative changes, particularly of the patellofemoral joint. A silhouette "skyline" view is very useful for assessing patellar pathology. Oblique views are useful in condylar problems, particularly damage of the anterior or posterior segments. Stress films have been supplanted by arthrography and arthroscopy, although they may be useful in the acute situation, especially in the adolescent, in order to differentiate a Salter I fracture of the distal femoral epiphysis from a ligamentous injury. Marshall's description of the one-shot knee arthrogram often goes far in elucidating internal knee problems.[5] Neither technique should replace a careful history and clinical examination.

Return to Play

Marshall's clinical research[5] has shown that the following conditions prohibit return to play after an acute injury:

1. Severe pain
2. Dislocated knee/patella
3. Acute instability/swelling
4. Excessively limited motion or locking

The physician should be capable of making a rapid, thorough "sideline" assessment. If the extent of injury is unclear from the clinical exam, the player should not be returned to the game.

Return to competition following surgical repair or injury rehabilitation should be predicated on the following parameters:

1. Equal flexor/extensor strengths when compared to normal side; muscle circumferences essentially equal (+ 1 to 2 centimeters)
2. Athlete able to do figure-of-eight in either direction, start and stop quickly, run in place symmetrically, and hop well on the injured leg

Contusions

The superficial anterior portion of the knee makes it vulnerable to contusive forces. Treatment is as previously detailed and consists of ice, rest, elevation, protection from further injury, and the appropriate analgesics. The conditions most likely to be confused with simple contusion are partial sprains of ligaments attached to the tibia or femur, on the medial or lateral side, strains of the quadriceps mechanism, and early apophysitis of the patellar tubercle.

Strains

The complex construction of the quadriceps muscle (medialis, intermedius, lateralis, and rectus portions) in addition to its three aponeurotic attachments medially, laterally, and inferiorly predispose it to muscle-tendon stretching anywhere along its mechanism (biker's or jumper's knee). One cannot predict where the weakest point will be at any particular moment. The medialis, lateralis, rectus femoris, or patellar retinaculum can be torn. Careful examination of the knee for trigger points, assessment of active and passive range of motion of the quadriceps mechanism, and a detailed review of the mechanism of injury are usually sufficient for diagnosis. Treatment of the acute injury consists of the RICE regimen (Chapter 12), and a progressive rehabilitation program within the limits of pain is mandatory. Strains of the knee flexors are very common and often present diagnostic dilemmas. For example, the biceps muscle-tendon unit attaches to the fibular head, injury to which must be distinguished from sprain of the fibular collateral ligament. Active biceps contraction or passive stretch of the muscle produces pain whereas lateral stress of the leg and thigh causes ligamentous tenderness. Hamstring strain may also occur at the pes anserinus and must be distinguished from tenosynovitis and bursitis, which often complicate the initial injury. The gastrocnemius and popliteus can also be torn in the region of the posterior capsule or femoral condyles. Treatment of first- and second-degree strains is conservative with sufficient time allowed for complete healing. Very often moderate or grade II strains require some form of splint for the first 3 to 4 weeks. Third-degree strains usually mandate surgical repair to prevent knee joint function and stability from being compromised.

Bursitis

There are a number of bursae surrounding the knee joint some of which are constant whereas others are adventitious. Those on the anterior aspect of the knee prone to inflammation are the infra-, pre-, and suprapatellar bursa. Direct trauma or repeated irritation from overexertion, as in running or jumping, can produce inflammation. Symptoms usually include variable amounts of pain and difficulty bending the knee. The examination may be remarkable for overlying erythema, palpable tenderness, and variable amounts of edema and effusion. Protection from further trauma, rest, local heat, and splinting produce good results. Large effusions should be tapped and the fluid removed. The anserine bursa lying between the long fibers of the medial collateral and upper tibia and the attachment of the pes anserinus hamstrings (sartorious, semimembranosus, gracilis) provides free-sliding mobility of the tendons along the tibial periosteum and the collateral ligament. Thus, functional forces are often responsible for inflammation though it is possible that a direct blow can initiate the process. "Snowball crepitation" is diagnostic although, more often than not, the injury must be differentiated from medial collateral sprains. In the case of anserine bursitis, the tenderness is located underneath the unattached portion of the ligament and not at the attachment site. Treatment is usually supportive.

The most common form of bursitis on the posterior aspect of the knee is a Baker's cyst—a catch-all term including synovial hernias as well. Very often the player complains of a long-term, dull,

aching heaviness behind the knee in association with a feeling of fullness. Baker's cyst must be differentiated from other posterior fossa masses such as popliteal artery aneurysm, A-V (arteriovenous) fistulas, or other soft tissue tumor including hypertrophied muscle or overredundant fat tissue. Ultrasound evaluation may be helpful in such cases. An effort at conservative management should be attempted, although large amounts of effusion and interference with knee motion should prompt surgical excision and repair of the cyst. There are numerous other bursae associated with the fibular head, popliteal space, lateral region of the gastrocnemius, and in the vicinity of the popliteus insertion.

Sprains

Ligamentous sprains of the knee are secondary to stress on the ligament from abnormal motion of the joint beyond its normal limit.[5] Motion may be in any direction (extension, flexion, internal or external rotation, abduction, or adduction) or in combination with one another (see Tables 18-1 to 18-4). The most commonly injured ligament in athletics, particularly in football, is the medial collateral followed by the anterior cruciate. Rotation in a semiflexed position, as in the case of an athlete who suddenly changes running direction with a planted foot produces tearing of the anterior cruciate due to the forced rotation in semiflexion. Hyperextension or a force directed in the AP plane against the tibia with the knee flexed catches the posterior capsule and cruciate ligament. A classic example of serious ligamentous injury is the "unhappy triad" caused by a clipping force or lateral blocking in football, the cutback motion of running, or the forward motion of a skier while the ski is planted in external rotation. In this particular situation there is spraining of the medial collateral and anterior cruciate ligaments as well as damage to the medial meniscus. (Table 18-1).

First-degree sprains are characterized by less than 25 percent of ligamentous fibers being torn. The athlete may complain of some localized pain and swelling, but there is no reduction in strength, stability, blood in the joint, effusion, or locking. In fact, most of these athletes (75 to 80 percent) are capable of normal ambulation. Treatment is conservative, consisting of the application of cold packs, compression, rest, and an early active rehabilitation program as immobilization produces unnecessary joint stiffness.

Second-degree sprains representing anywhere from 25 to 75 percent rupture of the fibers are characterized by definite strength loss and localized tenderness. When present, it usually indicates internal knee derangement. There is abnormal mobility and the athlete often complains of swelling and pain on rotational motion of the knee. Sterile aspiration should be performed for significant effusions and should be repeated as often as necessary if the fluid recollects. A hemarthrosis with a negative x ray is highly suggestive of anterior cruciate tear although the differential should include osteochondral fracture, peripheral meniscus tear, or a ligamentous tear. Hemarthrosis requires consultation and possible arthroscopy for accurate diagnosis. Treatment of a second-degree sprain is primarily protective and includes, in addition to the usual modalities, progressive application of a posterior splint or compression dressing for 3 days with ice and elevation. A cylinder case in 20° to 30° of flexion for 4 to 6 weeks is then applied. Orthopedic consultation is advised. Isometric quadriceps exercises may be started in the reliable, non-weight-bearing patient with a compressive dressing or knee immobilizer. Thereafter, progressive resistance exercises can be initiated with return to play allowed only after complete recovery of function and strength is achieved. It is most important to note that such ligamentous injuries often require a long time for complete recovery (6 to 8 weeks).

Severe ligamentous rupture (grade III injuries) produces immediate disability and severe pain with large amounts of bloody effusion and swelling, the diagnostic finding of abnormal mobility, and a positive stress film. However, some athletes with serious knee joint derangement have little pain. Treatment should be prompt, early surgical repair of the torn ligament as nonsurgical modalities are inappropriate. Repair must be meticulous and done by a surgeon well versed in the technique. It has been clearly shown that the percentage of recovery for cruciate injuries, particularly those of the "unhappy triad" is highest if surgery is performed early (suc-

cess rate approaching 85 to 90 percent). Late reconstructive procedures produce poor outcomes in 30 to 40 percent of cases. The majority (80 percent) of severe ligamentous injuries occur under 25 years of age; 60 percent occur under 20. However, it is not uncommon for middle-aged athletes also to rupture supporting knee ligaments and surgical repair should also be performed in such cases. Not all knee sprains fit neatly into a category. In fact the physician may at times be concerned about the accuracy of the diagnosis and the wisest course to follow. Perhaps the best rules of thumb to follow are serial examination of the injured joint and consultation with a specialist. Warning flags which should prompt re-evaluation include:

1. A stable initial examination but severe symptomatology
2. The presence of muscular spasm during the first exam
3. The diagnosis of a hemarthrosis
4. A history of a snap, pop, or click at the time of injury
5. Mechanism of injury suggesting a more severe injury than is evident on initial exam and
6. All grade II injuries.

Return to play following knee ligament injuries frequently presents a quandary for the physician. There is no question that the decision must be tailored to the individual player. First- and second-degree sprains with complete anatomic and functional healing and return of preinjury strength allow return to full play. Similarly, athletes who have required surgical repair of more severe sprains and who have normal function and strength following rehabilitation should be allowed to return to their chosen sports activities. The major problem is the athlete who does not achieve preparticipation function levels despite a complete rehabilitation program. For the athlete who is not committed to a particular sport or competition there is usually no difficulty modifying the sports prescription. For the athlete who strongly desires to return to the sport responsible for the injury, a serious discussion should center around potential complications and dangers of reinjury. If the athlete is absolutely adamant—

such that the psychological damage of prohibiting participation is greater than return to play—a custom-tailored knee orthotic from aluminum, steel, or similar material (Lenox Hill orthotic) can be designed to support the injured joint during play.

Meniscus Injuries

The fact that the medial meniscus is attached to the medial collateral via the coronary ligament often predisposes it to shearing forces when the collateral is stressed.[6] It may tear transversely but more commonly splits along its periphery. If the tear is within its substance, no healing will take place; if it tears at its attachment, healing may occur. The only reliable clinical finding associated with meniscus tears is knee joint locking ("trick knee"), which is present in only 30 percent of such cases. The locking may be complete or incomplete; that is, some extension against a spongy resistance may be present. However, if the physician waits for repeated locking in order to make the diagnosis of a fractured meniscus, many tears may be missed. Repeated locking has been shown to have a definite deleterious effect on the articular cartilage, so surgical intervention is wise after the first episode of locking. Occasionally, if one is fortunate to diagnose a peripheral tear following an acute injury in which there is no locking (by arthroscopy or arthrography), traction and careful manipulation may reduce the displacement. Careful follow-up is necessary in order to assess rehabilitative as well as further injury potential.

The loose redundant attachment of the coronary ligament to the lateral meniscus, plus the facts that the lateral meniscus is not attached to the fibular attachment and that the lateral ligament is infrequently damaged by lateral stress, are responsible for its infrequent tearing. On the other hand, prolonged repeated trauma (as in power squatting) or hyperflexion (as in deep knee bends or duck waddling in conditioning exercises) can produce this injury. Although these general guidelines are useful in the majority of cases there may be an occasional anatomic variant in which the anterolateral portion of the meniscus attaches firmly to the iliotibial band so that, on forced adduction of the leg on the thigh, tearing of the cartilage follows.

In summary, most meniscal injuries can be diagnosed by a history of knee locking or the "knee giving way," joint-line pain, and swelling. Remember also that, although it is important to be familiar with the various stress manipulation tests, they are only confirmatory and not specific. Point tenderness along the anteromedial joint line that is increased with internal tibial rotation and extension indicates medial meniscus injury (Bragard's sign). Pain produced by pressure on the knee joint in a patient seated cross-legged suggests injury of the posterior horn of the medial meniscus (Payr's sign). Pressure over the anterolateral joint space eliciting tenderness during internal rotation is associated with lateral meniscus tears, whereas pain during external rotation in the anteromedial joint space indicates medial meniscus damage (first Steinman's sign). The displacement of point tenderness from the anterior joint line posteriorly toward the collateral ligament as the knee joint moves from full extension to full flexion supports the diagnosis of a cartilage lesion and not a ligamentous tear (second Steinman's sign). Occasionally, neither the history, clinical exam, nor radiological exam is indicative of knee joint pathology.

However, every effort should be made to distinguish ligamentous from meniscal injuries. In the acute situation of meniscus tear, any effusions should be aspirated, a compression dressing or splint applied, and locking reduced. The initial injury should be re-examined in 24 hours in order to exclude any occult ligamentous damage. Meniscal tears without associated ligamentous sprains should be managed with a non-weight-bearing posterior splint and active quadriceps exercises. The worsening or recurrence of symptoms should prompt a more extensive evaluation (arthroscopy, arthrography) and consultation with a specialist, particularly in the competitive athlete. A longer interim period of conservative treatment and active physical rehabilitation is recommended in the noncompetitive athlete—the bottom line being the inability of the knee to achieve preinjury function and strength. Casts, if employed, should extend from the inguinal crease to the superior malleolar area.

Pellegrini–Stieda Disease

Partial avulsion of the adductor longus tendon or sprain of the medial collateral tendon at its femoral condyle attachment occasionally causes the formation of a calcium placque along the region of medial femoral condyle and the symptoms of knee sprain. The condition, termed Pellegrini–Stieda disease, should be recognized and known by the physician. It is usually of no consequence as surgical removal is rarely indicated; symptomatic therapy in conjunction with a good physiotherapy regimen is sufficient.

Patellar Malalignment Syndrome and Patellar Dislocation

Internal angulation of the femur in conjunction with a wide pelvis, more common in the female, predisposes the patella to premature cartilage softening, subluxation, and dislocation.[7,8] Genu valgus in either gender is also a predisposing factor. On clinical examination, there is often a high-riding patella (patella alta) which assumes a lateral posture on full knee extension, passive hypermobility of the patella on palpation, prominence of the lateral quadriceps tendon, dysplasia or atonia of the vastus medialis, and an abnormal Q angle (greater than 20°), although it is probably a secondary factor. The Q angle is formed by a line drawn across the mid patella to the tibial tuberosity and its intersection with a line drawn along the quadriceps to the mid patella. The female athlete usually complains of the knee having given way or the kneecap snapping or popping.

With time, subluxating forces stretch the medial portion of the patellar retinaculum until either a minor blow or fall in extension produces dislocation. The history usually reveals that the athlete strongly contracted the quadriceps while the knee was flexed and the foot was externally rotated. In the acute state, the athlete usually presents with knee painfully flexed resisting any manipulative attempts, the tibia abducted, and swelling from a hemarthrosis evident. Most cases of dislocation, however, usually present after spontaneous reduction. A useful historical fact is when the distal portion of the thigh was dislocated medially, which is due to the change of the anterior knee contour as the patella slid out of its groove. The patellar apprehension maneuver (Fairbanks test) should be performed by simply attempting to push the patella laterally. If positive, the sensation of an impending dislocation causes the athlete to grab for his or her

knee. The silhouette or "sunrise" view of the patella confirms the diagnosis of an acute dislocation. AP and lateral films should also be reviewed in order to assess the anatomy of the lateral femoral condyle and patellar groove. It is important that a dislocation be distinguished from meniscal damage as the two are often confused. Once the diagnosis of primary patellar pathology is made, it is important to decide whether it is a result of repeated episodes of acute subluxation/dislocation or secondary to some congenital anatomic predisposition—the treatments are different.

The patellar malalignment syndrome should be treated conservatively with salicylates or similar anti-inflammatory agents, progressive resistance exercises, especially for the vastus medialis, and perhaps the prescription of a light-weight knee orthotic in order to prevent subluxation and further damage during play. Chronic cases that lead to repeated dislocation and/or degenerative changes should be seen in conjunction with an orthopedic surgeon.

Acute lateral dislocations must be reduced immediately by hip flexion and gentle valgus pressure on the patella while extending the knee. Superior, horizontal, and intra-articular dislocations usually require surgery. After reduction, consultation is advised. Many orthopedic surgeons apply a long leg cast for 6 weeks in full extension.[9] Others surgically repair even the first dislocation.[10] Most surgeons recommend surgery for dislocation associated with osteochondial fractures.

Knee Dislocations

Tibiofemoral dislocations are very rare secondary to marked traumatic forces and easily diagnosed clinically at the time of occurrence. Primary consideration in a dislocation must be for the vascular status of the leg. Anterior dislocations are more common but posterior ones are usually complicated by tearing of the popliteal artery. Remember to assess the neurovascular status of the leg (e.g., looking for diminished or absent pulses, abnormal sensation, coolness, pallor, motor weakness). A vascular catastrophe can occur 10 to 14 days after the traumatic result. It goes without saying that any form of dislocation of the joint is often associated with severe and catastrophic ligamentous damage. Immediate reduction is the first priority and should be performed when it occurs. Gentle progressive traction in the line of the extremity usually effects relocation, with reduction easier the more complete the ligamentous disruption. Simple extension of the leg usually reduces anterior dislocations and gentle rocking of the tibia with traction reduces lateral and posterior positions. Pronounced muscle spasm, severe pain, and edema usually mandate anesthesia, which should be done at the earliest time.

Fractures

A brief mention should be made of fractures in and about the knee joint. Perhaps one of the most commonly missed fractures of the knee is one involving the articular cartilage. Direct stresses as well as strains can produce chondral fractures. Symptomatology often mimics joint strains or meniscal tears. There may be vague knee pain or limitation of joint motion in one or more direction. The patella followed by the two femoral condyles are the most vulnerable areas for such fractures. On examination there may be "snowball" or grinding crepitation on movement of the patella; rarely is there actual catching or locking of the knee. A differential diagnostic point distinguishing distal femoral epiphyseal fractures from collateral ligament strains is the fact that in the former the swelling is above the knee, involving the distal thigh as well as the knee, and the disability is moderate to severe; whereas in the latter, swelling directly involves the knee joint and disability is less. A high index of suspicion prompts an early diagnosis and a trial of protective immobilization should be made acutely in order to allow healing. Since most diagnoses are made after other injuries have been ruled out and there has been a significant lapse of time, surgery is definitive. Very often, years have passed since the original injury; the fragments within the joint are then termed "joint mice."

True fracture of the patella is less common than chondral fractures and is usually due to direct contusive blows rather than straining or spraining forces. The physician should recognize the normal bi- or tripartite patella. Because of the usual associated displacement secondary to tendon pull, open surgical reduction is mandatory for the best result.

Fractures and dislocations of the fibular head

should signal two warnings: (1) consider peroneal nerve injury; (2) the injury is often due to rotatory forces so that the ankle may also be damaged (Maisonneuve fracture—proximal fibular fracture with sprain of the medial ligaments). Treatment is usually conservative unless there has been tearing of the tibiofibular ligaments with resultant instability. Epiphyseal fractures in adolescents are often diagnosed as "sprains." There is usually localized pain, and stress in any direction aggravates the symptoms. Treatment should be conservative if there is no or minimal displacement, although surgery is reserved for complete avulsion or wide displacements. In investigating knee pathology, the fabella, a sesamoid found in the lateral head of the gastrocnemius tendon, should not be mistaken for a foreign body or fracture fragment. Although it is rarely injured, point tenderness and pain in that region of the gastrocnemius should prompt careful bilateral comparative x rays as a bipartite fabella can occur. If it is fractured, surgical removal is wisest.

Water on the Knee

A common athletic complaint is "water on the knee," a chronic synovial effusion. All too often a nonspecific diagnosis, treatment depends on identifying the underlying etiology. After a careful history and physical, it is wise to aspirate the joint and analyze the fluid including microscopic and bacterial analyses. Multiple aspirations may often be necessary in conjunction with protection from further injury, rest, and immobilization if necessary. Compression with an elastic wrap or neoprene sleeves is most useful in preventing the recurrence of an effusion. An active physical therapy program including diathermy, paraffin packs, and whirlpool are indicated. The amount of exercise should be carefully prescribed as any motion irritates the synovium, producing more fluid accumulation.

Iliotibial Band Syndrome

The iliotibial band, a thick strip fascia lata which extends from iliac crests to the lateral tibial tubercle and includes a portion of the tensor fasciae lata and gluteus maximus, is often injured through overuse primarily in distance runners. The band basically acts as a stabilizing ligament between the lateral femoral condyle and tibia, locks the knee into extension, and contributes to the pelvic slouch, thus allowing one to rest while standing. With overuse there is frictional inflammation of the band over the lateral femoral condyle so that activities that repeatedly flex the knee lead to chronic inflammation. The athlete complains of pain on distance running, climbing stairs, or repeated backward kicking in mushing a dog team (musher's knee). There is palpable tenderness in the region of the condyle but the rest of the functional exam is within normal limits. Renne's creak sign may occasionally be demonstrated.[11] In addition to the usual conservative modalities of standard treatment it is important to reduce the distance run by the patient. The majority of runners respond to this program, though occasionally the band must be surgically split in refractory cases.

Osgood–Schlatter's Disease

Osgood–Schlatter's disease represents quadriceps tendonitis with heterotopic bone formation at the site of the tibial tubercle but is often confused with bursitis of the infrapatellar tendon and aseptic necrosis of the patellar tubercle epiphysis. Infrapatellar bursitis lies at a point slightly higher than the tubercle and is usually not associated with tumorous swelling as in aseptic necrosis or true epiphysitis. The latter two conditions often produce marked painful swelling with sharp limitation of motion in all directions due to incomplete separation of the cartilagenous link between the patellar tendon and the tibia. The disease may be bilateral and usually remits by 18 years of age when the apophysis fuses to the tibia. The condition is self-limiting being treated conservatively with rest, activity reduction, ice, analgesics, anti-inflammatories, and reassurance. Those activities requiring forceful knee extension, such as running or jumping, should be curtailed. The use of a cylinder cast for immobilization is seldom necessary; one should be applied for only 3 to 4 weeks. Rarely, it may be necessary to remove the necrotic fragment surgically or trim down the bony–cartilagenous mass. Thereafter, a month of immobilization and several weeks of exercise training provide complete recovery.

Chondromalacia Patellae

Chondromalacia patellae (runner's knee) is premature softening of the patellar articular cartilage, or *malacia,* most commonly in young adults, particularly females.[12] Degeneration usually begins by the age of 30 and, in the majority of cases, remains asymptomatic. The disorder can be secondary to:

1. Excessive knee strain
2. Direct blow
3. Patellar malalignment with recurrent subluxation/dislocation[12]
4. Congenital patellar or femoral groove anomaly
5. Metabolic disease
6. Inadequate nutrition

The athlete typically presents with a history of deep aching in the knees without a history of recent trauma. Strenuous activity or prolonged sitting worsens the pain, which is localized to the kneecap or surrounds the medial aspect of the knee. Eventually the athlete complains that slight exertion (stair or hill climbing) exacerbates the pain. The production of the characteristic pain by firm compression of the patella into the medial femoral groove while the knee is in slight flexion is essentially pathognomonic. The patella is often flattened, roughened, and irregular and on glissement produces crepitus and tenderness. Further confirmation can be obtained by producing pain when the patella is held firmly against the femoral condyles with the knee extended while the quadriceps is actively contracted (patellar inhibition test). The Q angle should be measured in order to assess whether malalignment is present. Finally, the course of the patella should be observed through full range of knee motion. Normally the patella moves vertically and slightly medially as full extension is achieved. Wandering, high-riding, or hypermobile patellae are predisposing factors. X rays are of little diagnostic value except in the late stages where there may be sclerosis and osteophyte formation. The differential diagnosis should include a torn medial meniscus, prepatellar or anserine bursitis, and osteochondritis dessicans. The majority of these cases can be treated conservatively with reduction of activity, analgesics, anti-inflammatory agents (therapeutic salicylate levels for 3 to 4 months), and ice-cold water packs before and after sports activities. Steroids are not recommended as they may increase the rate of degeneration. The prognosis is generally good. Progressive resistance quadriceps exercises should be prescribed, though the final 15° to 30° of knee extension should be avoided initially, as should squatting, running, kneeling, and stair climbing. Casting is contraindicated. It should be noted that O'Donoghue and others recommend surgical management of chondromalacia by shaving, drilling with trephine, facetectomy, or in extreme situations, patellectomy.[13] Remember that with underlying intrinsic pathology the prognosis is comparatively affected.

Popliteal Artery Entrapment Syndrome

First described among army recruits, this syndrome consists of popliteal artery compression by a cyst, aberrant fibrous band, or the congenital deviation of artery from its normal course (looping around the medial or lateral head of the gastrocnemius muscle).[14] The condition is bilateral in at least 25 percent of cases, becomes symptomatic before the age of 30, predominantly in young men, and is rarely recognized before permanent arterial damage has occurred. Symptoms include intermittent claudication relieved by rest and the diagnosis is made by the absence or diminution of peripheral limb pulses. Passive dorsiflexion of the foot with the knee extended combined with active plantar flexion diminishes the pulses. Ultrasound of the popliteal fossa and arteriograms are confirmatory. The treatment of choice is surgical bypass or entrapment relief. The prognosis is good.

LEG

Contusion

The superficial nature of the anterior tibia predisposes it to easy abrasion, laceration, and contusion (barked shin) especially in sports such as field hockey, martial arts, and soccer. Very often such contusions are associated with a subperiosteal hematoma. The usual treatment modalities are indicated including

aspiration as necessary. There are two complications of contusive blows with which the physician should be familiar. First, contusion of the peroneal nerve causes paresthesias and pain most commonly due to small amounts of hemorrhage and fluid transudation with edema. Nerve function usually returns to normal following lessening of the congestion. More severe injury is accompanied by the initial symptoms which often disappear by variable time periods only to recur with increasing severity. Eventually hypesthesias and paresis of foot dorsiflexion intervene. Anesthesia and foot drop are characteristic of neural rupture. Chronic long-term fibrotic scarring can also produce the same symptoms. Partial or complete recovery may occur at any time and may be assessed by eliciting distal tingling on percussion (Tinel's sign), which indicates functional recovery. Intractable pain, immediate paralysis, or the development of later paralyses should prompt surgical explanation and repair if possible.

Compartment Syndrome

The tight lacing of skates can occasionally compress the medial and lateral dorsal branches of the superficial peroneal nerve causing an entrapment neuropathy (roller disco neuropathy).[15] The condition is reversible once the diagnosis is made and cause removed. Another important complication of severe contusions is development of the anterior compartment syndrome.[16] The tibialis anterior, deep peroneal nerve, anterior tibial artery and vein, extensor digitorum longus, and hallux longus muscle are tightly encased in a thick nonelastic fascia and together constitute the anterior compartment. With a direct blow or vigorous exercise in the unconditioned athlete there can be rapid compartment swelling with neurovascular compromise and muscle ischemia. Clinically the condition is manifested by observation of the five Ps: (1) pain, which is the most reliable, (2) pallor, (3) pulse diminution, (4) paresis, and (5) paresthesias. Definitive diagnosis is made by manometric studies. Early aggressive treatment with ice and elevation should be followed by surgical release of the fascia if there is no immediate improvement. Complete recovery is usually the rule, if surgery is done early.

Strains

Muscular strains of the calf are common particularly in the track events.[17] Careful review of the mechanism of injury in conjunction with a good clinical examination usually clinches the diagnosis. Treatment including adhesive strapping suffices in the mild to moderate strains. The foot is placed in a Gibney-type basket weave (Fig. 18-6) which prevents dorsiflexion of the foot. With the foot in mild equinus the strapping begins above the calf bulge and passes directly behind the back of the leg over the heel and the foot sole to the toes. The strapping should be supplemented with a heel orthotic designed to elevate the calcaneus about $\frac{1}{2}$ inch in order to provide further calf relaxation.[18] More serious strains should be treated with a walking cast and slow rehabilitation within the confines of pain over a 4 to 6 week period. Complete muscular ruptures

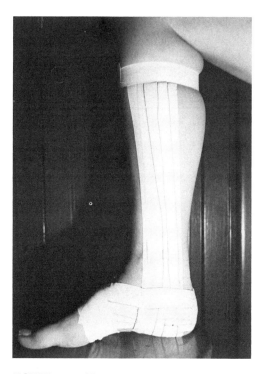

FIGURE 18-6. Gibney interlocking adhesive strapping.

require surgical repair with a 6-week healing period before active physiotherapy is pursued. It is common in certain sports (e.g., racquet games) to rupture the plantaris muscle. "Tennis leg" results from a strain of the plantaris or possible tear of the soleus or gastrocnemius muscle. The athlete often mentions being "shot" in the calf after a hump or cut and then complains of a dull deep calf ache. As the muscle is of little functional import, a relatively short period of protection and reassurance facilitates recovery. Of course it is important to distinguish plantaris rupture from grade III strains of larger muscles or the Achilles tendon (see Foot section). Fascial hernias, especially those of anterior fascia, periodically afflict the athletic population. Their symptoms are similar to those of "shin splints" or a simple contusion. A mass may be palpated. Treatment is similar to that for thigh fascial hernias.

Shin Splints

Shin splints or periostitis of the tibia is a multifactorial diagnosis.[19] There may be irritation of the posterior tibial attachment along the posterior tibia producing a periostitis. Diagnosis is by palpating direct tenderness along the posteromedial aspect of the tibia and the production of pain on contraction of the posterior tibial muscle. At other times there may be actual detachment of the posterior tibia or irritation of the interosseus membrane. Both conditions produce deeper lying diffuse calf pain. Occasionally the anterior tibialis muscle at its anterior or anterolateral insertion becomes inflamed. A stress fracture may masquerade as a shin splint.

Basic therapeutic interventions include rest, local heat, and removal from the precipitating problem. It is imperative that an anterior compartment syndrome be ruled out as heat markedly worsens this condition. Analgesics and anti-inflammatories may be useful supplementary methods. In terms of specifics, every effort should be made to identify the underlying etiology. A careful review of the athlete's ankle and foot, particularly for those involved in track events, should be made in order to assess the presence of excessive pronation or supination which could chronically stress the leg muscles.[16,17] Overfatigue can also be secondary to arch problem. Many times, simply changing the athlete's footwear and providing a simple office orthotic alleviates the problem. Strapping and elastic wrapping, on the whole, are not useful as the condition is most often due to muscle overuse. Finally, since the condition is most often due to a poorly conditioned athlete running for prolonged periods on hard surfaces or stretching overvigorously, some form of preventive education is mandatory for the treatment of this condition.

Fractures

Whereas tibial fractures are a rare though serious athletic injury, fracture of the fibula is not infrequent but, with few exceptions, not substantial. The most common form of fibular fracture is due to stress (runner's fracture) and in this respect is second only to metatarsal fracture. The player may complain of dull, aching soreness with minimal disability located near the fibular neck.[16] There is usually no history of trauma, although there may be a heavy training or exercise period within the preceding several weeks revealed on careful questioning. Initial x rays are often negative, but repeating films in 2 to 3 weeks may reveal a transverse linear line with possible callus formation. Radionuclide bone scanning is very useful in the diagnostic evaluation. Taping and gentle muscular rehabilitation is all that is necessary in accompaniment with analgesics. The tibia occasionally can be stress fractured for similar reasons and can be treated with a walking cast for 3 to 4 weeks. Complete fibular fractures can be treated with a 2- to 3-week walking boot followed by strapping and careful muscle physiotherapy. Participation in contact sports is not advisable for 6 to 8 weeks. Of course, the most important measure in evaluating a possible fibular fracture is to ensure the integrity of the ankle joint. Distal fibular fractures can involve the inferior tibiofibular ligaments and produce significant ankle instability.

Comminuted fractures of the tibia and fibula secondary to a high-speed forward spill as in ski racing (boot top fracture) is a serious injury requiring specialist consultation for early accurate report. Complications such as the compartment syndrome should be recognized early.

ANKLE

The ankle, functionally a hinge point, is capable of motion in only the plane of flexion and extension. Due to its unique construction of mortise and tenon it has considerable inherent stability. The medial malleolus, undersurface of the distal tibia, and lateral malleolus constitute the mortise; the body of the talus forms the tenon. Because the talus is wider in its anterior portion, dorsiflexion is very stable as the talus is forced between the malleolus in a wedge-like fashion. There tends to be some lateral instability in plantar flexion as the narrower posterior portion of the talus moves into the mortise. This is particularly true when the foot is placed in equinus. Additionally joint stability is secured by the extensive ligamentous reinforcement. The anterior and posterior tibiofibular bind the distal tibia and fibula so, with the exception of small amounts of motion at the syndesmosis, there is complete stability between the two bones. The deltoid ankle ligament is very strong, having a broad attachment to the medial malleolus and extending downward to the arch ligaments of the foot, thus stabilizing the medial aspect of the ankle as well as supporting the arch. The lateral ligament is divisible into three components: the anterior and posterior talofibular, and the calcaneofibular ligaments. Each also fuses with the various lateral ligaments of the foot which extend forward onto the fifth metatarsal and cuboid bones. The two malleoli are subcutaneous and in close association to the posterior tibial and flexor hallucies tendons medially and the peroneal tendons laterally.

Contusions

Contusions of the malleoli are common due to their superficial location, although it is important to bear in mind that the pain of ankle sprains is often referred to the malleoli. Therefore, range of motion must be checked in every ankle injury no matter how simple the history or obvious the injury. Occasionally direct blows can injure the Achilles tendon producing tenosynovitis as well as strain or dislocation of the peroneal tendons. Treatment of simple contusions is detailed in Chapter 12.

Strains

The ankle joint is perhaps the most common site for strains in the active athlete due to its role in weight bearing as well as being the focal point of a number of dynamic forces in most sports. The Achilles tendon may be strained at its musculotendinous insertion or at the site of its attachment to the calcaneus. In addition the anterior tibialis tendon may be strained at its medial foot attachment area or the posterior tibial where it inserts at the navicular tuberosity or under the navicular arch of the foot. Just the simple switch from street shoes to competitive athletic footwear can produce a static strain which may be difficult to manage. The treatment of strains of a mild to moderate degree has been detailed in Chapter 12. As in knee injuries, it is imperative that the athlete not be allowed to play until the healing process is complete. Very often, a felt-pad orthotic fashioned in the physician's office takes the stress off a strained muscle and allows a moderate degree of activity. Adhesive strapping to prevent hyperdorsiflexion is also useful although full athletic activity should not be allowed until maximum pain-free motion of the ankle is achieved.

Tenosynovitis. Tenosynovitis can often complicate strain injuries and can be caused by direct blows. The typical symptoms and signs ("snowball" crepitation) have been detailed in Chapter 17. Treatment is in the usual fashion and includes rest, protection from further injury, and the alternate application of cold packs and heat. Tenosynovitis of the Achilles tendon is common in unconditioned runners; usually a 10- to 14-day walking boot with rest provides good functional recovery and early return to training. Supplementation with adhesive strapping in plantar flexion usually prevents recurrence.

Peroneal Tendon Injury. Blows to the posterior portion of the lateral malleolus while the foot is actively contracted in dorsiflexion and eversion can produce subluxation or dislocation of the peroneal tendons. A palpable snap may be heard or felt by the player and spontaneous reduction usually recurs. A careful examination reveals tenderness over the peroneal tendons and, in combination with a good history, should rule out ankle sprain or tenosynovitis. Treatment for both acute and chronic subluxation/dislocation is surgical repair.

Sprains

Classification. Sprains of the ankle are classified as either first-, second-, or third-degree injuries based on the clinical presentation and the functional instability demonstrated by stress testing. In *first-degree* sprains there is mild to moderate pain on stress, no abnormal motion, minimal swelling, little or no functional loss, and slight point tenderness at the injured site. *Second-degree* sprains are characterized by pain on normal motion, moderate to severe pain on stress, immediate postinjury pain, edema with local hemorrhage, a moderate degree of functional loss, and the presence of an egg-shaped swelling within 1 to 2 hours after injury. Complete *(third-degree)* ruptures may be painless, though they usually cause severe pain.

Mechanism of Injury. Lateral stress forces in eversion or inversion and less commonly hyperextension/hyperflexion are responsible for the majority of ankle injuries. Most commonly such injuries are due to a combination of these forces, the classic being plantar flexion, internal rotation, and inversion of the foot. With gradually increasing forces there is sprain of the anterior talofibular ligament which then involves the calcaneofibular and eventually with progressive force, the posterior talofibular ligament.

Eversion Injuries. Eversion forces, usually in conjunction with dorsiflexion, produce straining of the deltoid ligament initially and, with more violent forces, straining of the anterior inferior tibiofibular ligament or interosseous membrane. Injury due to pure dorsiflexion alone is uncommon and usually occurs with some degree of eversion and external rotation. There is rupture of the distal tibiofibular ligament.

Diagnosis. The diagnosis of each of these sprain injuries consists of elucidation of the mechanism of injury followed by a careful clinical exam. Gentle but meticulous palpation of the entire ankle area should be supplemented by examination of the active and passive ranges of motion in order to determine whether there are any trigger points, palpable defects, swellings, or instabilities. Occasionally, particularly with dorsiflexion injuries, localized swelling may not be manifest due to the deep lying nature of hemorrhage and inflammation. Anterior–posterior stress should be performed on both ankles in the form of a drawer test with the leg fixed. A difference of 5 millimeters is suggestive of ligamentous disruption; 10 millimeters is diagnostic. A talar tilt test should also be performed comparing the normal and injured ankle. A difference of 5° to 10° or an absolute value of 20° to 25° is highly suggestive of ligamentous disruption. In order to perform stress tests properly in the acutely injured ankle, xylocaine infiltration may be required (opposite to the side of the injury). Radiologic evaluation should then follow, with standard views being

supplemented with stress films with unstable ankles.

Treatment. Because ankle sprains are associated with a significant degree of morbidity (30 to 60 percent symptom-free in 1 to 4 years with an average disability of 5 to 26 weeks) due to inadequate treatment, it is important that the therapeutic goal be twofold: maintenance of mortise integrity and complete re-establishment of weight bearing on the fibular and tibia.

First-degree sprains are treated with the RICE regimen (Rest, Ice, Compression, and Elevation for 72 to 96 hours). A *firm* ankle support (Richard's

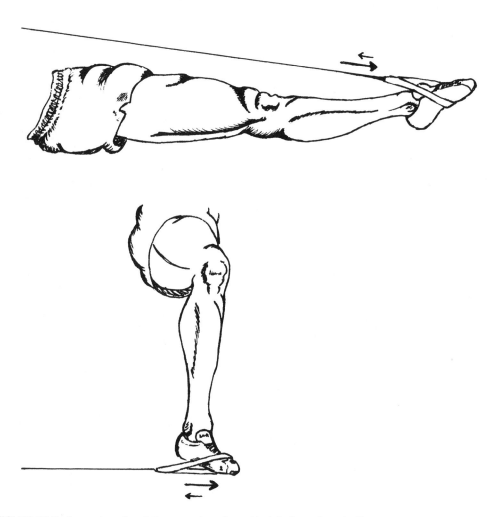

FIGURE 18-7. Examples of resistive exercises for ankle injuries using elastic gauze or wrap.

Ankle Support or Unna Boot) is useful. Adhesive strapping as outlined by Gibney is also useful (see Fig. 18-6). Progressive resistance exercises should be started immediately and continue within the confines of pain (Fig. 18-7). Elastic strapping does not provide good support. Return to play should be allowed only after the establishment of full functional ability and preinjury strength.

Second-degree sprains are also treated with the RICE regimen and a posterior splint for 72 to 96 hours. The ankle should then be re-examined. If a second-degree sprain is confirmed, cast immobilization in the neutral position for 3 weeks is recommended by some authorities. If the degree of injury is unclear, an orthopedist should be consulted. Rehabilitation should begin after resolution of the acute phase, remain within the confines of pain, and involve progressive resistance exercises.

Third-degree strains as established by stress testing and/or arthrography should be handled in consultation. For instance, calcaneofibular and anterior talofibular ruptures are often surgically repaired in the young athlete. In the older adult, posterior splinting followed by cast immobilization is often chosen. Early mobilization with physiotherapy is recommended by some.

Tip-offs to inadequately treated ankle sprains include ankle instability (feeling of insecurity and weakness), recurrent sprains, and peroneal subluxation or dislocation.

Fractures

Perhaps the biggest error to be made in ankle injuries of the sprain–dislocation–fracture group is to overlook one of the components after making an obvious diagnosis. For instance, severe inversion injuries can lead to vertical fracture of the medial malleolus along the tibial shaft (ski fracture) whereas severe eversion forces can fracture the distal fibula. Inversion injuries can produce an avulsion fracture of the lateral malleolus, particularly in the older population where the bone is more brittle.

Fracture of the lateral malleolus can accompany rupture of the tibiofibular ligament whereas distal fibular fractures should prompt consideration of fractures of the medial malleolus or rupture of the deltoid ligament (Pott's fracture). More proximal fractures of the fibula should suggest an investigation for ruptures of the tibiofibular ligament and medial collateral ligament in conjunction with medial malleolar fracture. There may be a bimalleolar fracture with ligamentous sparing.

Perhaps the biggest oversight is the negative x ray and the missed rupture of the lateral collateral, tibiofibular, or deltoid ligament. Until the diagnosis is made, it is best to err on the conservative side with aggressive nonsurgical treatment and weekly serial examinations for range of motion and strength recovery.

Chondral Fractures. Chondral fractures of the ankle joint are probably as common as those of the knee, but are often overlooked. The same forces that produce sprain, strain, and fracture can damage the articular cartilage of the talus, distal tibia, or fibula. Such fractures are often responsible for "chronic ankle sprains" and their subsequent disability. The medial, lateral, and inner surfaces of the fibula and the superior surface of the talus are the areas most frequently involved. If the diagnosis can be made early on, surgical repair provides the best results.

Exostoses

The successive irritation of talotibial exostoses, particularly of the anterior tibial or superior talor surface flexion (Fig. 18-8) causes the piling up of a bony protuberance which can be the cause of significant disability during weight bearing and motion. The most common mechanism of injury is the "drive phase" during sprinting or a football tackle in which there is direct trauma to the anterior tibial margin due to forced dorsiflexion of the foot. The player complains of the inability to "go all out" or is asymptomatic. Clinical diagnosis is made by tenderness in the direction of dorsiflexion of the foot or pin-point pain directly over the spur. Radiologic examination confirms the diagnosis in the asymptomatic competitive or weekend athlete; reassurance and periodic rest from weight are all that is necessary for symptom relief. In the highly competitive athlete, careful consideration should be given to surgical excision of the mass.

Rupture of the Achilles Tendon

This is a serious injury. Risk factors include increasing weight, height, and age (most common

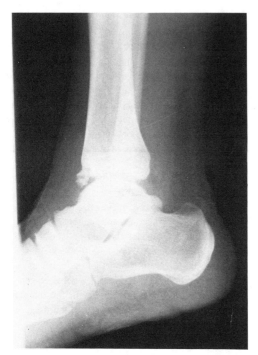

FIGURE 18-8. Painful exostosis in a martial arts athlete who presented with a history of "recurrent sprains."

between ages of 40 and 50) in association with a long foot. Chronic strain with gradual weakening of the tendon in the older athlete is a frequent contributing factor. Basic injury mechanisms include:

1. Direct trauma to a taut tendon
2. Forced dorsiflexion with the ankle in the relaxed state
3. Further stretch of a taut tendon

The athlete complains of severe pain in the lower aspect of the calf as well as difficulty ambulating. On examination there is marked plantar flexion weakness and, in the case of rupture, the Thompson test is positive; that is, normal plantar flexion is absent on squeezing of the calf belly while the patient is supine. Misdiagnosis of a strain occurs in 20 to 30 percent of cases due to a poor history, little pain, or plantar flexion being achieved by the

posterior tibialis muscle particularly in the young athlete. The site of rupture most commonly is 2 inches above the site of its calcaneal attachment. Treatment in the young adult is surgical, though immobilization with an equinus walking boot for 8 weeks followed by a 1-inch heel for another 4 weeks has been successful in the older adult.

FOOT

The complex structure of the foot, which consists of 26 bones and an impressive array of supporting muscles, tendon, ligaments, nerves, and vessels, in combination with its primary function of support and stability and secondary role of propulsion, makes it extremely vulnerable to a variety of traumatic forces. For a number of cultural reasons, the feet are often not treated with the same care as the hands, and a sense of false security is gained by the wearing of a protective shoe. Unfortunately, the foot can be directly contused, twisted, lacerated, or otherwise injured. In fact, many podiatric injuries are due to overuse and/or improper footwear.

Overuse Injuries

Overuse injuries occur under vigorous or excessive training conditions in the poorly trained athlete or one with improper training techniques.[12,14] Microtrauma in the form of friction and irritation at a particular pressure point leads to acute inflammation (erythema, edema, warmth, and tenderness) and possible blister or vesicle formation. With chronic inflammation, particularly of the ball of the foot or in the region of the hallux valgus, there is reactive hypertrophy of the skin in the form of a callus, if a diffuse region is involved, or the formation of a corn in more defined pressure point areas. Very often a bursitis accompanies a callus. Repeated microtrauma to the medial plantar nerve produces burning heel pain often referred to as "jogger's foot." Chronic reinjury can lead to neural entrapment contusion. Chronic irritation of the dorsum of the foot can lead to tenosynovitis, periostitis, and even stress fracture.

Because of the subcutaneous nature of the dorsum of the foot, the complications of a contusive blow are often more significant than the actual contusion. There may be a secondary neuritis, tenosynovitis, phlebitis, or hematoma following the dropping of a heavy weight or trampling by a cleated foot. Even the thick subcutaneous tissue of the plantar surface of the foot is not immune to contusive injury. Inflammation with secondary subcutaneous fat necrosis and fibrosis in the form of a "stone bruise" can occur if a thick sock is wrinkled or a spike or cleat is loose. This can be particularly aggravating in the high-arched foot with a tight heel cord since there is marked stress placed in the metatarsal heads, particularly the first, where forefoot stresses the two sesamoids underlying it. The same form of stress produces marginal spurring of the cuneiform bones, and at the junction of the metatarsal bases. In addition to the usual modalities in managing contusions it is particularly important to address the varying etiologies responsible for the injury. Very often an interim orthotic (pontoon or donut) should be fashioned in the office in order to hasten healing and prevent reinjury.

Strains

Strains of the foot usually involve the anterior or posterior tibialis, the peroneals, and the toe flexors. A more thorough discussion of their diagnosis and management can be found in the ankle section. The most important feature of the management of such strains is the elimination of the stress source via the preparation of a heel pad, adhesive strapping in dorsiflexion, or similar device. In the young athlete, strains of the Achilles tendon may be associated with apophysitis of the calcaneus. The athlete is usually without complaint during regular ambulation but, in running or jumping, pain at the heel occurs. Clinical examination reveals point tenderness over the calcaneus and perhaps along the Achilles tendon attachment. The apophysitis is pathologically a form of aseptic necrosis but, unlike in the hip or knee, is not usually significant. Adhesive strapping in plantar flexion for several weeks is usually curative. Bursitis of the foot, though uncommon, occurs in the region of the head of the first metatarsal (medial sesamoid), between the most inferior portion of the Achilles tendon and the calcaneus (retrocalcaneals bursitis) or between the

Achilles tendon and the overlying skin (posterior calcaneal bursitis). The latter conditions must be distinguished from plantar fascial strain, calcaneal epiphysitis, painful heel pad, "jogger's foot," or heel spur/apophysitis. Repeated superficial irritation to the distal Achilles tendon from poorly fitting footwear can produce characteristic "pump bumps." Removal of the aggravating etiology is often curative though large lesions do not completely defervesce.

Ganglia

Ganglia of the feet are second in frequency only to those of the hand. These synovial hernias can occur from any of the tarsal or tarsal–metatarsal joints, peroneal, or exterior tendon sheaths. They may be idiopathic or secondary to trauma. (See Chapter 17, section on Hand, for details.) Surgery is reserved for large, recurrent, painful ganglia and is best performed under anesthesia and meticulously, followed by immobilization in order to prevent recurrence.

Morton's Toe

Fibrotic thickening of the junction of the medial and lateral digital nerves between the third and fourth toe is termed *plantar neuroma* or *Morton's toe*. Though the athlete may complain of a "sprain" of the anterior arch, the condition is a static one often due to the lateral displacement of body weight secondary to a long second metatarsal. In addition, splaying of the forefoot due to intermetatarsal ligament laxity is a predisposing factor. The presenting complaint is usually severe, lancinating or burning pain of the lateral foot which may radiate to the dorsum of the foot. The "electric shock" feeling is intermittent and spontaneous, often not in association with motion. Careful palpation elicits point tenderness between the third and fourth metatarsal head when directed from the plantar surface or by mediolateral compression of the entire forefoot. This tenderness may be associated with a click. Careful preparation of a metatarsal bar or similar adhesive felt pad usually provides a gratifying and useful means of allowing the athlete to finish the season. The pad should be cut so that pressure is taken from the second, third, and fourth metatarsal heads and placed under the head of the first. Surgical excision is necessary for most neuromata.

Sprains

Because of the number and array of foot ligaments as well as the forces applied and the various ranges of motion possible, sprains are common. The physician should be familiar with the more common foot sprains. Sprains may be either dynamic or static in origin. The first cuneiform bone and medial malleolus are anchored to the cuboid bone by the cruciate ligament. Sprains of the lateral ankle also involve the cruciate. There is edema, pain, and tenderness along the course of the ligament on the instep of the foot. Adhesive strapping for 2 weeks is usually sufficient to produce good healing. Vigorous running in the poorly conditioned athlete, or repetitive running on a hard surface, can strain the intermetatarsal ligaments. Circular adhesive strapping over the metatarsal heads produces a good result in a short period. It is important that the circumferential taping be done with the foot at rest without tension and that the taping not extend completely around the foot so as to constrict the tissue. Hyperextension of the first toe can often sprain the metatarsal–phalangeal joint. This can occur during the violent push-off in sprinting on artificial turf ("turf toe") or from a blocked kick in the martial arts.

During the acute injury phase, weight bearing should be prohibited and adhesive strapping employed in order to prevent further plantar flexion. Once walking with taping is pain free, slow progressive jogging should be allowed. Sprains of the arch and plantar fascia can be due to trauma as well as static forces. Violent eversion and inversion can damage the plantar ligaments. Pain may be localized to the particular ligaments involved, though in a static injury there is usually pain along the plantar ligament from its attachment to the metatarsal heads posterior to the calcaneus. Plantar fascia sprains often occur at the beginning of the season when the athlete resumes wearing flat athletic shoes after an entire winter of shoes with good arch support. The careful preparation of arch support or similar orthotic devices, followed by rehabilitative foot exercises within the limits of pain, is usually satisfactory, though recovery from such sprains may

often be prolonged. A long period of minimum weight bearing or none at all may be required in association with analgesics and anti-inflammatory agents.

Dislocations

Dislocations of the foot bones, although less frequent than ankle dislocations, must be treated with early reduction and further evaluation for complicating fractures. The reduction technique must be chosen with some amount of discretion. For instance, dislocation of the small toes, while incapacitatingly painful, can be treated with ringside reduction, adhesive strapping to an adjacent digit, and return to play. Such dislocations are common in full-contact martial arts where an improper kick in combination with a forceful downward block can hyperextend the phalangeal joint resulting in dislocation (Fig. 18-9). An infrequent, newly recognized foot dislocation has been termed the *locked cuboid* or cuboid syndrome.[20] Approximately 4 percent of athletes with foot injuries have this diagnosis. Individuals with pronated feet are at risk because with this pedal configuration the peroneus longus exerts greater mechanical tension on the cuboid as a fulcrum than in the nonpronated foot. With increased activity the lateral aspect of the cuboid is pulled dorsally while the medial aspect moves in a plantar direction. Locking in this position occurs such that normal foot motion is inhibited. General foot pain and referred pain along the course of the peroneus longus tendon produce diagnostic confusion. Direct palpation of the cuboid along its peroneal groove elicits pain and tenderness in the athlete with this condition. Sharp downward thrust with the thumbs in a posterolateral direction with respect to the calcaneous reduces the dislocation. Thereafter adhesive strapping or a cuboid orthotic can be used especially in chronic cases. However less common dislocations involving the metatarsals or the first and second cuneiform bones usually require open reduction and internal fixation in order to prevent posttraumatic arthritis and aseptic necrosis. Following reduction and first aid, the athlete should be advised that it takes 4 to 5 weeks for a toe dislocation to heal properly provided that further injury does not occur; then, rest, elevation, and the usual supportive therapies are applied. It is well to pre-

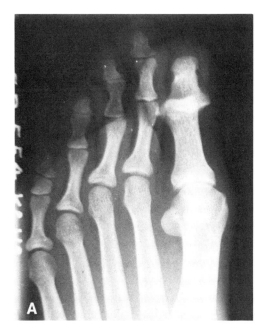

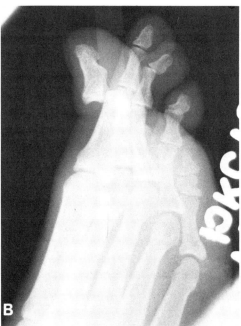

FIGURE 18-9. First toe dislocation following a blocked front kick in a karate tournament. **A.** AP film. **B.** Lateral film.

scribe a carefully fitted shoe with a firm, inflexible sole.

Fractures

With the exception of fractures of the small toes of the foot, proper treatment of foot fractures invariably requires the application of cast and the restriction of weight bearing for variable periods. Missed jumps, as in pole vaulting or high jumping, can cause compressive fracture forces in eversion, inversion, adduction, abduction, flexion, or extension on the calcaneus and talus. Because of the complex nature of some of these fractures, their management should be done in conjunction with a specialist for best results.

The central portion of the foot, consisting of the cuboid and cuneiform bones, is usually fractured in association with sprains and dislocations of the interconnecting ligament rather than by direct compression. The choice of closed or open reduction depends on the size and degree of displacement of the avulsed fragment. Regardless of choice, once reduction has been achieved, immobilization in a plaster cast that maintains reduction perfectly and does not allow weight bearing should be used for 2 or 3 weeks; a walking cast is acceptable thereafter. Eventual adhesive strapping in conjunction with a tailored arch orthotic and progressive rehabilitation within the confines of pain are the standard fare. The most common fractures of the foot involve the metatarsals and phalanges. In particular, the single most common fracture is of the base of the fifth metatarsal, which can occur with forced inversion and adduction. Symptomatic support is for the most part sufficient, though good results can be also achieved by closed reduction, immobilization, and the application of a posterior splint for 2 weeks, followed by a walking cast for another 2 to 3 weeks. Adhesive strapping has alternatively been employed. Forced plantar flexion can fracture–dislocate the other metatarsal bases. There is usually localized tenderness and x rays often reveal the avulsion fracture. Because joint integrity is essential for normal foot motion, careful consideration must be made concerning surgical fixation should the bone not easily be held in place. Fracture of the metatarsal shafts can follow a direct crushing blow to the dorsal surface of the foot or repeated microtrauma as would occur from running for prolonged periods on a hard surface. The "karate foot" is a fracture of the fifth metatarsal from a poorly aimed side kick meeting an unyielding olecranon. The more obvious fractures are easy to diagnose. Treatment consists of reduction and immobilization. The athlete who complains of dull aching pain over the foot dorsum, localized to 1 or 2 metatarsals for several weeks and especially aggravated by running or jumping, should be more thoroughly evaluated for a stress or "march" fracture. Often, such athletes have already been under a physician's care for a "foot sprain." Serial x rays may note the faint development of a tell tale callus or linear fracture line. Occasionally it may be necessary to do a bone scan. Rest, preferably with no weight bearing until the symptoms subside, is the preferred course. Often, this is difficult for the eager and active athlete, so it is wise to prescribe an alternative interim set of training exercises—e.g., swimming or upper-body weight training.

There are a number of accessory bones of the foot (accessory navicular and medial sesamoid of the first metatarsal) that can be fractured. Forceful eversion or vigorous contraction of the posterior tibial muscle can pull the accessory navicular from its attachment. Forced dorsiflexion in accompaniment with a traumatic blow to the ball of the foot can fracture the medial sesamoid. In either case, further activity requiring the use of the foot is prohibited. An immobilization cast for several weeks can produce good results providing early diagnosis was made; late diagnosis often requires removal of the sesamoid.

Fractures of the first or great toe deserve special consideration in that this toe is an important element in normal mobility—it assists in walk-over from heel to toe and, through marked dorsiflexion, aids in propulsion—and balance. The toe can be injured on the playing field (often from stubbing on artificial turf or crushing from a cleated opponent's foot) or off the field (should a piece of heavy locker-room equipment or bench fall on the unprotected foot). A good procedural guideline is that fractures of the distal phalanx can be treated in the same manner as fractures of the small toes—i.e., relative immobilization by taping or splinting to an adjacent

member followed by rehabilitation within the confines of pain. Fractures of the proximal phalanx or the metatarsal–phalangeal joint should be treated vigorously in terms of accurate reduction and adequate immobilization. Sometimes surgical fixation is necessary for a good result.

Miscellaneous Conditions

The primary care physician should be familiar with a variety of other foot conditions. Various combinations of extensor tendon contractures produce hammer-toe deformities (e.g., figure skater's foot). Usually the metatarsophalangeal joint is held in extension and interphalangeal joints are in flexion. The dorsum of the distal phalanx becomes chronically irritated, resulting in corn formation. If recognized and treated in the early stages, surgical repair can usually be avoided. The simple construction of a makeshift orthotic can go a long way in relieving the player's symptoms as well as effecting early return to sports participation. Subungual exostoses, particularly of the first toe, typically develop after repeated trauma (basketball stuffing with toe smash). The exostosis, which extends under the nail, can be very painful and sensitive to pressure or direct force. Surgical removal is indicated provided the condition has been differentiated from ingrown toenail, contusion with hematoma, or malignant tumor.

Ingrown Toenail

An ingrown toenail (unguis incarnatus) is a very painful condition which may involve any of the toes, most commonly the big toe. Successful treatment usually results in an eternally devoted patient. In the initial stages, therapy should be conservative and directed at the underlying inflammation and edema. If there is an associated paronchyia, incision and drainage should be performed. Simple podiatric measures such as trimming the nail edge and cleaning the ungual gutters, followed by packing with a cotton wick soaked in an antibiotic or iodinated ointment, go a long way in preventing further inflammation and infection. Occasionally, if the deformity persists and infections are recurrent, surgical excision of the offending portion of the nail should be performed. It is not necessary to remove the entire nail; a simple "straight-back" procedure of the offending side suffices. Though there are predisposing hereditary factors for the condition, improper footwear which is too tight or constricting can also instigate it. Therefore, it is imperative that the athlete's social as well as competition shoes be reviewed in order to prevent recurrence.

Hallux valgus can occur for genetic as well as environmental reasons, such as tight fitting narrow pumps. It occurs in association with bursitis of the metatarsal–phalangeal joint (bunion). Repeated episodes of irritation lead to bone hypertrophy and callus formation at the "bunion joint," with gradual lateral abductive deviation of the first toe. There are variable amounts of functional disability. Best treatment is early recognition and modification of shoes and other predisposing factors and the preparation of an adhesive donut surrounding the bunion in order to alleviate pressure from the joint (Fig. 18-10).

Common Foot Deformities

Finally, the physician should have a working knowledge of common foot deformities and their relationship to malfunction and overuse syndromes associated with the biomechanics and kinematics of walking and running.[21] The normal nonrigid foot consists of the calcaneus functioning around a perpendicular 5° valgus position when standing. When there is eversion of the foot (valgus) to between 5° and 10°, there is moderate flatfoot deformity; when deviation is beyond 10°, flatfoot deformity is se-

vere. Opposite degrees of deformity are referred to as arching of the foot. Inversion (varus) attitude is moderate if 5° or less and is usually a flexible deformity as the calcaneus can be pronated well beyond the perpendicular. An inability to pronate beyond the perpendicular produces a moderate to severe *cavus* deformity. The forefoot may also be everted or inverted. It is important to bear in mind that the flexible deformities must be preventively managed since recurrent secondary "microsubluxations" can result in arthritic changes over the years. Additionally, rear-foot varus is associated with an increased tendency toward hamstring strains and buttock–hip joint problems. Cavus foot, on the other hand, is predisposed to medial calcaneus contusions, possible subsequent development of an accessory bursa, and traumatic fibroma. Moderate cavus pathology predisposes the foot to plantar fascial sprains and callus formation under the metatarsal head and metatarsalgia. Ankle sprains are common as there are poor shock-absorbing properties in this foot. Finally, hammer toes and talar exostoses present as part of this foot deformity. (The reader is referred to a standard text on pedal biomechanics and pathology for a more detailed description.)

Remember also that the athlete's footwear should be thoroughly inventoried, including noncompetition, social shoes which may be responsible for the underlying pathology. All shoes should be carefully examined especially in the area of the player's complaint: there may be a rip, tear, deformity, or protruding edge that is irritating the foot. Additionally,

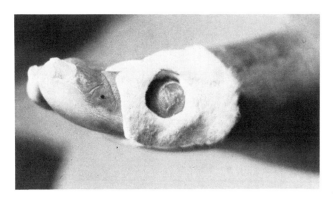

Figure 18-10. An example of an easily fashioned adhesive felt device for bursitis of the first MP joint.

the sole of the shoe may belie underlying foot deformity—excessive pronation or supination represented by frictional abrasion. Important clues may often be gleaned from such a thorough exam and provide the actual etiology for what would otherwise appear to be a secondary or unrelated factor.

A good progression for rehabilitation of ankle/foot injuries is as follows: bearing of weight and walking when there is no pain; jogging when there is no limp on simple ambulation; running thereafter; and return to full competitive activities when sprinting, cutting, and abrupt starts and stops can be performed without difficulty.

REFERENCES

1. Beaulieu JD: Developing a stretching program. Phys Sports Med 9(11):59–69, 1981.
2. Gold S: Unicyclist's sciatica. N Engl J Med 305(4):231–232, 1981.
3. McConnell RY, Rush GA: Mechanical bull syndrome. South Med J 75(6):681–686, 1982.
4. Hoppenfeld S: Physical examinations of the knee joint by complaint. Orthop Clin N Am 10(1):3, 1979.
5. Marshall JL, Rubin RM: Knee ligament injuries. Clin Orthop 123:115, 1977.
6. Noble J: Lesions of the menisci. J Bone Joint Surg 59(4):480, 1977.
7. Goodfellow J: Patello-femoral joint mechanics and pathology. J Bone Joint Surg (Br) 58(3):291, 1976.
8. Haycock CE: Sports related problems of women. Mod Med (July) 7:56–64, 1981.
9. Cofield RH, Brian RS: Acute dislocation of the patella. J Trauma 17(7):526–531, 1977.
10. Percy EC: Acute dislocation of the patella. Can Med Assoc J 105:1176, 1971.
11. Renne J: The iliotibial band friction syndrome. J Bone Joint Surg 57:1110–1111, 1975.
12. Insall J: Chondromalacia patellae: Patellar malalignment syndrome. J Bone Joint Surg (Am) 10(1):117, 1979.
13. O'Donoghue DH: Treatment of Injuries to Athletes. Philadelphia, WB Saunders, 1976, pp 672–678.
14. Rudo ND, Noble HB, Conn J: Popliteal artery entrapment syndrome in athletes. Phys Sports Med 10(5):104–114, 1982.
15. Dewitt L, Greenberg H: Roller disco neuropathy. J Am Med Assoc 236(8):836, 1981.
16. Brody DM: Running injuries. CIBA Clin Symp 32(4):19–20, 1980.
17. Clement DB, Tauton JE, Smart GW, et al: A survey of overuse running injuries. Phys Sports Med 9(5):47–58, 1981.
18. Eggold JF: Orthotics in the prevention of runners' overuse injuries. Phys Sports Med 9(3):124–131, 1981.
19. Slocum DB: The shin splint syndrome. Medical aspects and differential diagnosis. Am J Surg 114:875–881, 1967.
20. Newell SG, Woodle A: Cuboid syndrome. Phys Sports Med 9(4):71–76, 1981.
21. Subotnick SI: The flat foot. Phys Sports Med 9(8):85–91, 1981.

19
Common Skin Problems of Athletes

Richard B. Birrer

In general the dermatologic illnesses that affect athletes are similar to those in the general population. However, there are certain skin diseases peculiar to the athletic population with great impact not only on the individual athlete but also partners, opponents, and teammates.[1,2] It is always important to bear in mind that a variety of these skin conditions may produce a significant amount of morbidity for the athlete and, to a large degree, limit participation in sports. The majority of sports-related skin problems are due to infective agents or physical factors. A variety of bacterial, fungal, viral, and parasitic organisms can produce skin infections in the athlete. The physician must become familiar with these lesions in order to diagnose and treat the individual athlete so as to facilitate early return to the sport, as well as prevent epidemic spread to others in the competition. Contact sports, especially wrestling and the martial arts, provide a significant opportunity for the epidemic dissemination of these infections; thus, the temporary removal of an athlete from active sports participation is often mandatory as part of the treatment modality.

BACTERIAL INFECTIONS

Group A β-hemolytic *Streptococci* and coagulase-positive *Staphylococcus* cause *impetigo* which is contagious and characterized by an initial small, pus-filled blister. This rapidly breaks, leaving an erythematous weeping ulcer which then becomes covered by a honey-golden crust. The staphylococcal variety tends to produce a flaccid blister which becomes cloudy and is rapidly replaced by a thin, scaly crust. The warm environments of gymnasiums, saunas, and steam rooms, poor personal hygiene, and ancillary skin illnesses such as atopic or contact dermatitis or scabies can contribute to the development of impetigo. Treatment consists of administration of streptococcal and staphylococcal systemic antibiotics (penicillin or penicillinase-resistant penicillin, or erythromycin for allergic patients) and mandatory discontinuation of all sports until the condition clears.

Staphylococcus is also responsible for folliculitis, furuncles, and carbuncles. Predisposing factors include maceration of the skin secondary to training mats or certain forms of weight-lifting equipment (bench press), occlusive clothing (abdominal belts or wet suits), poor hygiene, and frictional trauma (athletic supporters, protective pads). Involvement of the superficial portion of the hair follicle by a pustule constitutes *folliculitis,* whereas deeper involvement produces a *furuncle,* which may or may not be accompanied by local cellulitis. Because of the superficial nature of folliculitis, topical antibiotics and antiseptic cleansers are usually sufficient. Deeper infections—particularly *carbuncles,* which consist of a number of furuncles—should be treated primarily with incision and drainage and may require systemic antibiotics if there are constitutional symptoms (fever, chills).

Pseudomonas species, and occasionally streptococci and staphylococci, are responsible for *external otitis* or swimmer's ears. Although the treatment is topical application of polymyxin, colistin, and neomycin, it is very important to treat the primary underlying etiologic factor: the mascerating effect of water. Necrotic debris within the canal should be manually removed with an ear curette for the best results. The presence of systemic signs or symptoms such as fever, anorexia, and malaise can accompany external otitis although examination should be made for further etiologies.

Corynebacterium can produce two forms of dermatologic pathology. The first is *pitted keratolysis,* which consists of the formation of uninflamed, discrete pits in the stratum corneum of the soles and occasionally the palms. The punctate erosions often become discolored by dirt, producing a brown or tan appearance. Predisposing factors include the presence of water, especially hyperhydrosis of the foot, in combination with pressure; thus the sole in the heel and ball areas is most prone. Treatment should therefore include elimination of water and the topical application of gentian violet or 5 percent formalin solution or topical administration of erythromycin.

Corynebacterium minutissimum produces a well demarcated, finely scaled, erythematous to brown, dry epidermal infection, termed *erythrasma,* of the intertriginous areas: the inner gluteal folds, inframammary regions, axillae, groin, and digital web. Diagnosis can be easily made by the coral orange to red fluorescence under a Wood's lamp. The condition commonly occurs in warm moist environments; treatment therefore should consist of dry loose clothing and the application of keratolytic agent such as 3 percent sulfur and salicylic acid ointment. The treatment of choice however is 500 milligrams erythromycin for 7 to 14 days. Uncommon bacterial infections include the following:

- *Swimming pool granuloma,* caused by *Microbacterium marinum* and characterized by erythematous violaceous nodules which may occasionally ulcerate or become verrucous and are derived from swimming either in pools or in salt- or fresh-water sources
- *Erysipeloid,* secondary to *Erysipelothrix rhusiopathiae,* which occurs in individuals handling fish or shell fish and appears on the hand as a red or purplish urticarial plaque and can be accompanied by systemic symptoms
- *Tularemia* caused by *Francisella tularensis,* which can be acquired by hunters who handle cottontail rabbits, although occasionally the infection can be transmitted from arthropod bites (i.e., ticks)

Further discussion of rarer skin diseases is handled in standard medical/dermatologic textbooks.

FUNGAL INFECTIONS

The ubiquitous nature of dermatophytes and such common predisposing factors as heat, friction, occlusive athletic wear, adhesive tape, and maceration are in large part responsible for the frequent occurrence of skin infections. The typical forms of these infections include tinea pedis (athlete's foot), tinea cruris (jock or judo itch), tinea corporis (ringworm), and intertrigo. Since the various tineal infections frequently coexist, an athlete with one variety should be examined for occurrence of the others. Infections may range from completely asymptomatic to very gross symptomatology including pruritus and painful weeping lesions which may become secondarily infected. The lesions of tinea cruris often spare the genitals but symmetrically involve the groin and upper/inner thigh areas. Tinea pedis, on the other hand, can take a variety of distinctive forms. One type entails just simple inner digital toe-web involvement characterized by thick scaling, fissuring, maceration, and variable amounts of erythema. The second variety, known as the vesiculobullous type, can involve the instep and can be remarkably erythematous, often resembling cellulitis. Redness, scaling, and remarkable thickening of the stratum corneum of the entire sole characterizes the third form of tinea pedis and is referred to as hyperkeratotic. Though diagnosis is most conveniently made by physical examination, it is wisest to take a scraping of the lateral active border of the lesion for simultaneous examination under a microscope and culture on special media (DTM or Sabourand's medium).

Treatment is twofold. First, topical therapy consisting preferably of miconazole nitrate or clotrimazole two to three times daily for 2 to 4 weeks is usually adequate. (The author feels that tolnaftate is not as effective.) Hyperkeratotic lesions should be trimmed or treated with keratolytic agents, whereas vesiculobullous infections respond well to astringent compresses (Domeboro's solution). Secondly, preventive measures are indicated, such as good hygiene, liberal use of drying powders (talc with anhydrous aluminum chloride), drying of the intertriginous areas after exposure to water, and application of loose soft cotton socks. It is important to continue these general prophylactic measures because of the ubiquitous nature of fungi as well as their ability to survive for many months after rigorous laundering and hygienic methods.

Intertrigo is caused by the yeastlike fungus *Candida albicans* and is characterized by beefy-red, macerated lesions in the intertriginous folds of the body. It may be accompanied by various forms of scaling at the margins as well as erythematous, papulopustular satellite lesions. Warmth, moisture, darkness, and maceration are predisposing factors to the infection. Once again, therefore, treatment consists of removing the predisposing factors as well as the application of specific anticandidal medication (clotrimazole or miconazole nitrate) applied three or four times daily are necessary. It is questionable whether direct contact, as would occur in wrestling, could possibly transfer dermatophyte or candidal infections under normal conditions. However, if predisposing factors such as those mentioned are present, it is possible that the conditions would be suitable for transfer of the infective agent.

Rarely, *onychomycosis* can occur, usually secondary to tinea pedis, though candida is often the cause of the infection on the fingernails. Because of the chronic nature of a fungal nail infection and its deep-seated location, topical measures are useless. Long-term administration of griseofulvin is indicated; occasionally, surgical removal of the nail must also be performed. Finally, extensive corporeal infections due to dermatophytes often respond best to systemic administration of griseofulvin.

Tinea versicolor, common in swimmers and divers especially in the tropics, is a chronic superficial asymptomatic fungal infection usually at the trunk, consisting of pink to tan or white finely scaled macular patches that often collect to larger areas.

Diagnosis can be confirmed by culture or orange fluorescence with a Wood's light. Treatment is with selenium sulfide suspensions which are best applied after an evening shower and left on overnight for each day of the first week; the following week there is no treatment and the third week the treatment is repeated. Unfortunately, recurrence is high and retreatment several months down the line becomes necessary.

An unusual deep fungal infection that may be seen in hunters and fishermen is that caused by *Sporotrichum schenckii* known as *sporotrichosis*. The ulcerated, painless nodule that develops at the inoculation site can spread along the local lymphatic vessel. It is best treated with a supersaturated solution of potassium iodide.

VIRAL INFECTIONS

A variety of viruses can produce skin infections, the most characteristic of which is the *papova* group. This DNA virus produces common warts, plantar warts, flat and filiform warts which are generally asymptomatic—though, when in a particular location or of certain size, they can become quite painful. The virus is transmitted by contact (direct or indirect) as well as autoinoculation, though studies have shown that transmission among athletes does not appear to be a problem. Diagnosis is clinical and such characteristics as pain on lateral compression and capillary bleeding or the presence of thrombosed capillaries on paring with a scalpel or razor are useful. Because the optimal performance of the athlete is affected, warts must be eradicated. Treatment modalities include chemical cauterization [topical retinoic acid or salicylic acid plasters (Duofilm)] surgical removal (electrocautery or scalpel), or cryotherapy (liquid nitrogen). Surgical excision is usually not performed on the sole of the foot because of the potentiality for painful scar formation. On the other hand the DNA-containing pox virus that causes molluscum contagiosum is contagious through direct human contact. This is particularly the case among weight lifters, gymnasts, and wrestlers. The discrete flesh-colored or pearly white dimpled papules can be treated with cryotherapy, curettage, or the application of cantharidin.

The most common viral skin infection is due to herpes simplex and can be either primary or secondary. Approximately 85 to 90 percent of individuals have a primary infection by the end of their adolescence. It has been noted that approximately 75 percent of these individuals later have a recurrent episode which represents reactivation or recrudescence of an established latent infection. The site of recurrence is typically the site of the primary infection, though it is possible for certain individuals to develop a new primary infection at a different site, usually due to cutaneous inoculation of the virus. The new primary infection is clinically and symptomatically indistinguishable from a typical recurrent episode. The primary infection can be moderate to severe with extensive, painful cutaneous lesions associated with systemic toxicity (fever, malaise, fatigue, localized adenopathy). Recurrent infections, however, tend to be mild, localized, and not associated with systemic illness.

Recurrent herpes, particularly of the lip, is often precipitated by sunlight, menses, stress, and recurrent viral illness with a fever. Thus, athletes who are in noncontact sports but exposed to sunlight are at high risk for this problem. On the other hand, inoculation herpes is common in such contact sports as wrestling, martial arts, or rugby and is often referred to as herpes gladiatorum.[3] In both instances, the clinical picture is one of small, clustered erythematous-based vesicles which rapidly become cloudy and purulent, then dry and crust usually in a week's time. Occasionally, under conditions of poor hygiene, the clustered vesicles can become superinfected with streptococci or staphylococci, forming one large eroded area. Any area of the body can be involved, though in wrestlers it tends to be the cheek or the inside of the arm which contacts the face. It tends to be the scalp in rugby players, the knees, shoulders, and elbows in basketball players, and the posterior shoulder in judo athletes.

It is mandatory for the physician to identify and remove the individual at once from continued competition. The infected athlete should be benched for at least 5 days (120 hours) after the initial vesicles appear, or perhaps until the lesions crust over and heal. Teammates with known atopic dermatitis are at high risk for herpetic infection, particularly

for generalized infections. Treatment of herpes infection includes the application of astringent compresses (Domeboro's solution) and the use of antibiotic ointment (bacitracin or povidone). Newer agents such as acyclovir (Zovirax), are specific for the treatment of herpes and are definitely indicated in active infections. The most feared complication of any herpes simplex infection concerns ocular involvement. Typified by a characteristic dendritic corneal ulceration, this requires immediate aggressive treatment by an ophthalmologist and typically involves such antiviral agents as idoxuridine, adenine arabanoside, and acyclovir.

Recently endemic percutaneous transmission of the hepatitis virus has been described in wrestlers.[4] Close contact among the same athletes in association with minor scrapes and cuts appears to be a significant risk factor. Echovirus has been reported to cause aseptic meningitis outbreaks particularly in team sports.[5]

ARTHROPOD INFECTIONS

A variety of arthropods can cause skin lesions in humans. The arachnids of medical importance include mites (scabies), ticks, spiders, and scorpions. The insects of importance are mosquitoes, bees, wasps, ants, lice, fleas, and flies. Infestations with the itch mite (*Sarcoptes scabiei* var. *hominis*) and bloodsucking lice *(Pediculus)* are the two major organisms that affect the athletic population. Scabies is an extremely pruritic condition acquired primarily through close personal contact, though it may be transmitted by fomites such as linen, towels, clothing, and equipment. The female itch mite can survive from 1 to 3 days in a variety of uniform items and other commonly used protective gear and among athletes who share common locker facilities, towels, or showers. Characteristic symptomatology includes pruritus, particularly at night, and the principle findings on physical exam are the scabetic burrow (a thin, discolored, S-shaped line $\frac{1}{2}$ to 2 centimeters in length) and, possibly, various associated papules, excoriations, vesicles, or nonspecific eczematous patches. These lesions are most commonly located in the inner digital webs of the hand, the anterior surface of the wrist, elbows, nipples, lower abdomen, genitalia, inner gluteal cleft, and umbilicus. The definitive diagnosis is made by microscopic examination of the mite from scrapings taken from the burrow vesicle, papule, or eczematous patch. Eggs and fecal material can also be considered diagnostic and, in the absence of any microscopic findings, the clinical picture usually is sufficient to make the diagnosis.

The treatment of choice is gamma benzene hexachloride lotion (Kwell, Lindane, or Scabene) applied to the entire body from the neck down and washed off after 12 to 24 hours. It is a good idea to repeat the treatment in 1 week in order to destroy any recently hatched nymphs or larvae. In addition, topical steroids and antihistamines are useful in supportive therapy for the pruritus and systemic allergic component. It is important for the primary care physician strongly to consider treatment of immediate family, close friends, sexual contacts, and other team members in order to prevent reinfection and small epidemics. Finally, all clothing, linens, and protective gear, which could harbor the infective mite, should be specially washed in very hot water or dry cleaned. It is not necessary to treat furniture, rugs, bathrooms, or other such objects with specific insecticidal poisons.

Lice are bloodsucking organisms that parasitize man in three forms: the head louse *(Pediculus humanis)*, the body louse *(Pediculus humanis,* var. *corporis)*, and the pubic or crab louse *(Phthirus pubis)*. The epidemiologic considerations presented for scabies are applicable to lice infestations. Thus, small epidemics can easily occur in team sports. In particular, the head louse is usually transferred through shared uniforms or brushes; the body louse through bedding and uniforms; and the pubic louse by personal contact and occasionally fomites such as uniforms, athletic supporters, bedding, or towels. The primary symptom of lice infestation is pruritis. The skin findings are often minimal, but when present are notable for the presence of nits on the hair shafts, possible secondary infections from chronic excoriations, hives, and perhaps persistent papules and chronic eczematous changes. With a large number of organisms, it is possible on occasion to ob-

serve with a magnifying glass adult organisms on the hair shafts in the axilla, on the head, in the pubic area, or even on eyelashes. The treatment of pediculosis is the same as for scabies except that the γ-benzene hexachloride lotion should be applied only to the infected areas. Towels, linen, clothing, uniforms, and protective gear should be washed in very hot water or dry cleaned. Lice on eyelashes can be treated with physostigmine ophthalmic ointment, although petrolatum ointment is just as effective and is cheaper and less toxic. It is easiest to remove nits with a solution of vinegar and warm water followed by the application of a fine-tooth comb. Remember to treat all family and team contacts of the infected athlete. For an unknown reason, the head louse does not affect blacks.

Numerous other stinging and biting insects can produce dermatologic as well as a general allergic response. *Hymenoptera* bites (bees, wasps, yellow jackets) are adequately described in Chapter 13. Certain outdoor sports, particularly hunting, can expose the unwary to tick bites, which are painless. The risks from such bites include the production of Rocky Mountain spotted tick fever and the Lyme arthritis syndrome (erythema chronicum migrans). Local tick-bite granulomas can also occur. Removal of the tick should be done carefully and nonforcibly. The application of such substances as mineral oil, rubbing alcohol, or gasoline aids in the easy removal of the tick, which should be accomplished with a pair of forceps. It is most important to remove not only the body but also the proboscis of the insect. It is most unusual for a competing athlete to suffer scorpion or spider bites, particularly of the variety *Latrodectus mactans* (black widow) or *Loxosceles* (brown recluse). Such bites can produce allergic or toxic reactions and need to be treated aggressively (see standard medical textbooks).

Preventive measures are probably the most important step regarding insect bites. Diethyltoluamide-containing insect repellents are quite effective against a variety of fleas, flies, and mosquitoes, but often require frequent application, particularly in hot, windy weather. This substance can also be used for treating clothes, tents, nets, and other sleeping equipment. Unfortunately, there is no insect repellent useful against the *Hymenoptera*.

AQUATIC INFECTIONS

Certain forms of reptilian and aquatic life can produce a variety of dermatologic lesions (see Chapter 25). Brief mention should also be made of *sea bather's eruption,* which typically occurs in salt-water swimming areas, particularly in Florida and the Caribbean. It is a self-limited pruritic, papular lesion of unknown etiology which requires only symptomatic treatment. *Swimmer's itch,* on the other hand, is caused by the penetration of schistosomal cercariae and is characterized by pruritic papules resulting from inflammation at the point of penetration. Swimmer's itch can be acquired in small freshwater lakes in the midwestern United States and its course is typically self-limited, requiring only symptomatic therapy. Prolonged exposure to swimming pool water can produce bleaching effects on the hair due to the excessive amounts of chlorine, as well as "green hair" due to certain high levels of chemicals in the pool; simple shampooing can prevent the latter condition. Finally, *salabrasion* is caused by the combined action of friction due to tight swimwear or wet suits and the abrasive action of the salt. The lesion is directly related to the amount of time spent in salt water and the fit of the swimwear.

PHYSICAL FACTORS

Physical factors causing skin diseases can be subdivided into mechanical, environmental, and chemical conditions. Prolonged horizontal shearing forces can produce prickle cell necrosis resulting in the accumulation of fluid within the epidermis, producing what is commonly known as blisters or vesicles. Frictional forces are increased if the skin is moist but are decreased if the skin is dry, greasy, or very wet. With the exception of such underlying diseases as epidermolysis bullosa and the Weber Cockayne syndrome, the prevention of blisters in athletes is directly related to the reduction of frictional forces. Therefore, footwear should fit well. Petrolatum emollient, talc, adhesive tape, or thick socks can be used to reduce frictional pressure over areas that rub against the skin. First aid for blisters

requires the multiple aspiration of fluid during the first 24 hours with preservation of the vesicle top: this produces the least amount of pain and the most protection from secondary infection.

The chronic prolongation of friction or pressure on the skin produces tylomata or *calluses.* These hyperkeratotic reactions typically occur on the weight-bearing sites or on the hands of weight lifters. They are usually asymptomatic but can be markedly painful. Diagnosis can be easily made by the simple paring of the callus in which the normal papillary skin-line pattern is preserved in calluses, whereas it is disrupted in warts and corns. Furthermore, lateral pinching pressure on a callus/corn does not produce pain (but produces exquisite pain in a wart), whereas vertical pressure does produce pain. Treatment of tylomata is twofold: First, the lesion(s) should be pared down with a No. 15 scalpel blade or via use of 40-percent salicylic acid plaster. The plaster should be applied daily over a week's time in order to remove as much of the callus as possible. The resultant whitened and soft skin is easily removed with pumice stone or callus file. Secondly, every effort should be made to identify the etiology: improperly fitting shoes, any inherent biomechanical problems, or anatomic malformations. The most common cause is a poorly fitting shoe, which often is not the competition footwear but rather a dress or a work shoe. Therefore, all the athlete's shoes should be carefully examined for pressure points. When a particular set of footwear is identified as the problem, then either the footwear can be discarded or modified or an orthotic device can be prepared for the affected foot. A pontoon, horseshoe, or other similar adhesive felt device can be easily molded in the physician's office (Fig. 18-10).

Helomata or *corns* are similar in etiology, presentation, and treatment to tylomata. They tend to occur almost exclusively on the plantar surface of the feet and are usually more painful than calluses. Although they can occur at the site of any excessive pressure, common points are the metatarsal arch and the fourth interdigital web space as the result of pressure from the head of the proximal phalanx of the fifth toe and the base of the proximal phalanx of the fourth toe. Unlike calluses, corns on paring can be seen to interrupt the normal papillary skin line; corns also have a central translucent core. A surgical scalpel blade or 40-percent salicylic acid plasters are used for initial paring down of the lesion combined with pontoons, donuts, or similar adhesive felt pads for long-term management. Chronic frictional pressure should be relieved and the corn allowed to heal. The combined approach often does not necessitate the removal of the entire central core of the corn.

Striae distensae or *stretch marks* are of unknown etiology and are responsible for a considerable amount of worry in the athletic population. Striae are two and a half times more common in females than in males, tend to occur in areas where mechanical stresses stretch or distend the skin, are often associated with significant weight gains (body builders), and are typified by initially erythematous or somewhat dusky blue, linear, serpiginous depressions in the skin. Microscopically, the epidermis is shown to be atrophic. The lesions typically develop in gymnasts, weight lifters, and body builders, most commonly over the lower back and lateral thighs, buttocks, and anterior shoulders—in all cases perpendicular to the direction of skin tension. Though it is common knowledge that systemic glucocorticoidal excess as in Cushing disease can cause stretch marks, the regular use of topical steroids, especially the fluorinated ones, can also produce striae, particularly in the intertriginous or occluded sites such as the groin. With the exception of avoiding extreme weight gains or tension in the tissues, there is no known treatment for striae.

Subungual, splinter-like hemorrhages beneath the toenails occur in those sports in which horizontal and upper shearing forces on the distal nail plate are generated by abrupt stopping of the forward thrust toe against the tip of the shoe. The condition is commonly referred to as "tennis toe."[6] It is peculiar to those sports in which abrupt stopping is the rule: racket sports, basketball, and certain forms of martial arts. The typical distributions of the lesions are 25 percent in the first toe, 25 percent in the second, and the remaining 50 percent in both the first and second toes. Treatment includes cessation of the predisposing activity as well as the proper fitting of shoes.

Repeated minor trauma associated with sudden stops has been known to produce small punctate hemorrhages in the heel called calcaneal petechiae (black heel).[7] This condition may also be caused by sudden shearing forces or traumatic pinching of the heel skin. It is characterized by an area of spotted, bluish-black discoloration of the heel in the superficial dermis and overlying epidermis. The condition is also seen in toes and fingers and has been encountered in many sports, e.g., weight lifting, volleyball, racquet sports, running, chinning, football, basketball, baseball. It is more common in those sports played on hard surfaces. Because the condition is painless, has no complication, and resolves spontaneously, it is important to diagnose the condition properly to avoid unnecessary therapy, particularly surgery. The keynote is preventive care, which includes proper fitting of all footwear, wearing thicker socks, and the preparation of a piece of adhesive felt for the heel of the shoe.

Biochemical stress has been noted to cause loss of hair—*traumatic alopecia*—though it is commonly recognized in those individuals using tight hair curlers or certain hairstyles, such as ponytails, braids, or tight buns. It has been observed with the use of the balance beam due to repeated handstands and rollovers[8] and in the use of improperly fitted headgear in boxing and hockey. Treatment is simply the avoidance of the particular activity that resulted in the traumatic alopecia and use of properly fitting headwear.

Perhaps the most common dermatologic injury in sports medicine is the common *abrasion,* in which a certain amount of skin is mechanically scraped off the body (strawberry). Though the etiology of most abrasions is self-evident, there are occasions when the physician has to examine more carefully and interview the athlete for the etiology: mat burns in wrestlers or judo athletes; midtibula abrasions from rigid, poorly fitted ski boots; or shoulder burns from improperly fitted football shoulder pads. The treatment of abrasions is handled in Chapter 12.

Environmental factors are primarily related to extremes in temperature and the presence or absence of moisture. The mildest form of cold injury, referred to as *pernio,* occurs on the extremities, particularly the hands or feet and occasionally on the face, in a symmetrical fashion. It is characterized by erythematous bluish discolorations, some edema, nodule formation, and rarely vesiculobullous and ulcerative lesions.[9] There may be some burning and pruritus upon rewarming as well as nodular tenderness. Though the pathogenesis of the condition is unclear, both cold and wet conditions are necessary for pernio to occur. Prevention involves waterproof covering; treatment, warm bed rest and elevation of the involved extremity. With the popularity of such winter sports as skiing, hockey, ice skating, backpacking, mountain climbing, snowshoeing, and snowmobiling, plus the perennial addiction of running (jogger's penis),[10] the frequency of frostbite has increased. The most common injury seen on ski slopes, *frost-nip,* occurs typically on exposed surfaces of the body (ears, cheeks, chin, nose, face, and the digits); the skin tends to be white and numb. Rapid rewarming of these various areas is essential. It is best accomplished in a progressive fashion indoors. Recooling, preservation in snow or ice, rubbing, or the use of nicotine or alcohol are all prohibited. The application of certain facial creams prior to the sports activity is also useful in preventing frost-nip. More serious degrees of frostbite do occur in a variety of sports and are related to increased durations of exposure and lower temperatures (see Chapter 10). Finally, *angular cheilitis,* erythematous scaling and fissuring of the angles of the mouth, occurs from a combination of the cold and sun with the wind. The condition is prevalent in skiiers who would be best protected by using petrolatum-based lip screens, particularly on the corners of the mouth.

Though heat exhaustion and heat stroke are the most important environmental heat-induced disorders, there are several other conditions in the athlete which primarily relate to eccrine or sweat gland function. Excessive sweat gland function or *hyperhidrosis* not only can cause competitive embarrassment but also can limit optimal sports performance, predispose to the development of a variety of cutaneous fungal and bacterial diseases, and aggravate eczema and contact dermatitis. Emotional stress is a normal aspect of all sports competition and is usually reflected in palmar, plantar, and axillary

hyperhidrosis. Certain grip aids or gloves usually ameliorate the palmar condition and the use of 20 percent aluminum chloride and 80 percent absolute anhydrous alcohol solution, when applied to absolutely dry skin, is very good in reducing the amount of hyperhidrotic skin surface area. The solution is best used with a plastic wrap which is left in place for 6 to 8 hours; this is used daily until the desired effect is achieved. Anxiolytic agents, sedative drugs, and anticholinergic systemic medications are of limited value and should be discouraged. A 2 to 5 percent solution of formaldehyde is useful in treating plantar hyperhidrosis, as is appropriate footwear and a frequent change of cotton socks. The most common causes of hyperhidrosis are dehydration and the more dangerous conditions of heat stroke and heat exhaustion (see Chapter 10). Once the state of hydration of the athlete is guaranteed, attention should be turned to possible underlying neuropathic sweat gland disturbances and certain congenital and miscellaneous idiopathic diseases.

When sweat becomes trapped within the skin, miliaria or *heat rash* occurs. Miliaria can occur in three forms: *miliaria crystallina,* which occurs when sweat is trapped within the stratum corneum; *miliaria rubra* or prickly heat, which occurs when sweat is blocked in the deeper vital portion of the epidermis; and *miliaria profunda,* which occurs when sweat is blocked within the upper dermis. Miliaria crystallina is usually seen in mild sunburn; the vesicles appear most commonly on the exposed portion of the body, particularly the face. The condition is asymptomatic, subsiding rapidly when the sweating ceases or the damaged stratum corneum is lost. Miliaria rubra is an erythematous papulovesicular, occasionally pustular lesion located on portions of the body that are covered by clothing. The condition occurs in hot, humid and hot, dry climates, tends to be nonfollicular in distribution, and causes burning, pruritic, stinging sensations, which fade after several days unless excessive sweating occurs. Miliaria profunda occurs after recurrent episodes of miliaria rubra. It is characterized by a whitish papule similar to that of gooseflesh, is asymptomatic, and can become chronic in nature as a form of heat intolerance. Treatment for all three conditions is a cool environment, adequate ventilation, and light-weight cotton clothing plus the use of such ancillary techniques as anhydrous powders and lotions (calamine) which may absorb some of the excess sweat and afford symptomatic relief.

Erythema ab igne is an irreversible erythema which has a reticulated appearance and is often associated with hyperpigmentation and telangiectasia. It is caused by prolonged exposure to intense local heat and can be seen in athletes who, having exercised in cold environments, placed themselves (particularly, their legs) in front of an open fire or electric radiator.

Dermatologic conditions related to exposure to the sun are discussed in Chapter 25.

A variety of irritants in sensitizers can produce *contact dermatitis* in athletic activities. Two types of reaction can result: primary irritant contact dermatitis and allergic contact dermatitis. The most common form, *irritant dermatitis,* is commonly due to repeated or prolonged contact with particular kinds of cologne, detergent, soap, or solvent and may in fact result from excessive hygienic measures. *Allergic contact dermatitis,* though less common, can result from use of rubber and leather products (pads, straps, bands, sneakers, hand grips, adhesive tapes, swimming equipment, rubber balls, shoes, jackets, chin straps, gloves), grip aids (beeswax, rosin, benzoin), topical medications (anesthetics, antibiotics, liniments, certain forms of rubbing compound and moisturizer), and plants (poison ivy, poison oak, and poison sumac). Both irritant and allergic dermatitis produce a nondistinguishable eczema: vesiculation, crusting, weeping erythema in the acute phase, followed by lichenification, scaling, fissure, and dry skin in chronic phase. The diagnosis is clinched, however, by noting the distribution and configuration of the lesion; the lesion tends to be confined to the area of contact, may have sharp borders and acute angles, and appear artificial at times. Treatment includes removal of the offending agent, application of astringent soaks (Burrow's compresses), and the use of topical steroid creams with the fluorinated varieties being reserved for the most refractive cases. In very severe cases of contact dermatitis, systemic steroids such as prednisone

should be used at a dosage of 50 to 60 milligrams daily, being tapered over 2 to 3 weeks. If it is unclear as to what the offending agent was, patch testing should be considered as well as a consultation with an allergist. Finally, ancillary contributing factors such as friction, moisture, and heat should be eliminated or minimized.

MISCELLANEOUS

There are several common pre-existing dermatologic problems that can be exacerbated by concurrent athletic activities. Some of the more important ones include physical urticarias, xeroderma, acne, atopic dermatitis, dyshidrotic eczema, and Raynaud's disease and phenomenon. The detailed description of these individual pathologic states is reserved for standard medical texts. However, it should be noted that common sports conditions such as wind, humidity, heat, and cold, often exacerbate them and, together with such individual athletic problems as friction, pressure, occlusion, clothing (especially wool), equipment, solvents, and detergents, can compound the problem. In particular, irritation from padding in football or rugby (footballer's acne) or weight-lifting equipment, such as the bench press or the bar in squatting (lifter's acne), can cause an acne flare. Its treatment, in addition to the regular dermatologic regimen, includes removal of the offending irritant.

REFERENCES

1. Houston SD, Knox J: Skin problems related to sports and recreational activities. Cutis 19:487–493, 1977.
2. Spoor HJ: Sports identification marks. Cutis 19(4): 453–456, 1977.
3. Porter PS, Baughman RD: Epidemiology of herpes simplex among wrestlers. J Am Med Assoc 194(9): 150–151, 1965.
4. Kashiwagi S, Hayaski J, Ikematsu H, et al: An outbreak of hepatitis in members of a high school sumo wrestling club. J Am Med Assoc 248(2):213–214, 1982.

5. Baron RC, Hatch MH, Kleeman K, et al: Aseptic meningitis among members of a high school football team. J Am Med Assoc 248(14):1724–1727, 1982.
6. Gibbs RC: Tennis toe. Arch Dermatol 107:918, 1973.
7. Verbov J: Calcaneal petechiae. Arch Dermatol 107:918, 1973.
8. Ely PH: Balance beam alopecia. Arch Dermatol 114:968–970, 1978.
9. Short JM: Frostbite, pernio, immersion foot, in Dennis DJ, Dobson RL, McGuire J (eds): Clinical Dermatology. New York, Harper & Row, 1979.
10. Hershkowitz M: Penile frostbite—An unforeseen hazard of jogging. N Engl J Med 296:178, 1977.

20
Special Considerations in the Injured Child

Richard B. Birrer

PREPARTICIPATORY EVALUATION

Of overriding importance in the management of children participating actively in sports programs are the regular and thorough consideration of growth and development, proper assessment that carefully matches players according to their athletic ability, psychological maturity, and physical size, attention to any underlying medical conditions, and keynoting prevention through continual education (proper conditioning and equipment).[1-3] Every preadolescent and adolescent athlete should have a careful anthropomorphic assessment consisting of height, weight, and overall habitus. The results should be tabulated and a physical growth chart placed in the athlete's record. A sexual maturity rating should also be determined according to the Tanner scale, with which every primary care physician should be familiar. Finally, some reasonable attempt should be made to determine psychological readiness and coordination for the sports under consideration.

Even though the growth and development of an individual child is along a physiologic continuum, there is no standard sequence or particular pattern applicable to all child athletes. Examples of mismatches might include:

- Two children who lie within the same normal physical growth range, one weighing 52 pounds and the other weighing 108 pounds

- Two children of the same height and weight one of whom is Tanner stage 1 and the other is Tanner stage 5
- One child who is small in terms of height and weight but is well coordinated and another who is much larger by height and weight but is not as coordinated
- A child who is psychologically prepared for a particular sport event as compared to another child who is participating in a sport due to parental pressure

Performance in a sport, therefore, depends on many athletic skills including muscle power, coordination, size, and aerobic capacity as well as the psychological readiness to participate. As there is no standard formula relating one factor to another or predicting the comparability of one child athlete to another, it is the physician's responsibility to synthesize these factors thoroughly in the final sports prescription and counsel the young athlete.

OVERGROWTH SYNDROME

The injuries most common in the young athlete are results of the overgrowth syndrome.[1] Due to rapid increases in body size, a child's flexibility is actually decreased particularly in the lower back, ankle, foot, and knee; as a result, sprains and strains are common. When combined with inadequate warm-ups and improper training, children are at significant risk for many adult injuries. On the other hand, a variety of sports can be safely played by the young athlete on a regular basis. One large study of pre-adolescent wrestlers showed, with the exception of one metacarpal fracture, the minor nature of 21 injuries over 190 consecutive matches.[4] This particular study reaffirmed the importance of careful evaluation of the young athlete and proper warm-up and training.

EPIPHYSEAL INJURIES

Epiphyseal injuries are a major concern in the active young athlete and have been classified according to the work of Salter and Harris.[5] A common example of such an injury is Little Leaguer's elbow—osteochondritis dissecans of the capitellum (most commonly) or of the radial head.[6] As the elbow joint is extended in the final phase of throwing, acceleration, and follow through, the pronounced forces of valgus stress and rotatory compression from the medial to the lateral side of the joint can produce several pathologic processes involving the epiphysis. Bony avulsion of the medial epicondyle is a more common problem although epicondylitis, ulnar neuritis, olecranon spurring, and straining of the flexor forearm muscles can also occur. Acutely, medial epicondyle avulsion or a flexor muscle mass strain results, though chronic repetitive stress causes articular surface damage with formation of inter-articular "joint mice" and progressive fragmentation of the articular cartilage with arthritic spurring. In the growing athlete these pathologic changes can produce significant growth abnormalities of the elbow; sequelae include articular deformity and functional instability.

Diagnosis of an acute elbow injury is made by the symptoms of pain along the epicondyle which can be aggravated by gripping and resisted wrist flexion if the medial epicondyle is involved, or resisted wrist extension if the lateral condyle is involved. Localized tenderness can be palpated along the injured epicondyle or upward along the supercondylar ridge for a short distance. The treatment of epicondylitis is discussed in Chapter 17 (section on the Elbow). All epicondylar fractures should be

replaced surgically even when the avulsion is simply of a muscle detachment with a small splinter of bone: direct surgical fixation permits more rapid establishment of motion and more complete rehabilitation. If the fragment is not reattached, muscular pull tends to rotate it so that the cortical surface is toward the humerus and the fractured surface is toward the skin. As a result, nonunion is frequent and, in the young athlete, growth disturbance inevitable.

Undisplaced fracture of the proximal humeral epiphysis with widening of the proximal humeral epiphyseal line (Little League shoulder) can occur from forceful pitching activities. Treatment can be conservative with sling and swathe if separation is minimal; otherwise consultation is essential.

In terms of prevention it should be emphasized that, for any young athlete who has open epiphysis, the Little League regulations should be followed for limited pitching. Although it is true that an individual player's skeletal maturation and development are related to the age limits of pitching, it is impossible to find this precisely. Furthermore, the risk of impairment is directly correlated to the number of innings pitched by a child with open epiphysis. A good rule of thumb is to counsel the athlete to pitch no more than six innings every 4 days with appropriate modification based on the recurrence of symptoms.

Occasionally the epiphyseal plate of the femoral neck can slip because it is unfused in most adolescents.[7] In the male it fuses between the ages of 17 and 18; in the female between the ages of 16 and 17. Usually secondary to a minor trauma, slipped capital femoral epiphyses are more common in the endomorphic obese athlete. Typically the child complains of pain in either the knee or hip, with hip pain being referred to the knee. A high index of suspicion and careful x rays, particularly the lateral view, are necessary to make the diagnosis. A patient with a slipped epiphysis should be immediately admitted to the hospital and taken off weight bearing. Because time is of the essence, consultation should be sought as soon as possible and a decision made as to whether manipulation in combination with internal fixation should be performed. Because there is a significant incidence of bilateral involvement (25 percent) particularly in the individual with an endomorphic habitus, prophylactic pinning may be indicated.

Fracture of the femoral epiphyseal plate is a serious injury and requires early adequate treatment.[7] Similar to the case of a femoral neck fracture, the patient complains of severe hip pain and the limb is externally rotated, abducted, and shortened. Because the fracture may be incomplete, the characteristic position may not be assumed but rather resemble that of a dislocated hip. Before any manipulation is performed, a careful x-ray study must be made. Since the epiphysis reaffixes early onto the femur, it is imperative that surgical reduction and internal fixation be performed as early as possible.

PERTHES' DISEASE

Perthes' disease (osteochondritis juvenilis dissecans), although not specifically secondary to sports injury, is mentioned because it should enter diagnostic considerations in any adolescent with hip or knee symptomatology. It is a disease of unknown etiology but can result in significant epiphyseal necrosis of the femoral head with subsequent deformity and degenerative osteoarthritis particularly in the adolescent. In a large study by Foster and Bowen, five factors were shown to be of prognostic significance[8]:

1. Age—the younger child has significantly less deformity of the femoral head since the potential for remodeling is high. Under the age of 6, 15 percent have poor results, whereas older than 9 years, 70 percent are left with some residual deformity.

2. Degree of epiphyseal necrosis—grade 1 injuries heal well, whereas grade 4 have 50 to 60 percent poor results. The larger the area of necrosis, therefore, the higher the probability of a poor result.

3. X-ray findings—lateral calcification of the epiphysis, a horizontal physeal line, lateral subluxation of the epiphysis, Gages sign, and extensive metaphyseal reaction are associated with severe disease course and a poor outcome.

4. Premature proximal femoral epiphyseal arrest.

5. Marked joint contracture, prolonged hip stiffness, and recurrent hip pain.

Early preventive treatment in Perthes' disease is critical. Most patients should be treated even before the degree of epiphyseal involvement and the prognostic risk factors are clearly identified. First the patient should be placed at bed rest to alleviate hip symptoms. Thereafter physical therapy involving passive and active range of motion is incorporated into the patient's care as well as the use of Buck's traction in order to maintain an abduction. The use of a Toronto brace, Petrie cast, or Scottish Rite orthosis is used to maintain abduction and contain the necrotic epiphysis in a viable acetabulum. Should the patient not be able to tolerate the brace, surgical fixation should be strongly considered. An active physical therapy program in conjunction with those sports that allow full range of motion and maintain the abduction and internal rotation of the hip is encouraged [swimming and upper-extremity exercises, such as archery and table tennis (using the sitting posture in the latter)]. Once femoral head reossification begins, the brace can be removed and the sports activity rapidly progressed, though contact sports, jumping, or prolonged running are not recommended until the subcondral bone of the epiphysis is well formed.

REFERENCES

1. Rosegrant S: Boston sports medicine: Helping the young athlete. Phys Sports Med 9(10):105–107, 1981.
2. Garrick JG: Sports medicine. Pediatr Clin Am 24(4):737–747, 1977.
3. Sports in childhood. A round table symposium. Phys Sports Med. 10(8):52–60, 1982.
4. Hartmann PM: Injuries in preadolescent wrestlers. Phys Sports Med. 6(11):79–82,1978.
5. Salter RI, Harris WR: Injuries involving the epiphyseal plate. J Bone Joint Surg (Am) 45:587–622, 1963.
6. Tullos HS, King JW: Lesions of the pitching arm in adolescents. J Am Med Assoc 220:264–271,1972.
7. Ogden JA: Skeletal injury in the child. Philadelphia, Lea & Febiger, 1982.
8. Foster BK, Bowen JR: Perthes' disease: Returning children to Sports. Phys Sports Med 10(6):67–74,1982.

21

Athletic Participation in the Presence of Chronic Disorders: Asthma, Obesity, Diabetes, and Seizure Disorders

Mark F. Sherman, John P. Reilly, Joel R. Bonamo, and Richard B. Birrer

The tremendous increase in athletic participation in the United States has made our society quite conscious of the benefits of physical fitness. However, it has become apparent that as sports participation rises, the individuals becoming involved vary in their preconditioning status. The "healthy" individual usually has freedom of choice with regard to which sport to practice, but his or her profile (flexibility, strength, agility, endurance, etc.) greatly influences the incidence of injury in the various sports attempted. For an athlete with underlying medical problems, exclusion from athletic participation is no longer an acceptable alternative. The psychological affects of the inability to be involved in some form of sport can be permanently devastating. Choosing the appropriate sport for an individual with a chronic disease is very satisfying for both the physician and patient, and the long-term benefits are well worth the efforts.

Much of the attention and discussion as well as the glamour has been directed toward the orthopedic problems of sports participants. There is a more fundamental and more far-reaching role for the physician; that is, evaluating each patient's health and providing safe guidelines for those who have identifiable medical disorders. In our sports-minded society, it has become important for all participants to feel as "normal as possible" in order to prevent many of the psychological effects of feelings of inferiority or imperfection. With this in mind, this chapter discusses the management of different disorders in school-age children. The responsibility and goal of the physician is to evaluate each patient completely not with the purpose of excluding the patient from sport, but rather to make sure that no patient is excluded without a good reason. Thus, when confronted with the question, "My son is a diabetic, can he play football?", physicians may have more information in order to make an educated decision as to what limitations, if any, should be imposed.

ASTHMA

The asthmatic has historically been an outcast from athletic participation. Thanks to the recent research and improved pharmacologic approaches, the benefits of sports for the asthmatic are now appreciated.

Asthma is a leading cause of chronic illness in childhood, responsible for a considerable portion of lost school time. Recent estimates indicate that somewhere between 5 and 10 percent of all school-age children have at some time during childhood signs and symptoms compatible with asthma.

Although there is no completely acceptable definition of asthma, it may be regarded as a diffuse, obstructive lung disease, with hyperirritability or hyperactivity of the airways to a variety of stimuli. Asthma has a high degree of reversibility of the obstructive process, which may occur spontaneously or as a result of treatment.[1]

Symptoms and Pathophysiology

As a rule, exercise-induced asthma (EIA) or bronchospasm occurs at a predictable time after starting exercise in cold air (temperature relative to the lung), though exercise is an extremely common if not universal factor in all forms of asthma. Other forms include extrinsic (infectious) and intrinsic (allergic) varieties. The symptoms commonly seen include: (1) dyspnea, (2) bronchospasm, (3) increased mucus production, (4) choking, (5) fatigue, (6) chest pain, and (7) wheezing.[2]

Although the etiology and mechanism of EIA remains obscure it appears not to be caused by atopic mediators. Hyperventilation, metabolic acidosis, respiratory acidosis, arterial hypoxemia, lung deformation, autonomic imbalance, and β-adrenergic blockade have all been proposed, though no single mechanism has clearly been delineated. Sixty to 80 percent of individuals with allergic respiratory disease experience this prolonged exercise-induced response; the remaining subjects show no significant alteration.[3] The trigger of asthmatic attacks is not the exercise itself but the resultant cooling of the bronchi, with the degree of cooling being inversely related to the humidity and temperature of the ambient air and directly related to the respiration rate.

Brief exercise for 1 or 2 minutes has been shown to decrease airway resistance (obstruction) as measured by forced expiratory volume (FEV-1); however, exercise continuing for 4 to 12 minutes increases the airway obstruction. Should asthmatic children therefore be excused from gym, or should they be encouraged to play active sports?

Recommendations

All children including asthmatics benefit by exercise and need good programs of general physical education. As a benefit of recent research including pharmacologic intervention and prophylaxis, both children and teenagers with asthma can now be encouraged to participate in most activities. Proper exercise prevents asthmatics from being left out of a sport, which can make them feel isolated and inferior. Taking into consideration the alterations of pulmonary physiology in EIA, one can suggest activities in which strenuous exercise is limited to 5 minutes. Such sports which can be recommended include baseball, short distance running, and swimming.[4] To be discouraged and avoided are basketball and long distance running. Those athletes with allergic etiologies can enjoy most sports in the "off seasons" but require careful follow-up and medication during the pollen periods. Infectious causes must be treated vigorously in order to minimize time lost from sports activity. Regardless of etiology, the asthmatic athlete can markedly improve his or her aerobic capacity over the years.

As noted, pharmacologic intervention has begun to play an important role in the daily management of the asthmatic child. It is only natural that its uses be carried over into the area of prophylaxis prior to exercise.[2,3,5–7] Historically, isoproterenol (Isuprel) has been shown to be most useful in preventing EIA when administered 5 minutes prior to exercise, with its effects lasting 2 hours. More recently, cromolyn sodium (Intal) inhalation has been shown to inhibit the exercise-induced asthmatic response.[8] The wearing of a simple surgical mask has also been demonstrated to relieve exercise-induced asthma markedly. Regularly prescribed medicines such as theophylline and ephedrine sulfate preparations should be taken and periodically checked for effectiveness (serum levels). Children should be allowed to take their medications to school. A point that is still somewhat controversial pertains to amateur sports and the use of medications before competition. It is the unanimous opinion of the American Academy of Allergists, as well as the American Academy of Pediatricians, that these participants are to be allowed to compete and not be disqualified because of the use of therapeutic doses of drugs before or during competition with proper medical supervision. Finally, the state of hydration of an asthmatic should never be neglected.

OBESITY

Today, the United States has the dubious distinction of having the highest incidence of obesity in the world. As most observers easily admit, the problem has reached epidemic proportions and is present at all age levels. Most recent estimates indicate that one-third of all children under 18 are obese.

Obesity elicits differing opinions in all aspects of its multifaceted conception. These range from how exactly one defines obesity, to determining its causes and an adequate treatment program. Without help, the obese child or adult suffers from higher incidence of disease severity, experiences a decreased life expectancy, and suffers the psychological consequences of being considered a deviate in a society where "thin is in."

Definition

Initially, almost naively, one would assume that defining obesity would pose no real problem. Nothing could be further from the truth. Basically, we can define obesity as a chronic disturbance in homeostatic function—in this case, "excessive fatness." The controversy revolves around what characterizes *excessive*.

To some, the popular use of body weight standards or percentage overweight for height and age represents a gross oversimplification of the obese state (20 percent overweight = obesity; 50 percent = frank obesity; 100 percent = morbid obesity). It fails to take into consideration variations in

body type or *somatotype*. The body fat content may be too gross an index for purposes of assessing body composition (e.g., excessive fatness versus excessive muscularity). Several alternative methods have been proposed to assess body composition. The most clinically applicable of these techniques is caliper measures of the skin-fold fat. Obesity in childhood is the area to which valid principles of obesity recognition should be most carefully applied, especially when one notes the fact that 75 to 80 percent of children with juvenile obesity become obese adults.

Etiology

The etiology of obesity is multiple and complex, being both physiologic and psychological in origin and having its roots in regulatory, metabolic, nutritional, emotional, and even genetic disorders. To state simply that the cause of obesity is the intake of more calories than are expended misses the point entirely. Almost all patients who are obese are physiologically normal; however, their obesity may bring with it some metabolic differences, such as exaggerated insulin response. The decreased rate of glucose disposal found in many obese subjects, despite high levels of circulating insulin, suggests insulin antagonism probably at a tissue level. The prevalence of childhood obesity has been clearly linked to excessive weight gain during the first 6 months of life. This means that the earlier the onset of obesity, the greater the proliferation of adipose tissue cell number. When obesity is initiated at under 10 years of age, the child has as many as three times the normal amount of adipose cells. In contrast, when an adult becomes obese, it is a result of cellular hypertrophy and augmented lipid content per cell.

Aside from the biochemical data, evidence exists on a more clinical level that obesity is closely related to low energy expenditure in relation to food intake. For example, the obese are observed to be more energy conserving, spending many hours daily watching television, walking slowly, or riding rather than walking. They have been shown to expend less energy when participating in sports.

Obesity has been associated with sociopsychological maladaptation. For some patients, it is a method of coping with stress. There are often disturbances in body image, both in the way they perceive themselves and how they believe others perceive them. Curiously, obesity is not an affliction of the poor; in fact, there is epidemiologic evidence that an inverse relationship exists between obesity and socioeconomic status.

Need for Prevention

Numerous epidemiologic studies have been undertaken and have all indicated that obesity is associated with a wide variety of health hazards. The high mortality rate of overweight persons is most often attributed to cardiac dysfunction. However, there is also abundant evidence to indict obesity for increasing morbidity in hypertension and pulmonary disease, as well as aggravating and accelerating such conditions as degenerative osteoarthritis. As of yet, these causal relationships exist only for the obese adult. Concern for fat children is real because of the observation that they become fat teenagers and then fat adults. Dempsey queries, "Why is obesity, by statistical criteria incurable, when it is obviously controlled on the short term through the manipulation of one's environment?"[9]

An interesting point at least philosophically is whether the emphasis should be put on measures to correct obesity or to prevent it. Does it in fact make a difference? The argument for prevention should be overwhelming. There exists a firm metabolic, psychogenic, and actuarial basis for either avoiding the onset of obesity or controlling its progress at the time of onset. However, the cry for prevention is hardly unique to the problem of obesity, and attempts to educate physicians, public health personnel, and patients toward preventive action in such areas as cardiovascular and pulmonary disease have met with limited success.

Muscular exercise is an important deterrent in obesity, and it is important to develop and discover activities that can be enjoyed by the obese seeking weight control. Primarily, prevention of obesity should be attempted. This includes a good physical education program encouraging a broad range of activities. Even as a child, it is important to control two variables: (1) overeating and (2) underactivity. Every individual who grows to adulthood without some sport, game, or recreational activity is de-

prived of an enjoyable aspect of life and a valuable means of health maintenance. Treatment of the obese should be viewed as the least desirable method of solving the problem!

Strategies to be considered are as follow:

1. Consultations with parents of obese children
2. Parental cooperation with children's diets
3. Complete physical examination of all obese patients
4. Special classes for obese students providing them with education for a good nutritional and exercise program

Physical Education for the Obese

Physical education should be part of the curriculum for both the normal and obese child. Programs should be developed that consider individual differences and the needs of the obese, particularly in the terms of body build, stamina, maturation, coordination, nutrition, motivation, and limitations imposed by congenitally acquired defects, emotional disorders, chronic diseases, and recent illnesses or injury.

In general, the obese are poorly coordinated, awkward, and underdeveloped and may be sensitive about their appearance and performance. The obese adolescent is painfully aware of his or her status and society's judgment. Obese children should be given help to socialize more effectively in school and to improve their general comfort and function in the community. These patients may be very reluctant to participate in a regular physical education program of any type. They can, however, often accept a regular physical program if they are initially in a small class with a modified program, and with the proper help develop their physical abilities, self-respect, and peer relationships.

The most significant factor in good physical education for all obese patients is to choose activities that provide constant motion rather than those that involve standing and sitting.[10,11] A useful set of exercise criteria is as follows:

1. *Moderate intensity*—exercise with sustained heart rate of about 120 beats per minute.
2. *Duration*—activities that can be sustained for more than a few minutes.

3. *Utilization of the lower body muscles*—these muscles are active in locomotion and are essential in maintaining a prolonged activity level.
4. *Fun*—sports and activities cannot be presented as drudgery but rather as enjoyable.

Good examples include walking, hiking, bicycling, rope skipping, and swimming. In addition, the obese should be encouraged to develop specific physical attributes such as their strength, flexibility, and agility.[12]

Sports participation for the obese must be prescribed with care. The obese are painfully self-conscious and are usually reluctant to be exposed to an outward act such as athletic endeavors. They must be made to understand that a sport is one way of "burning calories," and at the same time establish some self-confidence. Jogging is often acceptable to the obese, since it is likely that they have already seen other obese people who are running with success. (The sweat suit is a good way to cover up body size.) However, running has the associated problems of traumatic arthritis secondary to excessive weight bearing on the joint surfaces, intertrigo, and increased severity of sprains and muscular strains. Swimming, on the other hand, may be less acceptable because of the more obvious body exposure. However, it is an excellent aerobic regimen for the obese and alleviates the sheer forces on the weight-bearing joint surfaces. Outdoor bicycling is usually difficult, whereas a stationary bicycle in the home is often quite appealing and readily accepted. Competitive team sports are the next step, and once the obese youth is able to function in this athletic mode, care is usually less difficult—they have already proven to themselves that they are able to cope with their condition. Once the motivation factor to participate is ignited it is not uncommon for the overweight individual to lose weight rapidly and become a frenzied physical fitness model.

DIABETES

Diabetes and exercise have long been a controversial issue.[13,14] Hypoglycemia related to exercise is easily avoided by not exercising, and this has been the acceptable and simple solution to this problem.

However, due to patient demand, it has become apparent that a diabetic can compete successfully.

Historically, muscular exercise has long been recognized as an important part of the management of juvenile onset diabetes mellitus.[15–17] Along with insulin and diet, exercise constitutes the "triad" of therapy. Yet, even with acceptance of this concept, the management of the patient's exercise program continues to be the part that receives the least amount of emphasis and is often neglected.

Much clinical and basic science research appearing recently, particularly from Scandinavia, has been directed to physical exercise and the diabetic.[18] The key word to the care of the diabetic is *control*. Exercise has been shown to have beneficial normalizing effects in diabetics who are in good metabolic control. For the diabetic with poor or no control, exercise aggravates the existing metabolic imbalances. Exercise has been clearly shown to decrease blood glucose levels in the diabetic with good control (nonketotic), whereas blood glucose levels increase in the diabetic with poor control (ketotic). Similarly, although blood levels of free fatty acids and ketones increase after exercise in the nonketotic diabetic, the increase has been shown to be less than in ketotic diabetics. In addition, exercise retards the appearance of diabetic microangiopathy by means of improving circulatory function. The proposed mechanisms include increased blood through the capillary system, improved oxygen transport, or the secondary effect of decreased lipid levels. Naturally, the concern with diabetes is whether or not exercise potentiates hypoglycemic episodes. The absorption of insulin is more rapid during physical activity when compared to rest. Usually this shows as only a marginal effect. However, when doing heavy muscular work (for example sports), absorption may be accelerated to such an extent that the major insulin effect occurs earlier than anticipated, hence producing the hypoglycemic episode.

The following steps can be easily taken to prevent hypoglycemia:

1. Change the site of injection to a location where blood flow is not maximally increased during exercise (e.g., abdomen for running sports, or thigh for upper body weight lifting).

2. Place diabetic on a strict and daily exercise schedule rather than allowing sporadic athletic activity.
3. Exercise should preferably be after meals.
4. Evaluate for possible adjustment in daily insulin dosage. It has been shown that if a diabetic is well controlled and under a well supervised exercise program, insulin requirements may be decreased by as much as 10 percent.
5. Educate the diabetic athlete regarding this potential problem so that he or she is always prepared to take steps to prevent the impending hypoglycemia.

When compared with nondiabetics, diabetic patients have been shown to be more inactive and reluctant to engage in many types of physical activity. Many reasons have been put forward for this. One is that these are "sick" children, and should be exempt from participation in sports. The fear of exercise causing hypoglycemia is another reason for the higher incidence of inactivity in these patients. It must be explained to the diabetic that exercise-induced hypoglycemia is caused by insufficient "fuel" and that, as diabetics, they should schedule their exercise program to fit their meal plan. The lack of spontaneous motivation for exercise has been observed in diabetics because they (especially teenagers) identify exercise as part of the therapy, which has a negative connotation as opposed to being a pleasant natural healthy activity.

Exercise is an integral component of growth and development. No form of exercise, including competitive sports of any kind, should be forbidden to the diabetic child, who should not be made to feel different or restricted. Before a program is recommended, good diabetic control should be maintained. Carbohydrate-loading diets should be discouraged. The exercise program should be started on a gradual basis and increase in activity by small increments, enabling the physician to make the appropriate dietary and insulin adjustments. Coaches and trainers must be made aware of the athlete's problem and should be instructed in the care of the hypoglycemic episode.

Thanks to the exposure of several professional diabetic athletes, the adolescent with diabetes no longer has to feel inferior to his or her peers. Athletic participation is physiologically and psychologically beneficial to these patients and should be strongly recommended.

SEIZURE DISORDERS

The stigmata attached to seizure disorders have long made this problem a direct contraindication to any sports activities. Because of society's attitude towards epileptics, the importance of "being normal" is of overwhelming psychological significance, and sports can be an excellent means to prove this equality.

The three main types of seizure are (1) grandmal, (2) petit-mal, and (3) psychomotor seizure. Although sweeping generalizations are to be avoided, several pertinent group rules are as follow:

1. An athlete can be considered safe for athletic activities if seizure free for 1 year while on medication.
2. Special head gear is mandatory if the seizure disorder is secondary to or was triggered by trauma.

In grand-mal and petit-mal seizures there is minimal risk from strenuous activity. Contact sports have not shown an increased incidence of seizure activity and, in fact, the psychological affects of leading a more normal life (by team participation) probably offset the stresses that induce the seizure disorder.

Psychomotor seizures require more sophisticated management. These are forms of abnormal behavior patterns which may be interpreted as warranting punishment. The seizure is characterized by a period of amnesia, tonic spasm, and occasionally muscular hyperactivity. Patients appear as if they are out of touch with reality. Because of their often bizarre behavior, such seizures are more often mistakenly labeled with a psychological diagnosis. Patients with this disorder do require restrictions from strenuous activities for the seizures are often triggered by such activities.[19]

As with diabetes, control of seizure activity is

the essential ingredient to treatment. Patients with poorly controlled seizure disorders should be restricted from potentially hazardous activities such as horseback riding, climbing, diving, and swimming if proper supervision is not available.[20]

The team approach is essential in the supervision of these patients. The individual athlete should be the one to decide whether the other teammates are to know about his or her disability. It has become quite apparent that the ability of a patient with a seizure disorder to participate in sports usually provides tremendous satisfaction for these patients. The ability to cope with a stress typically yields greater enthusiasm for other social activities, and often provides a major thrust for future success.

REFERENCES

1. Ellis E: Allergic disorders, in Nelson W, Vaughn VC, McKay RJ, Behrman RE (eds): Nelson's Textbook of Pediatrics, ed 11. Philadelphia, WB Saunders, 1979, pp 627–635.
2. Godfrey S: Exercise-induced asthma. Allergy 33:229–237, 1978.
3. Ghory JE, Bailet IW, Bierman CW, et al: American Academy of Allergy—Report of the Committee on Rehabilitation Therapy. J Allergy Clin Immunol 54(6):396–399, 1974.
4. Fitch KD, Morton AR, Blanksby BA: Effects of swimming training on children with asthma. Arch Dis Childhood 51:190–194, 1976.
5. Morton AR, Fitch KD, Hahn AG: Physical activity and the asthmatic. Phys Sports Med 9(3):50–61, 1981.
6. Godfrey S: Asthmatic children benefit from intermittent exercise. J Am Med Assoc 231:1017–1018, 1975.
7. Sly RM: Exercise and the asthmatic child. Pediatr Digest 14:42–49, 1972.
8. Morton AR, Fitch KD: Sodium cromoglycate (BP) in prevention of exercise-induced asthma. Med J Aust 2:158–162, 1974.
9. Dempsey JA: Exercise and obesity, in Ryan AJ, Allman F (eds): Sports Medicine. Englewood Cliffs, NJ: Prentice-Hall, 1974.
10. Dean RS, Garabedian AA: Obesity and level of activity. Percept Mot Skills 49(3):690, 1979.
11. Ragg KE: Exercise: A misused factor in weight control. J Sch Health 49:459–462, 1978.
12. Schwarzkopf R, Morris G: Obesity and the forgotten child. Phys Educ (Phi Epsilon Kappa Fraternity Publication) 34(1):12–14, 1977.
13. Vranic M, Berger M: Exercise and diabetes. Diabetes 28:147–163, 1978.
14. Johansen K: Physical training and diabetes mellitus. J Endocrinol Invest 1(4):367–371, 1978.
15. Costill DL, Cleary P, Fink WJ, et al: Training adaptations in skeletal muscle of juvenile diabetes. Diabetes 28:818–822, 1978.
16. Bennett DL: The adolescent and diabetes mellitus. Pediatr Ann 7:626–632, 1978.
17. Sperling MA: Diabetes mellitus. Pediatr Clin N Am 26:149–163, 1979.
18. Larsson Y: Physical exercise and juvenile diabetes—Summary and conclusions. Acta Paediatr Scand Suppl 283:120–122, 1980.
19. Korczyn AD: Participation of epileptic patients in sports. J Sports Med Phys Fitness 19(2):195–198, 1979.
20. Livingston S: Should epileptics be athletes? Phys Sports Med 3:67–72, 1975.

and passive movement to restore joint range of motion are initiated.

EVALUATION PROCESS

The steps in the delivery of physical therapy after injury are initial evaluation, goal setting, treatment planning, and treatment execution, including ongoing reassessment of the condition of the patient (follow-up).

The initial evaluation of the patient by the physical therapist begins with a *detailed history*. This most important step includes information concerning all previous medical problems, past injuries and surgeries, and a detailed account of the mechanism of injury for which treatment is being sought.

The *subjective examination*, the next step in the initial evaluation, reveals much about the severity of the injury to the patient. The therapist must systematically collect data on the nature of present pain (e.g., site, depth, constant, improving, shooting) and how pain behavior is related to posture and activity. Other symptoms, such as paresthesia, stiffness, dizziness, and bowel and bladder function, are explored at this time.

The *objective examination*, the third part of the initial examination, begins with an inspection of the injured part and related areas. The patient's posture is noted. The physical therapist examines the affected area for changes in skin color, moisture, and temperature. Changes in underlying muscle tone and soft tissue swelling are noted. Joint stability, available active and passive movement (range of motion), and manual muscle tests are performed. Special tests, such as appropriate neurologic tests or isokinetic evaluation, are performed when indicated. The integration of the data from the history and subjective and objective examinations, coupled with the diagnosis from the primary care physician, enable the therapist to arrive at an assessment of the condition of the athlete. Since the patient's condition changes as treatment progresses, the therapist selects key elements from the initial evaluation to be retested periodically to aid in determining progress and the efficacy of the treatment plan and rehabilitation.

From the assessment, the therapist sets long-

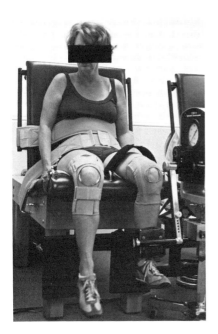
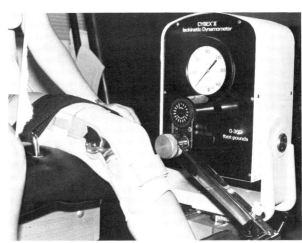

FIGURE 22-1. The Cybex II isokinetic device in operation.

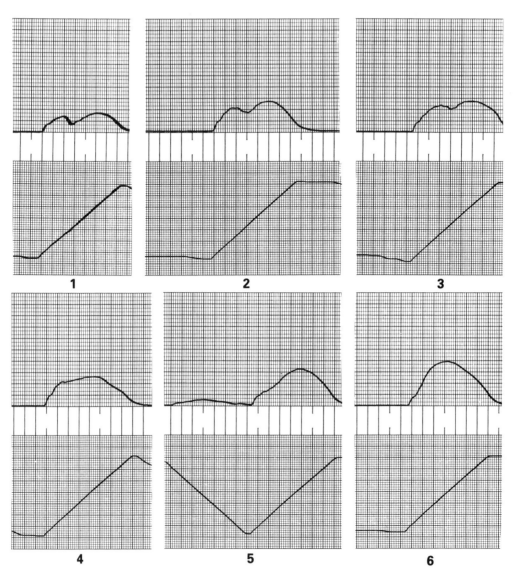

1   2   3

4   5   6

and short-term goals for the patient and arrives at a treatment plan.

TOOLS OF THE TRADE

The practice of sports physical therapy requires equipment that may not be necessary in other physical therapy practices. At the heart of most sports physical therapy practices today are *isokinetic test-*

ing and exercise units, such as the Cybex II Dynamometer (Fig. 22-1). As a testing unit, the Cybex II is used to measure torque development of an extremity joint at various speeds of movement. The speed range for testing and training is infinitely variable from 0°/second (isometric contraction) to 300°/second. A chart recorder is used to obtain a permanent record of the results of the isokinetic evaluation.

From the isokinetic evaluation, the physical

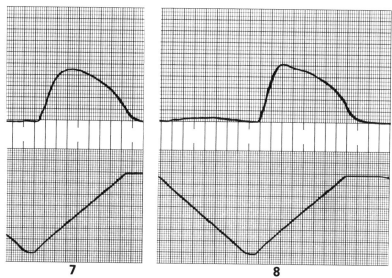

FIGURE 22-2. Sequential Cybex II printouts in the rehabilitative training of a grade II hamstring tear. Numbers refer to weeks post injury.

therapist can determine maximal peak torque at a given speed, time interval from initiation of movement to maximum torque, angle (the point in the range of motion) at which peak torque is achieved, endurance of the musculature tested, and percentage deficits in strength of the affected limb (by testing and comparing the contralateral, uninvolved joint musculature). The shape of the curve representing torque development in the affected limb shows the ability of the patient to develop torque without char-

acteristic "bumps" or "dips," which represent weaknesses or painful points within the arc of movement (Fig. 22-2). The isokinetic evaluation not only serves as a determination of the state of the affected limb, but is also a formidable tool in designing a specific rehabilitation program focusing on particular weakness(es).

Table 22-1 shows test results of the torque output developed by a patient with a grade II hamstring tear. As soon as the patient was able to tolerate resistance, an isokinetic evaluation was performed and the muscle group was tested every week for a period of 8 weeks. The first test shows a slow rise time in torque development with a characteristic dip in the curve where torque output is limited due to pain and weakness. As progress improves the "dip" disappears, and the ability of the patient to produce a high level of torque in knee flexion improves in both quantity (amplitude) and quality (fast rise time from zero to maximal torque with no dips or wavers).*

TABLE 22-1. ISOKINETIC EVALUATION FOR PATIENT WITH GRADE II HAMSTRING TEAR

Test No.	Weeks Post Injury	Maximum Torque (ft–lb)	Time From 0 to Maximum Torque (s)
1	7	30	1.0
2	8	50	1.0
3	9	50	1.1
4	10	48	0.9
5	11	59	0.8
6	12	70	0.7
7	13	81	0.5
8	14	92	0.4

A special device can be used to determine by integration the area under a curve. The result represents the work (foot-pounds) performed. This measurement is a highly accurate method for assessing rehabilitation.

The Cybex II and other isokinetic devices (e.g., Orthotron, Hydragym Powernetic Equipment, and Minigym) offer two distinct advantages over traditional progressive resistive exercise devices in neuromuscular re-education (Fig. 22-3). The first is that isokinetic devices offer perfectly accommodating resistance. The force generated by the patient while moving the limb through an arc at a preset speed is likewise matched by the resistance the device provides. If the patient moves slower than the preset speed, no external force is encountered by the patient (except for overcoming gravity and the weight of a portion of the movement arm of the device). The therapist cannot overload the muscle or the joint

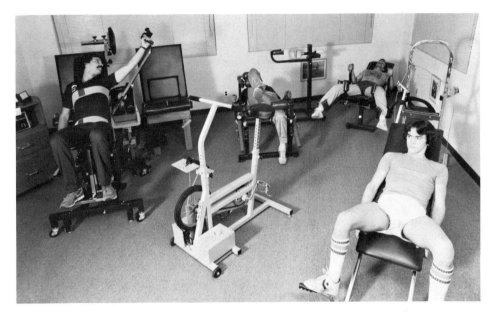

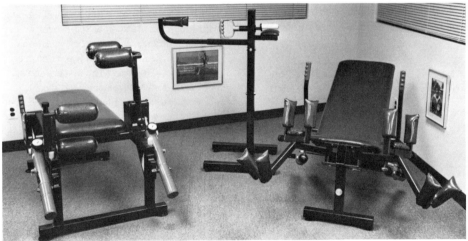

FIGURE 22-3. Additional examples of isokinetic equipment.

by asking the patient to lift more than he or she is capable of lifting. The second major advantage of isokinetic exercise is that the athlete can work toward developing torque at high speeds of movement. It is more important, for example, for the runner to develop a strong contraction quickly in the lower extremity musculature than to be able to lift heavy weights at a slow speed.

In addition to isokinetic devices, the sports physical therapist employs other resistive exercise devices in muscle strengthening and re-education. Wall pulley systems, Nautilus and Universal apparatus, as well as dumbbells and cuff weights are used in providing resistance in progressive resistive exercise programs.

Resistance exercises (isometric, isotonic, or isokinetic) can be prescribed when the patient can tolerate such activity. Joint swelling should be minimal or absent, and the patient should accomplish the activity with little or no discomfort. The goal of strengthening weakened musculature can only be attained when the structures involved (muscle, tendon, musculoskeletal attachment, and joint components) are capable of responding to the stress of resistance while maintaining their integrity.

The *treadmill* and *bicycle ergometer* are used mainly to improve the aerobic capacities of patients. This is especially important after an athlete has sustained an injury which decreases his or her activity level for a prolonged period. In an Achilles tendon strain, although the emphasis of the physical therapy program is return of range of motion and strengthening of the triceps surae, the deconditioning effect of the injury cannot be overlooked. While the athlete is recovering muscle and joint function, cardiopulmonary conditioning is begun. The athlete may begin stationary cycling with the uninvolved limb and, when sufficient function has returned to the affected limb, use both legs. The treadmill can also be used to retrain the patient in such ambulatory maneuvers as sidestepping, walking backwards, and walking uphill (forwards and backwards). The cycle ergometer can be used as an effective active assistive exercise device to increase range of motion in knee flexion. At slow speeds, the cycle ergometer can be used as a resistive exercise device.

Electromyographic (EMG) feedback is a valuable tool to enhance an isometric contraction, for example, when joint motion is contraindicated. It is also employed to assist the patient to voluntarily recruit more motor fibers in an active contraction. A third way the physical therapist uses EMG biofeedback is to have the patient accentuate a particular muscle or a portion of a muscle group during contraction when it is almost impossible without such feedback; e.g., when the therapist wants the patient to develop a stronger contraction from the vastus medialis portion of the quadriceps to accentuate terminal extension following muscle atrophy. Small surface electrodes are placed over the muscle which the patient is having difficulty contracting. The action potentials generated by the firing motor units are picked up by the electrodes and transformed (through preamplification and amplification) into usable auditory and/or visual feedback information. By providing the patient with continuous, proportional, and immediate knowledge of results of the muscle contraction, the motor learning process (voluntary control) is greatly enhanced.

Cryotherapy, the therapeutic use of cold, is one of the most important modalities to the sports physical therapist. The beneficial effects of local cooling are decrease of edema, local vasoconstriction, decrease of sensation over the area treated, and reduction of pain and spasm. Application is usually made by using crushed ice in a plastic bag or by the use of commercially available cold packs, stored in a special freezer. A cold, damp towel is placed between the patient and the ice bag, and optimal benfits are accrued with a 20-minute application (which may be repeated after 1 hour if necessary). The use of a vapocoolant spray, ethyl chloride, has tremendous value in the treatment of muscle spasm or painful trigger points. Cold application is prescribed during the first 72 hours following injury to reduce swelling and diminish pain. It is also used by the physical therapist following exercise to attenuate joint pain and swelling. It is used to lessen muscle spasm in thoracic and lumbar paraspinal musculature.

Moist heat can be applied superficially to the patient using commercially available hot packs or "hydrocollators." These are canvas-covered packs with silica gel inside, stored in special thermostatically controlled hot-water tanks at about 170°F. These packs are wrapped in terry-cloth covers and, when applied to the skin surface, produce a heating effect by conduction several millimeters into the subcutaneous tissue. The effects of superficial moist heat are muscle relaxation, promotion of healing, and increased local circulation. In sports physical therapy moist heat is especially useful before stretching tight musculature and in decreasing spasm in vertebral muscles. Application time is generally 15 to 20 minutes, with care taken not to overheat the tissue.

To aid in decreasing edema, the physical therapist employs an *intermittent pressure device*. The use of external pressure to control and reduce edema has long been recognized as beneficial. Devices currently available provide a sleeve or bag shaped for a specific extremity area to be treated. The therapist can adjust cycle time for pressure "on" and pressure "off," as well as the amount of pressure to be applied externally by the device.

The use of *whirlpool hydrotherapy* is widespread in sports injury care. In physical therapy, the whirlpool is generally used to restore active movement in the wrist, forearm, and ankle. Warm water (104° to 106°F) produces a vasodilatory effect, and the action of the water from the agitator has a relaxational effect on the patient.

There are several types of *electrical stimulation* used in physical therapy with application in sports medicine. *Transcutaneous electrical nerve stimulation* (TENS) is useful in the management of both chronic and acute pain. The anesthetic effect is accomplished by stimulation of the dorsal root through the peripheral nerve. Direct current, or medical galvanism, can be used with a positive ion under the anode or a negative ion under the cathode in *iontophoresis*—the introduction of ions through the skin and subcutaneous tissue by the repulsion of the ion under the similarly charged electrode. Anesthetics (procaine), vasodilators (histamine or carbachol), and medication to decrease edema (hyaluronidase) can be introduced into subcutaneous tissue by this method. Alternating current, either pulsed or surged, can electrically stimulate a muscle where the nerve supply is intact. Its therapeutic value is in increasing local circulation or in a muscle re-education program.

Ultrasound uses high-frequency (1 million cycles per second) energy which is converted by the body into heat. With a coupling agent used on the skin, the ultrasonic energy produces a local, deep heating effect, increases the permeability of semipermeable membranes, and softens scar tissue. *Phonophoresis,* the use of ultrasound for the introduction of medication through the skin, can be of great therapeutic value in the practice of sports physical therapy. For example, a 5- or 10-percent solution of hydrocortisone cream can be introduced to a specific area in the treatment of tendonitis and neurotis. Salicylates and local anesthetics can also be used in coupling agents via phonophoresis.

Massage is a highly skilled modality used by the physical therapist to increase local circulation, decrease muscle spasm, and reduce adhesions. Techniques used in therapeutic massage include *effleurage* or light stroking, *petrissage* (kneading and stretching), and deep friction massage.

SELECTING A PHYSICAL THERAPIST

The field of orthopedic and sports physical therapy is highly specialized, and the physician will derive the most benefit from the services of a physical therapist who has an extensive background in this area and the necessary space and equipment to provide optimum care. The physical therapist must be available for his or her patients, both providing office hours and being flexible enough to accommodate the athlete. The therapist must have the time and interest to spend with family, coaches, trainers, teachers, and—most important—the physician. It is also a definite plus if the physical therapist is involved in organized sports activities or affiliated with local organized groups, such as running clubs. The therapist who is involved with the school system by donating time to team practices or games or working with other health care professionals in preseason screening examinations provides a valuable community service while enhancing his or her own practice and those of associates.

Once the physician has located physical therapists within the community who can provide the necessary services, a meeting should be arranged to discuss patient care philosophy. Time should be taken to visit the facility at which referrals will be seen by the physical therapist. The team approach to patient care is best exemplified by the physician–physical therapist relationship. Medical care does not stop at the time of referral. The maintenance of the continuity of care provided to the patient is based on mutual respect and trust of the team members. Communication among the members of the health care delivery team enhances the level of care received by the patient. The patient is the ultimate benefactor of a careful selection of a physical therapist by the leader of the health care team—the physician.

CASE HISTORIES

Case 1. A 19-year-old college track athlete, Phil B., had suffered from chronic hamstring strains of the left leg during his high school athletic career which now plagued his freshman track season. Initial examination revealed a grade I hamstring strain, left leg. The patient's chief complaint was pain in the posterior thigh, more noticeable during and after sprinting. Objective examination revealed $-20°$ straight leg raise when compared to the right leg. Long-term goals for the physical therapy program were to increase functional use of the left hamstring group to tolerate high-speed activity (sprinting) and improve the pain-free range of motion of the left knee and hip in straight leg raise.

Initial treatment consisted of moist heat application, gentle massage, and gentle passive range of motion to tolerance to increase straight leg raise. Treatment was administered three times per week for 2 weeks. After 2 weeks, ultrasound was administered over the painful area to reduce adhesion buildup and aid in the stretching regime. Within a total of 4 weeks since the initiation of treatment, pain-free range of motion had returned to normal. An isokinetic evaluation revealed a 34 percent torque development of the left hamstring when compared to the right at a speed of 60° per second, and a 44 percent deficit at the high-speed test at 180° per second. The patient was trained on the Cybex II Dynamometer with

special emphasis on knee flexion torque development at high speeds. Within 7 weeks after isokinetic exercise was begun, the patient returned to active competition. Follow-up examination 6 months after discharge from the physical therapy program was quite satisfactory. This young, gifted, and diligent athlete ran pain free (and with much less psychological stress) for the first time in 3 years. He completed his personal best trials in several sprinting events, and was invited by a prominent national amateur organization to compete in Europe.

Case 2. Julie B., a 36-year-old woman, was referred to the physical therapist with a diagnosis of lateral epicondylitis of the right upper extremity. She had been playing singles tennis for about three 1-hour sessions per week. She had pain over the common extensor tendon in her right forearm, more pronounced on resisted finger and wrist extension. Range of motion was within normal limits but painful at the end of the range of finger and wrist flexion.

Initial treatment consisted of a 2-week rest from tennis, and thrice weekly hydrocortisone phonophoresis over the affected area for 2 weeks. After the first week, the pain in the forearm had subsided. After the fourth treatment with hydrocortisone, friction massage was begun over the wrist and finger extensors. She was symptom free after 2 weeks, and a precise strengthening program of progressive resistive exercise was begun to strengthen both upper extremities with special emphasis on the right forearm, wrist, and finger musculature. She returned to activity 5 weeks after initial treatment began. Unfortunately, her symptoms returned after her third tennis session. Phonophoresis treatment was resumed for 1 week. Since her symptoms had again subsided, the progressive resistance exercise (PRE) program was again undertaken. In addition, isokinetic exercise was instituted on the Cybex II Dynamometer to strengthen all forearm and wrist musculature. The therapist contacted the tennis pro where the patient played; he changed her racket and fitted her with a correct grip. The patient resumed tennis playing after 4 weeks of isokinetic exercise and is now playing pain free.

REFERENCES

1. Gould JA, Davies GJ: J Orthop Sports Phys Ther 1 (1):1, 1979.

2. Blackburn TA (ed): Guidelines for Pre-Season Athletic Participation Evaluation. Georgia, Diversified Printing Services, 1979, p 11.

3. American Physical Therapy Association: Why Physical Therapy? APTA, 1980, p 2.

4. Zohn DA, Mennell JM: Musculoskeletal Pain. Boston, Little, Brown, 1976, p 4.

23
Injection Therapy

Mark F. Sherman, Joel R. Bonamo, and Richard B. Birrer

The use of injections has aroused much controversy in the field of sports medicine. Public statements regarding the abuses of "cortisone injections" in athletes have given injection therapy an extremely poor reputation. Patients typically fear such injections and are reluctant to receive them even when indicated. Primary care physicians must thoroughly understand the proper usage of drugs for injection of sports injuries and be aware of the potential abuses that may develop.[1]

The sites for injection of medication typically are the common areas of inflammation; that is, the joints (synovitis), the various bursae (bursitis), the tendons (tendinitis), and the linings of the tendons (tenosynovitis). The drugs most commonly injected are the anesthetic agents (lidocaine hydrochloride, bupivacaine hydrochloride) and the numerous injectable steroid medications (e.g., methylprednisolone acetate, triamcinolone acetonide, hydrocortisone). The anesthetic agents are beneficial in that they offer initial pain relief from the injection itself, but are more useful for their diagnostic abilities (discussed below). The steroid preparations serve as anti-inflammatory drugs which tend to reduce the acute or chronic inflammatory process. Shorter-acting (quickly absorbable) preparations offer rapid but brief relief; longer acting preparations produce a more prolonged beneficial response.

INDICATIONS

The indications for injection therapy are both diagnostic and therapeutic. Diagnostically, an injection of an anesthetic agent in an area of suspected pain can be very helpful in pinpointing a diagnosis. A typical example would be a baseball pitcher with shoulder pain that has not responded to other conservative measures (i.e. rest, oral anti-inflammatory medication, exercise programs). In such a patient, the differential diagnosis includes the impingement syndrome (rotator cuff irritation leading to inflammation and resultant impingement, with pain on overhead activities) versus possible shoulder subluxation (slipping of the shoulder in and out of the joint). A subacromial injection of 5 cc of lidocaine (2 percent), which offers immediate and prompt relief, indicates that the patient's problem is more than likely an impingement syndrome. This diagnostic test is very helpful in the further treatment of the patient, for this condition may be alleviated by a steroid injection or possibly a surgical release of the impingement problem.

An anesthetic agent can also help distinguish sites of pain. For example, in the shoulder, the acromioclavicular (AC) joint is another typical site of shoulder pain. Arthritis in this joint from a previous traumatic injury can lead to a pain pattern similar to that of the impingement syndrome. An injection into the AC joint, which offers prompt relief, aids in discriminating the diagnosis. Relief due to such an injection can dramatically change the future course of therapy. The differentiation of ankle pain from pain in the subtalar joint is another similar diagnostic dilemma. A joint injection in the ankle offers the answer to where the actual source of pain is located. Again, diagnostically, this method is extremely effective.

The selective use of steroids for injection is indicated for both acute and chronic inflammatory

TABLE 23-1. INJECTION THERAPY—LOCATIONS AND INDICATIONS

Region	Diagnosis	Site of Injection
Shoulder	Impingement syndrome	Subacromial bursa
	Acromioclavicular arthrosis	Acromioclavicular joint
	Bicipital tendinitis	Biceps tendon
Elbow	Lateral epicondylitis	Extensor muscle origin
Wrist	DeQuervain's syndrome	1st extensor compartment
	Flexor carpi ulnaris tendinitis	Flexor carpi ulnarus tendon
Hand	Flexor tenosynovitis (Trigger finger)	Tendon sheath
Knee	_a_	Infrapatellar fat pad
	Iliotibial band tendinitis	Iliotibial band
		Insertion fibula head
Ankle	_b_	Retrocalcaneal bursa
Foot	Plantar fascitis	Calcaneal origin of plantar fascia

_a_Diagnosis is patella tendinitis. _Note_: Very rare to inject this site, since there is a significant potential for tendon repture (see text).
_b_Diagnosis is Achilles tendinitis. _Note_: Very rare to inject this site, since there is a significant potential for tendon rupture (see text).

processes that do not respond to other conservative measures.[2] Oral anti-inflammatory medications, proper exercise programs, and ice therapy, are typically the first line of treatment for most athletic inflammatory conditions. Common inflammatory disorders are listed in Table 23-1 with the appropriate site of injection.

The appropriate dose of drug to be used depends on the type of steroid preparation (Table 23-2) and the location of the injection. This information is usually available within the drug packaging, and recommended doses are given for the specific sites to be injected. Allergy to a steroid, though rare, is an obvious contraindication. Pregnancy is also a contraindication because of the water-retentive potential of steroid medication. The usual preference is for a long-acting steroid; the longer-lasting relief is obviously more therapeutic. However, the short-acting steroids are absorbed quickly, have less chance of side reaction, and are helpful if the patient is in acute pain. Often, a combination of short- and long-acting steroids are given, providing immediate short-term relief as well as the potential longer-lasting benefit. Generally, it is preferable to inject steroid medication along with an anesthetic agent. A typical combination of bupivicaine hydrochloride and methylprednisolone acetate gives the immediate long-lasting analgesic effect followed by the onset of the long-acting steroid. The dosage, again, depends on the site involved. It is important to be familiar with one or two medications in terms of dosage adjustment, side-effects, and duration of action.

TECHNIQUE OF INJECTION

Injection of bursae, tendon sheaths, and joints is considered a surgical procedure much like a lumbar puncture. Therefore, the site for injection is given a careful scrub with an iodine or hexachlorophene

TABLE 23-2. INJECTION THERAPY—TYPES OF CORTICOSTEROIDS

SHORT-ACTING
  Dexamethasone sodium phosphate
  Hydrocortisone sodium succinate
INTERMEDIATE-ACTING
  Betamethasone acetate
  Triamcinolone acetonide
LONG-ACTING
  Methylprednisolone acetate
  Prednisolone acetate
  Dexamethasone acetate

containing surgical solution for several minutes. Routine prepping of the area is done, and a sterile drape applied. The gauge of the needle to be used depends on the site to be injected. (Hand injections usually require a 25-gauge needle, whereas other joint injections usually require 22- or 20-gauge needles.) A 3- or 5-cc syringe is all that is necessary. It is not routine to give anesthesia to the skin; however, ethyl chloride spray or a small wheal of an anesthetic agent decreases the pain of the injection. A quick injection usually does not require an anesthetic agent. After injection, an adhesive bandage is applied. The patient should be told to move the injected extremity immediately. If an anesthetic agent is used, the patient should be taken through a complete range of motion to see if the injection was effective. This is extremely important for it is part of the diagnostic examination. Often, an athlete is sent home and told immediately to throw a ball or use an extremity while the anesthetic agent is in effect, to see if the injection has worked. However, overuse of an extremity, particularly after an intra-articular injection, may cause deterioration in excess of benefits gained. The patient must be warned that, after the initial anesthetic agent wears off, the pain of the inflammatory disorder may be intensified. This is probably secondary to the rapid inflammatory response to the injection itself. The long-term steroid usually takes 36 to 72 hours to become effective, and the patient should be aware of this. Ice is often effective in alleviating the acute pain after the injection. The patient must also be told that recurrence of symptoms is not uncommon after steroid injections. Depending on the state of the inflammatory process, steroids may not be the final cure.

In treating nonspecific tenosynovitis, care should be taken to ensure that the injection is made into the tendon sheath rather than the tendon substance. The tendon should be identified by careful palpation and by placing it on stretch. Epicondylitis may be treated by infiltrating the preparation into the area of greatest tenderness. Tendon sheath ganglia should be directly injected. Often the cyst disappears due to a single puncture; some physicians recommend multiple cyst punctures with aspiration after a single cutaneous puncture with anesthesia. A 20- to 24-

gauge needle is used to puncture quickly a bursa or joint after adequate preparation and anesthesia. The site chosen should be most superficial and free of large nerves and vessels. Fluid is aspirated into a dry syringe, thus confirming proper location. The aspirating syringe is then removed and a smaller one containing the desired dose is attached. The injection is performed carefully, periodically pulling the plunger outward in order to ensure its location in the bursa or synovial space. Treatment failures are most frequently the result of failure to enter the appropriate space or trigger area. The spinal and sacroiliac joints are not suitable for injection because they are anatomically inaccessible or devoid of a synovial space.

The major contraindications to injections are allergy to the steroid (quite rare) and the history of multiple injections in the past. Certain inflammatory disorders (e.g., Achilles or patella tendinitis) should rarely be injected. The steroid is catabolic to collagen substance of the tendon and can weaken the tendon's tensile strength.[3,4] These particular sites have been shown to have an increased incidence of rupture after injection (typically after multiple injection), so an ultraconservative approach is warranted in these regions.

Multiple injections of steroids become a "double-edged sword." Eventually with repeated injections, more harm than good is achieved. A good rule of thumb to remember is that after 2 or 3 injections of an area, it is probably better to switch to another therapeutic mode (e.g., surgery). With time the steroids seem to become less effective; there is enhanced potential of rupture, and there are systemic side-effects that may occur (i.e., water retention). Intra-articular usage of steroids is associated with cartilaginous degeneration.[5,6]

Steroids should not be used for the treatment of acute injuries. "Masking" the symptoms of an injury with an anti-inflammatory medication is *dangerous,* because pain is an essential feature of the body's early warning system against further injury. The days of getting an athlete back to a sport with a "steroid injection" are long gone, and the bad press that such injections received was certainly well warranted. The acute injury must be treated in an appropriate manner for permanent and functional healing of the damaged tissues. Furthermore, steroids or anesthetic agents injected into regions of acute injury may protract the healing process.

CONCLUSIONS

The success rate of a steroid injection usually depends on:

1. The physician's ability to inject the site properly
2. The proper indication for injection
3. The appropriate physical therapy program to follow the postinjection phase of treatment
4. The avoidance of contributing mechanical factors[7]

The athlete must be made aware that the condition can recur after these injections and that a steroid is not a panacea. A detailed training program for the prevention of further injury is the key to long-term treatment, and the patient must understand that the steroid is only one aid along the way.

The physician typically uses injectable steroids more for diagnostic knowledge than for therapeutic benefits. If used appropriately, the injection is a marvelous medication but, as with most good things, overuse leads to abuse. Today, joint pathology is rarely an indication for corticosteroid injection in an athlete: steroids have been shown to have deleterious effects upon the cartilage of joint surfaces. It is more important to define the source of pain in the joint rather than treat the joint with these nonspecific anti-inflammatory medications. For the most part, injection sites today are limited to the bursa and tendons.

Perhaps, future drug preparations will not have such harmful effects upon the joint surfaces, and yet will be able to reduce the inflammatory response to injury. Such medications, if produced, will be a major breakthrough in the injection treatment of athletic injuries.

REFERENCES

1. McCarty D: Arthritis and Allied Conditions, ed 9. Philadelphia, Lea & Febiger, 1979, pp 402–417.
2. Hollander JL, Brown EM, Jessar RA, et al: Hydrocortisone and cortisone injected into arthritic joints. J Am Med Assoc 147:1629–1635, 1951.
3. Ismail AM, Balakrishnan R, Rajakumar MK: Rupture of patellar ligament after steroid infiltration. J Bone Joint Surg (AM) 51B:503–505, 1969.
4. Cowan MA, Alexander S: Simultaneous rupture of Achilles tendons due to triamcinolone. Br Med J 1:1658, 1961.
5. Chandler GN, Wright V: Deleterious effect of intraarticular hydrocortisone. Lancet 2:661–663, 1958.
6. Mankin HJ, Conger KA: The acute effects of intraarticular hydrocortisone on articular cartilage in rabbits. J Bone Joint Surg (AM) 48A:1383–1388, 1966.
7. Leadbetter WB: Corticosteroid injection for the treatment of athletic injury. American College of Sports Medicine 1983 Annual Meeting, Montreal, Canada.

BIBLIOGRAPHY

Danyo JJ, Kruper JS: The Illustrated Handbook of Injection Techniques. Rahway, NJ: Merck, 1975.

24
The Runner: A Profile of Problems

Franklin E. Payne, Jr.

Americans of all ages have poured into the streets, roads, and byways by the thousands as a wave of interest in running has rapidly gained momentum. The Atlanta Peachtree Road Race grew from having a few hundred runners in 1974 to limiting its registration to 25,000 in 1980. Similar examples of road races are present throughout the country. The total number of runners is at least 20 million. Obviously, primary care physicians must be ready to face the medical problems of these new sporting participants.

Initially, the psychology of the runner should be understood. Gabe Mirkin states the runner's attitude:

> A jogger jogs because he feels it will improve or protect his health. A runner runs even if he thinks it might kill him.[1]

The distinction between a runner and a jogger is artificial and is not made here. As a generalization, however, there are two classes of runner: low mileage and high mileage. Those runners in the latter group run more than 10 miles per week and participate in races regularly. Both types frequently go to any length to be able to continue their running. Thus, a runner presenting with a problem or an injury related to running usually is resistant to any restriction of this activity, even when it appears to the physician that healing is not otherwise possible or further injury is probable. In addition, runners are reluctant to see physicians, whom they presume ignorant of sports medicine for runners because of

physicians' lack of direct participation. To some extent, this attitude is accurate. However, basic research broadly based in all sports is becoming available to primary care physicians. A debate continues between physicians and runners as to whether the orthopedist or the podiatrist is the better consultant. The runner probably considers the podiatrist first when an injury occurs; the primary care physician, however, may be the first consulted if known among the running population to be interested and possess expertise. Such initial contact may also occur due to continual care of the patient as the primary care physician.

Although many consider running to be the best mode of exercise in relationship to health,[2] the frequency of injuries that result should be appreciated. A *Runners' World* survey of 1000 runners in 1977 showed that 60 percent of runners experience injuries each year. In order of decreasing frequency by site, their injuries were of the knee, shin, Achilles tendon, forefoot, hip, thigh, calf, heel, ankle, arch, hand, and groin.[3] It is certain that some people are unable to run without being injured. If exercise is promoted for health reasons, running cannot be seen as the only alternative. Equivalent sports, such as swimming and bicycling, must be considered.

TREATMENT

Specific treatment of all injuries cannot be adequately presented here; yet a general approach can be developed that should solve many problems. Most injuries that occur in running are probably due to overuse since the runner's foot strikes the ground an average of 5000 times per hour at a force of three to eight times body weight. Few people have perfect alignment of skeletal structures, so the slightest malalignment can result in severe trauma when subjected to such repetitive impact for 4 to 7 days per week. Such malalignment may occur anywhere from the spine to the forefoot.[4-7] Indeed, the anatomical cause of the injury itself may be distant from the site of the injury.

A history should include specific questions that define the runner's recent program. These areas involve total mileage, type of terrain, interval (speed) training, upcoming races, recent increases in mileage, and warm-up and cool-down stretching. An excellent source of information are the soles of running shoes, which show areas of wear corresponding to the areas of greatest stress. Worn shoes and new shoes cause a change in skeletal alignment and should be considered the etiology if related in time to the injury. Although inflammation of musculoskeletal structures is usually the problem, the possibility of a stress fracture must be entertained if symptoms and physical findings are consistent with this diagnosis, or if symptoms persist in spite of appropriate treatment. Bone scans in addition to x rays may be necessary to make the diagnosis.[8]

In the treatment of running injuries stretching should be encouraged, if not already being done. A general program that concentrates on the hamstring and calf muscles, sites of frequent tightness, is usually adequate, but specific injuries may require a specific stretching prescription. Stretching should be vigorous to the point of mild discomfort.

Orthotics have a place in the treatment of runners' injuries. These devices are primarily indicated for malalignments of the foot, most commonly excessive pronation. In addition orthotics have been found to relieve many injuries of runners: knee pain, plantar fasciitis and arch strain, shin splints, Achilles tendinitis, and others.[9] However, orthotics may be abused if the biomechanics of the foot are not understood.[10] The primary care physician may prescribe a flexible orthotic (e.g., Sporthotic) that is preformed, or one made from Plastizote, which can be molded by a specialist who fits orthopedically designed shoes. Another option would be a temporary device of felt or foam rubber made by the physician, but care must be taken to prevent rolling or wadding when it is used. Molding and casting of orthotics should only be done by those who have had specific training. The patient should be cautioned to stop the use of the orthotic if improvement does not occur within 1 week or if the pain increases. Beyond this approach, further prescription of an orthotic should be referred to a podiatrist or orthopedist. Orthotics should not be prescribed as a preventive measure unless injury has already occurred. Many biomechanical malalignments may be well tolerated or cancelled by the body's own adjustments.

Available running shoes vary widely in cost and design. Selection of a shoe should be carefully pursued[11] with the following suggestions: Most name brands are quality shoes. Shoe surveys are helpful but cannot address individual fit, which is the most important consideration. The shoes should fit in the store and can be worn around one's house for several days for verification. The fit should be snug on all areas of the foot with approximately 1 centimeter of space from the longest toe to the tip of the inside of the shoe (toenails are commonly injured). The shoes should be comfortable on the first run, without their needing a period of being broken in; however, they should not be worn in a race the first time in use. Seams can result in blisters. Observation of shoes from behind when placed on a flat surface reveals any varus or valgus tilt that may require correction. Reputable shoe stores specializing in running usually do a satisfactory job in helping to select the proper fit. If a single style of shoe suits an individual, any change is made at some risk of injury or discomfort. The durability of soles can be increased, and injuries that result from excessive wear prevented, by the application of a synthetic glue available at shoe stores.

With quality shoes, the running surface of streets, i.e., concrete or asphalt, is preferable because of the even surface when compared with the irregular surfaces of dirt or grass trails. Of course, each runner may discover that one surface is better than another when based on individual considerations, such as total distance, speed, and musculoskeletal adaptation.

Nonsteroidal anti-inflammatory agents may be useful initially in the treatment of running injuries but should not be continued over long periods of time because of their side-effects (see Chapter 23). The use of these drugs should be accompanied by stretching techniques and a consideration of realignment of weight bearing. Ice and heat may be tried in various combinations; the advantages and disadvantages of each technique continue to be debated, with response probably being of an individual nature. Logically, ice reduces swelling and inflammation immediately after running, but does not increase blood flow as had been thought.[13]

The injection of steroids should be considered only after all modes of therapy except surgery have been attempted. Both runner and physician should be aware that tendon rupture is a possibility through weakening of collagen by the steroid.[12,14] This result is more likely in the Achilles tendon, which is subjected to tremendous stress in running.

If a swimming pool is available, water rehabilitation that results in reduced weight bearing allows maintenance of cardiovascular function with muscular action similar to that of running.[15] Muscle strengthening exercises locally increase support of injured structures. Examples include quadriceps-strengthening exercises for knee problems and dorsiflexion exercises of the foot for ankle and anterior compartment problems.

The usual approaches to sports injuries are applicable to runners but proper alignment of skeletal structures in runners is crucial. If runners are agreeable, mileage may be reduced and/or interval training ceased to aid the healing process. Frequently, however, healing occurs without any reduction in the training program when the above modalities are prescribed. An individual approach to each runner according to his or her psychology and the presenting injury must be made.

HEART, HEAT, AND HEMATURIA

Runners of all backgrounds, including physicians, may develop an attitude that they are invulnerable; still, some runners do die while running.[16] Severe problem areas are coronary heart disease, motor vehicle collisions, and weather. The attitude that marathon running prevents coronary heart disease is often promoted. Certainly, it is likely that an overall effect on populations is to forestall cardiac events with the direct enhancement of myocardial function and reduction in risk factors. The argument as to whether the fatal event is an infarction or an arrhythmia is irrelevant. Heart disease in runners is a real possibility, and symptoms referable to the heart should be evaluated appropriately. On the other hand, physicians should understand that coronary heart disease does not prevent long-distance running[17] and a very active lifestyle (see Chapter 7). Both runner and physician need to make such life and death considerations with mutual understanding.

When a runner is killed by a motor vehicle while running, either the driver or the runner may have been negligent.[18] This reality needs recognition by all runners. The euphoria which long-distance runners often describe and seek may be involved. Failure to observe traffic rules is definitely a factor, as every runner is likely to have violated a traffic law at some time. Incredibly, runners have described a feeling of invulnerability to tons of steel on the roads moving at high rates of speed. Stark statistics reveal their fragility.

Heat stroke is a constant threat to runners in hot humid weather (above 70°F) because running is frequently an intense exercise that is performed over several hours (e.g., marathons). The symptoms of heat exhaustion, which can rapidly become heat stroke, are virtually indistinguishable from extreme fatigue (see Chapter 10). By the time heat stroke is imminent, the sensorium is blurred and runners are not able to recognize their plight. Core temperatures of 104°F are common in runners finishing marathons normally.[19] Runners must be encouraged to ingest plain, cold water frequently in runs up to a marathon in length (longer runs require the addition of sugars and electrolytes). The recommended volume is 6 to 8 ounces every 20 minutes during the run, and twice that amount 15 to 20 minutes prior to the start. Runners must experiment during their training runs to determine the maximum volume that they are able to ingest without stomach discomfort. Solutions with sugars and electrolytes are also appropriate at the end of a run.

Physicians who attend races in warm or hot weather *must* be knowledgeable about the details of treating heat stroke and *insist* on large quantities of ice being available in which to pack afflicted runners. In addition, the American College of Sports Medicine has a set of official guidelines,[20] and other directions for the management of hot weather races are available.[21]

Dry, cold weather is not as dangerous, but deaths have occurred upon prolonged exposure during exercise in cold (2 to 3°C), wet, and windy weather.[22] On the other hand, in otherwise healthy people, cold-air inhalation does not result in injury to the bronchi or lungs even at temperatures far below zero.[23] Primary preventive attention should be directed toward the wearing of two or more layers of lightweight clothing with additional protection for ears, hands, and male genitalia.

In one series, 18 percent of runners after a marathon had gross or microscopic hematuria. All urines were clear after 48 hours.[24] A urologist found contusions of the bladder and related these findings to "a combination of exertional forces, intraabdominal pressure, and the repeated impact of the flaccid bladder wall against the bladder base."[25] Thus, hematuria that clears within 48 hours may be considered benign in the absence of other symptoms. It is recommended that runners not completely empty their bladder prior to participation, as the urine acts as a cushion between the bladder surfaces.

GI TRACT AND NUTRITION

Gastrointestinal problems are common to runners. Cramping pains may occur which exist only while running or may persist afterwards. Diarrhea, occasionally bloody with or without cramping, occurs.[26] Probably every long-distance runner has experienced the inconvenience of an imminent bowel movement while running. Thus, symptoms may range from mild to incapacitating. The explanation of these events is not yet known, but theories include increased parasympathetic tone and ischemia of the gut. Low-fiber diets have been advocated, but a high-fiber diet may allow a bowel movement prior to the run and thus prevent the symptoms. Each approach should be tried to determine which is in-

dividually effective. If the runner is a novice or has recently increased his or her mileage, symptoms may disappear with time. To date, however, no pathological changes have been identified that might seriously endanger the health of the runner.

Nutrition for runners is essentially no different from a basic, healthy diet. Runners often lose weight markedly and may have gaunt facies, but no detrimental effect of this change has been identified. Extra vitamins and other dietary extras have no proven benefit. Runners do need more carbohydrates because of their high mileage, but the amount is highly individual and only partially related to total distance. Carbohydrate loading—an extra long run followed by 3 days of carbohydrate restriction, then carbohydrate excess—is effective in prolonging muscular work. It is not, however, tolerated by everyone, and not a guarantee of better performance (see Chapter 11). Diabetics, with minimal adjustments in their routine, are able to run long distances on a regular basis.[27]

ADDICTION AND "ABNORMAL" LAB VALUES

Other than a higher proportion of introverts being present in marathoners, their personality profiles show essentially no differences when compared with the general population.[28] A frequent phenomenon, however, is an addiction to running.[29] Symptoms consist of a strong attitude that one cannot cope with living without running daily. Withdrawal symptoms occur if this pattern is not followed. The addictive process is similar to other addictions. Running becomes an increasingly higher priority than family, jobs, friends, or other values. The development of this addiction may be determined by observation that running is increasing in priority or by asking, "What would you do if you had to stop running?" Injuries may force a runner to stop, bringing the situation to a crisis; the physician and the runner then need to re-examine which values are most important.

Initial reports indicate that *endorphins* may play a role in these emotions and behaviors associated with running. Endorphins are peptides found initially to be secreted by the hypothalamus but more recently found in other sites, such as the gastrointestinal tract and elsewhere in the brain.[30] Findings have been consistent in showing marked elevations of endorphins during and following active exercise.[31,32] Since these peptides are known to have opiate-like analgesic and euphoric effects and to be blocked by opiate-antagonists, these substances may indeed play a role in the runner's "high," addiction, or withdrawal symptoms that may occur upon cessation of running. Experiments concerning the exact role of endorphins in running and other exercises are just beginning to be studied and remain otherwise inconclusive at this point.

All physicians should be aware that laboratory values deemed abnormal in most patients may be a direct result of physiological effects of running. These changes include ECG findings from a hypertrophied heart, arrhythmias, anemia from hypervolemia, and serum enzyme elevations from vigorous muscle activity. Of course, pathophysiology may be concurrent in a runner, but these values should usually be attributed to running. Unnecessary tests and inconvenience to the patient can thus be avoided. For more detail on these findings see Chapter 8.

As large numbers of runners continue their sport for many years to come, much more will be known about chronic effects and measurable benefits from long-distance running. Physicians must follow these findings as many of their patients are likely to be runners and may present with injuries or other related symptomatology.

REFERENCES

1. Mirkin G, Hoffman M: The Sportsmedicine Book. Boston, Little, Brown 1979, p 180.
2. Elrick H: Distance runners are models of optimal health. Phys Sports Med 9(1):67–68, 1981.
3. Sheehan GA: An overview of overuse syndromes in distance runners. Ann NY Acad Sci 301:877–880, 1977.
4. Klein KK: Evaluation of running injuries. Phys Sports Med 8(2):141–143, 1980.
5. Schuster RO: Foot types and the influence of environment on the foot of the long distance runner. Ann NY Acad Sci 301:881–887, 1977.
6. Subtonick SI: A biomechanical approach to running injuries. Ann NY Acad Sci 301:888–899, 1977.
7. Kristoff WB, Ferris WD: Runner's injuries. Phys Sports Med 7(12):55–64, 1979.
8. Norfray JF, Schulachter L, Kernahan WT, et al: Early confirmation of stress fractures in joggers. J Am Med Assoc 243:1647–1650, 1980.
9. Eggold JF: Orthotics in the prevention of runners' overuse syndromes. Phys Sports Med 9(3):125–132, 1981.
10. Subotnick SI: The abuses of orthotics in sports medicine. Phys Sports Med 3(7):73–75, 1975.
11. Dunn K: Choosing a running shoe: Science or subjectivity. Phys Sports Med 8(12):85–86, 1980.
12. Gottlieb NL, Riskin WG: Complications of local corticosteroid injections. J Am Med Assoc 243:1547–1548, 1980.
13. Knight KL, Londeree BR: Comparison of blood flow in the ankle of uninjured subjects during the therapeutic application of heat, cold, and exercise. Med Sci Sports Exerc 12:76–80, 1980.
14. Ford LT, DeBender J: Tendon rupture after local steroid injection. South Med J 72:827–830, 1979.
15. Cooper DL, Fair J: Rehabilitation through underwater exercise. Phys Sports Med 4(10):143, 1976.
16. Thompson PD, Stern MP, William P: Death during jogging or running: A study of 18 cases. J Am Med Assoc 242:1265–1267, 1979.
17. Kavanagh T, Shepard RH, Pandit V: Marathon running after myocardial infarction. J Am Med Assoc 229:1602–1605, 1974.
18. Insurance Institute for Highway Safety: When motor vehicles hit joggers: Analysis of 60 cases. Washington, DC, Insurance Institute for Highway Safety, 1980.
19. Maron MB, Horvath SW: The marathon—A review. Med Sci Sports 10:135–150, 1978.
20. American College of Sports Medicine: Heat peril in distance runs spurs ACSM guideline alert. Phys Sports Med 3(7):85–87, 1975.
21. Noble HB, Bachman D: Medical aspects of distance race planning. Phys Sports Med 7(6):78–86, 1979.
22. Pugh LGCE: Deaths from exposure on Four Inns Walking Competition. Lancet 1:1210–1212, 1964.
23. Claremont AD: Taking winter in stride requires proper attire. Phys Sport Med 4(12):65–68, 1976.
24. Siegel AF, Hennekens CH, Solomon HS: Exercise-related hematuria: Findings of a group of marathon runners. J Am Med Assoc 241:391–392, 1979.
25. Dunn K: Contusions may cause runner's hematuria. Phys Sports Med 7(10:)20, 1979.

26. Forgoros RN: "Runners trots": Gastrointestinal disturbances in runners. J Am Med Assoc 243:1743–1744, 1980.
27. Costill DL, Miller JM, Pink WJ: Energy metabolism in distance runners. Phys Sports Med 8(10):64–71, 1980.
28. Clitsome T, Kostrubala T: A Psychological study of 100 marathoners using the Myers–Briggs type indicator and demographic data. Ann NY Acad Sci 301:1010–1019, 1977.
29. Morgan WP: Negative addiction in runners. Phys Sports Med 7(2):57–70, 1979.
30. Krieger DT, Martin JB: Brain peptides. N Engl J Med 304:876–885, 944–951, 1981.
31. Carr OB, Bullen BA, Skrinar GS, et al: Physical conditioning facilitates the exercise-induced secretion of beta-endorphin and beta-lipoprotein in women N Engl J Med 305:560–563, 1981.
32. Letters to the Editor: Exercise and the endogenous opiods. N Engl J Med 305:1590–1591, 1981.

BIBLIOGRAPHY

Brody DM: Running injuries. CIBA Clin Symp 32(4): 1–36, 1980.
Cooper KH: The Aerobics Way. New York, M Evans, 1977.
Daniels J, Fitts R, Sheehan G: Conditioning for Long Distance Running. New York, John Wiley, 1978.
Jesse J: Hidden causes of Injury, Prevention and Correction, for Running Athletes and Joggers. Pasadena, Calif: The Athletic Press, 1977.
Milvy P (ed): The marathon: Physiological, medical, epidemiological, and psychological studies. Ann NY Acad Sci 301:1–1090, 1977.
Mirkin G, Hoffman M: The Sportsmedicine Book. Boston, Little, Brown, 1978.
Subotnick SI: The Running Foot Doctor. Mt View, Calif, World Publications, 1977.
Wenger NK: Exercise and the Heart. Philadelphia, FA Davis, 1978.

25

Special Problems of the Water Sports Participant

J. David Busby

Historically, water has been credited with medicinal properties. Biblically, water is allegorically associated with eternal life. The explorer, Ponce de Leon, searched for the fountain of youth. Many resorts and spas now center around hot and "mineral" springs in this country and on other continents. The concept of water's medicinal values may stem partially from an unconscious desire to return to the support, warmth, and protection of the womb.

BENEFITS OF WATER SPORTS

The physician and other specialists providing primary care have a unique opportunity to affect the long-term physical and emotional well-being of the individual and the family by encouraging recreational water sport activities, including the following:

- Water skiing
- Swimming (pool and nonpool)
- Diving
- Scuba diving
- Snorkeling
- Fishing (fresh and sea water)
- Ice fishing
- Canoeing/boating
- Sailing
- Rowing
- Yachting
- Water polo
- Hot-tub bathing
- Para-sailing

Water sport activities may build cardiovascular reserve and can be used as part of the exercise prescription for physical conditioning. Vigorous swimming allows the individual to approach more rapidly his or her physician-recommended maximum heart rate than does jogging. Swimming at 2 miles per hour has been reported to consume 7.9 calories per kilogram per hour[1]; swimming, therefore, can be considered as adjunctive therapy for the obese patient. The popularity of water sports is well documented: one eastern state has over 1 million pleasure boaters alone.[15] The variety of activities make water sports popular with the family. Water sports may be associated with group activity or may be enjoyed in solitude. Fishing alone in remote areas may be a form of escape for the individual caught in the hustle-bustle of the busy twentieth century. Water sports may be competitive, such as tournament fishing, collegiate rowing, swimming, diving, and water polo. They also appeal to those individuals who equate a bronzed body with beauty. For certain families, then, water is synonomous with recreation. Its appropriate benefits and risks, as one form of an exercise prescription, should therefore be well known by the primary care physician.

Water sports are associated with accidents that are preventable. Certain water sports have injuries peculiar to them; however, several common problems are associated with all such activities and may be prevented by simple education. Fortunately, most of these problems are minor; they are considered here, looking primarily at prevention and briefly at treatment. The greatest preventive measure is generic for all water sports—knowing how to swim. The primary care physician should take an active community role in urging swimming lessons for all persons of all ages.

SWIMMING

Swimming, the oldest and most popular water sports activity, is enjoyed worldwide. This vigorous physical activity can provide an alternative activity for those people interested in physical conditioning but unable or unwilling to walk, run, or jog. Swimming is excellent for the arthritic and elderly patient whose painful joints cannot absorb further wear and tear. The runner with stress fractures, sprains, or other running-related injuries may do rehabilitative exercises in the swimming pool. The runner may "run in place" in water while being supported by the buoyancy of personal flotation devices (life buoys).[2] The lower extremities have no shock transmitted if the runner is in 8 feet of water. Additionally, knee and back injuries secondary to a variety of sports (football, weight lifting, martial arts) can be rapidly rehabilitated by a swimming prescription, and cardiovascular fitness is preserved as well as muscle tone while the injuries heal.

Those patients being treated with anticonvulsants for epilepsy should be allowed to participate in swimming or other water sports activities under the following guidelines:

1. The patient with seizure activity in the past 24 months or with medication change or withdrawal should be involved in water sports activity only when a person trained in water rescue is immediately available.

2. The patient with no seizure activity in the past 24 months should be allowed to participate in water sports activities using the "buddy system."

SUN-INDUCED INJURIES

Sunburn is the most common injury seen in water sports. Most sunburns are first degree, i.e., causing only redness of the skin. Treatment consists of oral analgesics and/or over-the-counter topical anesthetics. Topical anesthetics, however, may sensitize the individual and perhaps later trigger allergic reactions during minor surgery or dental work. Oral analgesics and topical corticosteroid aerosols are preferred for first-degree burns. Second-degree burns, with blister formations, may require hospitalization if extensive. Skin grafting is rarely required. These burns are seen mainly in patients with light skin or those with no recent sun exposure.

Prevention of sunburn is relatively easy. The individual active in water sports activities should be instructed by the physician about the factors involved in sunburn. The likelihood of sunburn is increased at high altitude, on windy days, when the humidity is high, with certain medications, and between the hours of 10:00 A.M. and 2:00 P.M. Effective sunscreens are commercially available over the counter. Sun worshippers, those working in the sunlight, and all those involved in water sports activities should use the correct sunscreen, to be recommended by the physician after a careful discussion of sun exposure. Sunscreens are rated, with higher numbers indicating greater protection. As an example of this rating, SPF 8 means that the individual can tolerate eight times the amount of sunshine that normally causes him or her to burn. Sunburn is expected from UV-B light, which has a relatively short wavelength of 290 to 320 nanometers. It is also referred to as "erythema-range light."[3] Long-wavelength light, UV-A light, does not cause sunburn but does allow tanning and photosensitivity reactions. No epidermal damage occurs with UV-A light but dermal changes may occur over long periods. Such changes (e.g., wrinkling, senile keratosis, senile purpura due to thinning of the skin, and loss of elasticity) are minor compared to the epidermal changes that may occur with UV-B light. Sunscreens are made up of PABA derivatives, oxybenzone derivatives, or a combination of both. PABA blocks UV-B light, whereas oxybenzone derivatives block UV-B and UV-A light. In the photosensitive athlete, both UV-A and UV-B light must be blocked. Individuals allergic to PABA should use oxybenzone derivatives. Sunscreens are to be applied 30 minutes before entering the sunlight, upon entering the sunlight, and each time after leaving the water. The lips and nose should be protected as well as the rest of the body. At the beginning of each summer season, limited exposure (10 to 15 minutes) before 10:00 A.M. and after 2:00 P.M. is recommended with gradual daily increase in time exposure. Exposure increases are restricted to 5-minute increments with photosensitive patients.

With the increase in popularity of water sports activities, it is expected that there will eventually be an increase in the number of new skin malignancies in the form of actinic keratosis and basal cell epitheliomas. The question has not been definitely answered, but it appears that malignant melanomas may be increased with sun exposure. For patients with lightly pigmented skin there is a real problem. The physician must educate them because prevention is the best treatment.

SWIMMER'S EAR

Swimmer's ear is the most common form of external otitis and develops due to increased moisture and heat in the external auditory canal. This disease presents with pain in the ear, otorrhea and, in some instances, a decrease in hearing. The patient experiences severe pain with manipulation of the outer ear; this is helpful in distinguishing it from otitis media, which usually does not cause pain when the ear is moved. Swimmer's ear sometimes presents with obvious swelling of the external ear and face. The etiology of this illness is bacterial in the vast majority of the cases, with fungal infections causing only 10 percent of the illnesses. Treatment should

begin with debridement of the free material present in the external ear. Topical agents are the mainstay of treatment. Drops are most frequently used but are not as efficacious as the use of a wick saturated with an appropriate agent. Multipurpose creams such as nystatin are antibacterial, antifungal, and also anti-inflammatory. For pure fungal infections one of the acetic acid–propylene glycol preparations should be used along with debridement. Debridement is best performed by suctioning.[4] Swimmer's ear is quite painful and the physician should prescribe an appropriate analgesic. It can be prevented by drying the external canal immediately after water sports activities. The instillation of a few drops of rubbing alcohol in the auditory canal dries that area. Proper chlorination of swimming pools reduces the possibility of this infection, but obviously this is not possible in lakes or rivers where boating occurs.

CUTS AND PUNCTURES

As in other sports, *lacerations* are very common in water sports. Most result from falls, knives, broken glass, and so on. These lacerations should be closely monitored as many waters are routinely found to be colonized with various species of *Pseudomonas,* and some waters are contaminated with various strains of *Mycobacterium* that are difficult to treat. Appropriate debridement and copious irrigation reduces the possibility of infection. As with any other laceration, tetanus prophylaxis must be considered.

Imbedded fishhooks are often painful, but most are minor and leave no sequelae. Fishhooks may cause eye injuries that leave permanent visual defects and should be referred to an ophthalmologist. Removal of fishhooks in other areas may be accomplished by one of several methods:

1. The barb may be pushed through and cut off, allowing the hook to be removed by reversing its path.
2. The hook may be sharply excised under local anesthesia.
3. The eye of the hook may be cut off and then the hook is pushed forward along its path.

4. A string may be attached to the hook at its curve so that, while pressure is exerted on the eye, a sudden jerk of the string pulls the hook free.

Again, tetanus prophylaxis is necessary if the individual is not currently immunized.

BITES AND STINGS

Snake and insect bites are an unwarranted fear of many people who swim. In the United States there are only four snakes that are poisonous: the coral snake, the copperhead, the rattlesnake, and the cottonmouth (water moccasin). The coral snake is usually seen only in the Southeast. It is primarily a subterranean dweller and, hence, unlikely to be the source of bites of water enthusiasts. Rattlesnakes and copperheads are sometimes found near water, but only the cottonmouth is routinely found around water in the South and Southeast. According to Russell, there are 45,000 bites annually in the United States with only 6000 venomous bites being treated; less than 15 people die from these bites.[5] The majority of these deaths occur in the elderly and children: In 12 deaths reported by Ennik, six were in children younger than 4 and two were in people over 70. The majority of the deaths were due to rattlesnakes.[6]

Snakebite treatment remains controversial and each year there are usually two articles on treatment that contradict each other. With the low potential for harm from a venomous bite, and with the possibility of more harm from inappropriate first aid, first aid must be simple. Transportation to the nearest medical facility, with the victim in a neutral recumbent position, is the most appropriate emergency field care. Direct application of ice may cause injury if left for a significant period or if salt is added to the ice. The snake (dead) should be taken to the medical facility to aid in determining whether or not it was venomous. Antivenom should be reserved for those with grade II or higher envenomization. The grade descriptions are in the product insert (antivenin). A helpful poster is available through the American College of Surgeons, listing the grading of envenomization as well as treatment. The suggested treatment points out the controversy involved in snakebite treatment. It suggests that if the patient is treated within 30 minutes of the bite, suction should be applied after incision of at least full thickness skin. A second statement also suggests that some people with extensive experience recommend exploration of the snakebite to determine the depth of the tissue destruction. Serious allergic reactions are possible with the antivenom, and skin testing for allergic reaction is required. Those with less than grade II envenomization should be treated conservatively—analgesics and observation.

Ennik reported seven more deaths in California from insect stings than from snakebites (1960 to 1976). These fatalities are due to anaphylactic reactions.[6] Desensitization greatly reduces the possibility of death in allergic individuals, who should carry with them a kit containing epinephrine (1:1000) with a method of delivering it (e.g., EPI-PEN); for adults 0.3 to 0.5 cc subcutaneously repeated in 10 to 15 minutes if needed.

Water enthusiasts in coastal water ways may have problems from jelly fish stings, particularly the Portuguese man-of-war. These stings may occur in all oceans, but are most common in the South Asian and Australian waters. These coelenterates do not attack humans; they have no mechanism for doing so. One is harmed by coming in contact with floating tentacles. These tentacles can cause linear erythematous wheals associated with severe burning pain and may cause blister formations.[7] Some of these may be associated with systemic symptoms, primarily dyspnea, nausea, and muscle cramps. Local necrosis of tissue has resulted from a severe sting. If the tentacles are attached or adhering to the skin, they should not be removed until alcohol or meat tenderizer has been applied. The alcohol inactivates the nematocysts. If the tentacle is compressed or mechanically removed, it may cause injection of more venomous material. The treatment is basically conservative with antihistamines or analgesics for the pain.[8]

Some fish, such as the stonefish, lionfish, scorpionfish, and weeverfish, have venom-secreting glands that may be associated with spines on their fins. These primarily are shallow-water fish that tend to hide or be concealed in a crevice or sand. Individuals are injured accidently, either by stepping on them or by coming in contact with them as they swim. The stingray fish is distributed primarily in warm coastal waters, but may inhabit fresh water. These fish may be quite large: up to 8 feet in length and weighing up to 100 pounds. The secreting organs are located in the tail of the stingray and the individual may step on this fish or come in contact with its tail which can drive the stinger in. This may be associated with severe pain and edema at the area of injury. Systemic symptoms may include nausea, diaphoresis, and syncope. In the United States a report of a 5-year period detailed 1097 stingray injuries with 62 patients requiring hospitalization and two of these individuals died.[7] Minton has suggested that first aid be conservative and consist of irrigation of the area with salt water and removal of any part of the stinger that can be seen. Next, the injury should be washed with lukewarm water and the individual given tetanus prophylaxis. Rarely, the stingray may cause quite severe injuries, driving large spines into individuals, requiring surgical debridement.[7]

Shark bites receive a lot of publicity but are infrequent and, of course, occur in coastal waterways only. Fatalities and amputations may result. Prevention is critical and swimmers should heed shark warnings posted by various beach municipalities.

HOT TUBS

Hot tubs began as a fad in California within the past few years. The hot tub in California is a large redwood tub filled with tepid water and usually contains a whirlpool. The temperature of the water is generally at or just above 100° F. There have been two cases reported in California of individuals who died while they were in a hot tub. It was suggested that dehydration could have played a role here as well as the use of substances such as alcohol. Hot tubs have become a fad nationwide now and

have a potential danger. The temperature and the amount of time within the tub should be limited. The use of alcohol and narcotics should be discouraged as deaths from drowning or even heat exhaustion might occur. Folliculitis caused by *Pseudomonas aeruginosa* has occurred in hot tub and whirlpool users.[9]

WATER SKIING

Water skiing may be associated with peculiar injuries. Avulsions or amputations of fingers may occur when the ski rope becomes wrapped around the finger. Wedding or other rings increase this risk. The skiing "douche" may cause peritonitis, if water is forced into the peritoneum through fallopian tubes, as well as lacerations of the vagina and cervix. Rectal injuries are less common and occur when water is forced into the distal sigmoid—the skiing "enema."[10] An observer in the pull boat is mandatory and a wet suit or similar neoprene device can help prevent these injuries.

Cerebral concussions occur frequently to water skiers. Most of these are treated by observation and usually clear without sequela. Competitive and acrobatic skiers, as well as those that ski at high speeds, should consider using a lightweight cycling-type helmet. Serious intracranial injuries are not commonly seen in skiing. All injured skiers should be evaluated for possible neck and cranial injuries and treated appropriately.

Propeller injuries, caused by the individual being run over by the propeller of the boat, are common. Reports indicate that 1 out of 20 boating injuries may be due to the propeller (Fig. 25-1). Mann reported 32 cases of propeller injuries with 20 deaths. Several amputations and several *Pseudomonas* infections were reported.[11] Propeller injuries may be greatly reduced by a "kill" switch—one connected to the motor's electrical ground and to the boat driver by lanyard switch. When the driver is thrown out of the seat or the boat, the ground is broken and the motor and the propeller stop instantly. Skiing with an observer also reduces the frequency of propeller injuries as the driver can be instructed to stop

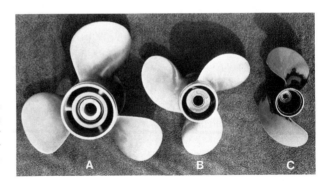

FIGURE 25-1. Propellers from pleasure craft. **A.** 13-inch-diameter stainless steel propeller for 150-horsepower motor. **B.** Stainless steel propeller for 100-horsepower motor. **C.** Aluminum propeller for 50-horsepower motor.

as soon as the skier loses the skis. This reduces the time that a skier spends in the water, perhaps in the path of another boat.

BOATING ACCIDENTS

Boating collisions may cause many of the same injuries seen in automobile accidents. Blunt trauma may occur when the individual is thrown from the boat, landing on the abdomen or the bony thorax. A 1979 collision accident in Pennsylvania resulted in two fatalities. The boats involved had very large engines.[12] Many pleasure jet boats and bass boats easily run 50 miles per hour (Fig. 25-2). At these speeds death is likely if collisions occur.

Kayaking and canoeing have seen a rapid surge in popularity in the past few years. They require skill and experience on difficult rivers, pitting humankind against nature. This activity requires vigorous paddling and may be part of the exercise prescription for physical conditioning. An inter-

national classification scale of white water rivers allows the physician to recommend specific levels of participation. Class I streams have only a few ripples and waves and are free of obstructions. Class VI streams are the most difficult to navigate, having long and rough rapids and obstructions with a critical hazard in the event of capsizing. These streams should be left to expert teams who know the risks and know the stream.[13] The physician must counsel patients about the perils as well as the pleasures of canoeing. Class I or II personal flotation devices are necessary and a lightweight helmet is recommended. Kayakers and canoeists face a great risk of drowning secondary to hypothermia due to rapid heat loss in the circulating water (see Chapter 10).

DROWNING

The major cause of death in water sports is drowning (Chapter 10). During the first half of 1980 in Arkansas, ten fishing deaths were reported.[14] In one

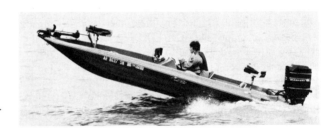

FIGURE 25-2. 18-foot "Bass" boat accelerating on take-off.

year the state of Pennsylvania reported 27 drowning deaths, 20 in boating. Chambers, in a review of the deaths in Pennsylvania, found a distinct pattern. Over half of the boating deaths involved boats less than 16 feet long and without motors. One-fourth of the deaths involved boats with motors under 10 horsepower. The water was most often rough, but no definite weather pattern was found.[15] The use of drugs and alcohol is well documented in many drownings.[16] Other common factors include improper boat loading and improper lookout.

The majority of drowning deaths in Pennsylvania were reported as occurring in the spring and fall. Hypothermia is postulated as the common factor. Survival in water between 32° and 40° F (0° to 5° C) is 15 minutes or less. With water temperatures of 60° F (16° C), survival time may be as long as 2 hours.[17] Heat loss is tremendously increased with vigorous physical activity in the water. A posture to reduce heat loss has been presented to prevent or retard body heat loss: HELP (Heat Escape Lessening Posture) may double the survival time in 60° F water.[18] This posture requires the knees to be flexed sharply upward toward the abdomen, the lower legs to be crossed and drawn to the hips, elbows at the side with the forearms flexed, the hands crossed, and the neck flexed. Victims of drowning in cold waters should have prolonged resuscitative efforts as cases of successful resuscitation after 30 minutes of submersion have been reported. The mammalian diving reflex has been suggested as the cause of this dramatic success. This reflex is thought to reduce the inspiration of water into the lungs, reduce the oxygen needs of the brain, and hence aid survival.[19] It is seen usually in water at temperatures less than 70° F, when the person's face was immersed first; it is most pronounced in the younger age group.

The most common factor in drowning is failure to wear personal flotation devices (PFD). These devices are required in most states for boaters and skiers. These devices are classified and approved by the U.S. Coast Guard. Type I and type II PFDs are both capable of turning the unconscious person to a vertical or slightly backward position from a downward one. Type III PFDs are more comfortable but do not turn the unconscious person. Type IV devices include throwable buoyant cushions or ring buoys.[20] The ski belt is not an approved device and the primary care physician should urge patients to use either type I or II PFDs. Type II devices are perhaps not appropriate for the high-speed skier as neck injuries may occur on impact with the water. They must be fitted to the individual. After each use they should be cleaned and dried. Each year they should be tested to see if they have lost any flotation capability. Most of all, they must be worn.

People for whom water recreation activities are prescribed should be instructed by their physician on how to reduce the possibility of drowning according to the guidelines provided:

1. Learn to swim or tread water.
2. Use the buddy system—do not swim alone.
3. Avoid the use of drugs and alcohol in water sports.
4. Wear the PFD.
5. Have boats inspected by the U.S. Coast Guard Auxiliary to determine if they meet minimum safety requirements.
6. If unexpectedly thrown into the water, remain calm and stay near the boat.
7. Choose one of the newer boats that has positive flotation and remains upright even if filled with water.
8. Be aware that water distances are not easily judged and it takes a good swimmer to swim 200 yards.

REFERENCES

1. Krause M, Mahon LK: Food, Nutrition and Diet Therapy. Philadelphia, WB Saunders, 1978, p 30.
2. Brody David M: Running injuries. CIBA Clin Symp 32(4):27, 1980.
3. Erythema range. Data on file. Dohme Laboratories.
4. Farmer HS: A guide for the treatment of external otitis. Am Fam Physician 21(6):96–101, 1980.
5. Russell F: Snake venom poisonings in the United States, in Greger WP (ed): Annual Review of Medicine. Palo Alto, Calif Annual Review, 1980, pp 247–259.
6. Ennik F: Death from bites and stings of venomous animals. West J Med 32:463–468, 1980.
7. Minton S: Marine venoms, in Beeson PB, McDermott W (eds): Textbook of Medicine. Philadelphia, WB Saunders, 1975, pp 92–93.

8. Keegan HL: Venomous marine animals, in Beeson PB, McDermott W (eds): Textbook of Medicine. Philadelphia, WB Saunders, 1979, pp 123–125.

9. Zacherle BJ, Silver DS: Hot tub folliculitis: A clinical syndrome. Western J Med 137:191, 1982.

10. Kaiser R, Armenia D, Baron R, et al: Waterskier's enema. N Engl J Med 302:1264, 1980.

11. Mann R: Propeller injuries incurred in boating accidents. Am J Sports Med 8(4):280–284, 1980.

12. 1979 Boating Accident Reports. Pennsylvania Fish Commission, 1979.

13. Canoe Safety. Pennsylvania Fish Commission, 1979.

14. Personal communication. Arkansas Fish Commission, 1980.

15. Chambers V: The common sense approach. Pennsylvania Angler 49(7):27–29, 1980.

16. Bullard J: Death in sports and recreation. Phys Sports Med 9(6):124–130, 1981.

17. Hypothermia and Cold Water Survival. Department of Transportation. US Coast Guard, 1977.

18. Survival in Cold Water. Pennsylvania Fish Commission, 1979.

19. Smith DS: Sudden drowning syndrome. Phys Sports Med 8(6):76–82, 1980.

20. Personal Flotation Devices. Pennsylvania Fish Commission, 1979.

BIBLIOGRAPHY

Coles KA: Heavy Weather Sailing. New York, John DeGraff, 1976.
  Most useful book for any sailor who may expect to encounter extremes of wave or temperature common to offshore sailing. Many useful survival hints.

Morris D, Strung N: Family Fun On and Around the Water. New York, Cowles, 1970.

US Coast Guard: Safety Standards for Backyard Boat Builders. CG-446, 1978.

US Coast Guard: Rules and Regulations for Recreational Boats. COMDTINST M16752.2, 1978.
  Useful guides on outfitting, equipping, and sailing a small boat.

26
Special Problems of the Hunter

J. David Busby

Old habits are hard to discard. Hunting is a habit that dates to the beginning of humankind. The unlucky animal not only provided meat for the early hunter, but also clothes, shelter, and tools or utensils made from bone. The hunt is no longer mandatory in this country as agricultural producers can supply adequate meat and vegetables for the American table; however, it persists.

The reasons for enjoying hunting are as varied as the individuals who hunt. Many hunt because it is a contest pitting human against animal; others simply because it is an activity that allows them to be outdoors; still others because of the social activities associated with hunting clubs. Some hunt because of the physical activity required.

Hunting is a traditional American pastime and, to a large degree, constitutes a frequent and acceptable exercise prescription by the primary care physician. It must be considered here because of the magnitude of the injuries and deaths associated with it. The number of accidental hunting deaths alone in one state during one hunting season is greater than the number of deaths in all levels of football during one season nationwide. The impact of the primary care physician in health maintenance through preventive medicine in this sport can be life saving. In addition, the physician must be knowledgeable about the pathophysiology of injuries and deaths in hunting activities. This chapter reviews the nature of this sport, highlighting its beneficial aspects as well as its risks.

HUNTING AS PHYSICAL ACTIVITY

The physical activity associated with hunting varies with the quarry and the terrain. *Still hunting* has the hunter walking to a spot thought to be traversed by the animals hunted. During the early autumn, the squirrel hunter walks to a tree producing nuts. These nuts are sought by the squirrels and the hunter waits expectantly out of sight. The caloric expenditure for this type of hunting could be considered somewhat greater than sedentary activities and perhaps 150 calories per hour are expended. *Bird* (nonwaterfowl) *hunting* requires walking great distances in flat terrain wearing light clothing and carrying a light shotgun. This moderate activity probably burns 250 calories per hour. *Big game hunting* may involve walking and still hunting. The terrain is usually rough and/or hilly and the hunter carries a heavy rifle. Big game seasons are during cold weather, and heavy clothing is required. Caloric expenditure may be greater than 400 calories per hour.[1]

Hunting should not be suggested by the primary care physician as a method of weight loss as it would take 2 hours of big game hunting just to burn up the calories of one large hamburger, french fries, and a cola. Hunting, being seasonal in nature, cannot be used alone as a continuing activity for developing stamina; however, the physician may recommend hunting for anxiety or similar stress states, as the activity required may be stress reducing. Because hunting conditions and locations vary so greatly, hunting may be recommended for many individuals who are unable to participate in other outdoor sports. The rheumatoid arthritic who needs exercise may have a prescription for hunting that requires walking on flat terrain during hunting seasons that are climatologically temperate. The osteoarthritic who has involvement of the hips, knees, or ankles probably cannot participate in hunting if the animal being stalked requires much walking; this individual should consider "still" hunting for deer and squirrel.

The seizure patient who is well controlled and has not had a seizure in the past 2 years should be allowed to hunt as any other individual. The seizure patient who is uncontrolled or who has had a recent

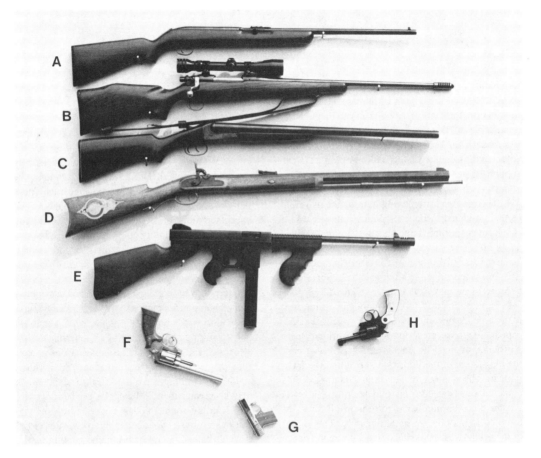

FIGURE 26-1. Guns used in hunting. *Rifles:* **A.** .22-caliber semiautomatic used for small game hunting. **B.** .3006 bolt action rifle used in big game hunting. **C.** 12-gauge double-barrel shotgun used for bird hunting. **D.** .45-caliber black powder (muzzleloader) used in special big game seasons. **E.** .45-caliber semiautomatic rifle. *Handguns:* **F.** .357 magnum revolver. **G.** .25-caliber semiautomatic. **H.** .22-caliber revolver, "Saturday Night Special."

drug change should not be hunting alone, and these individuals should avoid hunting that requires them to climb trees or cover dangerous terrain.

Paraplegics may be able to "still" hunt with appropriate help. They may be transported to an area and may hunt from a wheelchair, which may require modifications so that the hunter can have a stand or a support for the weapon. Amputees may be able to hunt depending on the terrain and the animal sought. Lower-extremity amputees with below-the-knee amputations of one or both legs may be able to hunt normally. Individuals with above-the-knee amputations in both legs may have difficulty in walking and may have to "still" hunt. The upper-extremity single-arm amputee may be able to hunt simply by modifying the weapon or choosing one that will allow firing with one arm.

HUNTING METHODS

Today hunting is a sport allowed in all states. Forms of hunting include:

- *Big game*—deer, elk, antelope, bear, and moose
- *Small game*—rabbit, squirrel, and raccoon
- *Bird*—quail, dove, pheasant, turkey, and grouse
- *Waterfowl*—various species of ducks and geese
- *Varmint hunting*—woodchuck, badger, and gopher

Most methods of hunting use the gun as the lethal agent (Fig. 26-1). *Rifles* are primarily used in big game hunting. These are large-caliber weapons with high muzzle velocities; hence, the projectiles have high kinetic energies. Bird and waterfowl hunters use the *shotgun*. These are large bore but have many lead or steel pellets in each shell (Fig. 26-2). Their range is rather limited but they are most effective at close distances. *Pistols* or handguns are often carried by the modern hunter as a throwback to the days of Matt Dillon and Jesse James. They are legal for hunting in some states but are infrequently used as accuracy comes only with extended practice.

Hunting today with the bow and arrow would be mind boggling to the Native American of the old West. The modern compound bow has 70- to 85-pound pull and is capable of sending a factory built and aligned arrow through a large deer. A few states allow the use of crossbows during selected times. These weapons, which have a bow attached to the stock of a gun and shoot a metal arrow, require a very strong individual to load. Bow and arrow sea-

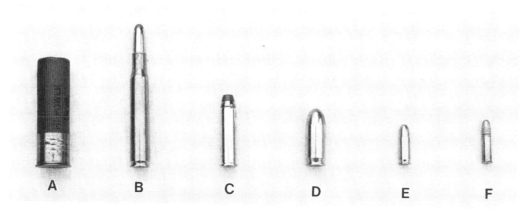

FIGURE 26-2. Hunting ammunition. **A.** 2 ¾-inch, 16-gauge shotgun shell. **B.** .3006 shell. **C.** .357 soft point lead. **D.** .45 caliber. **E.** .25 caliber. **F.** .22 caliber.

sons for big game are often longer than gun seasons and may allow the harvesting of animals of either sex. Bow hunters most often "still" hunt and usually climb trees. Sitting in a tree the hunter has a better view and is less likely to be seen or smelled by the big game.

TETANUS

Hunters are at a greater risk of developing tetanus than are other individuals and tetanus vaccination status must be assessed. All penetrating wounds occurring outdoors may contain the clostridial organism whose neurotoxins are responsible for this disease. Morbidity and mortality for tetanus remain significant: Even with appropriate treatment the mortality has been listed at 30 percent or more. The first symptoms of tetanus may be trismus and the development of the anxious expression (risus sardonicus). Shortly after this, perhaps 12 hours, spasms and sudden jerks may develop. With shorter incubation periods and more rapid development of these symptoms, the prognosis is worse. These severe spasms may stop respiration, resulting in death. The diagnosis is primarily clinical, but occasionally a bacterial confirmation is possible.

The prevention of tetanus must be aggressive and vigorous. All wounds should be treated surgically as appropriate. Penetrating "dirty" wounds, such as those from thorns, rusty nails, and dirty abrasions, should be debrided and generously irrigated with copious amounts of saline. Individuals who have had a primary series of tetanus vaccination and have had a booster within 5 years may not require any further booster. However, those individuals with "dirty" puncture wounds should have a booster. Individuals who have not had the primary series or who cannot document that they have had the primary series should be treated with tetanus immune globulin and tetanus toxoid. After an appropriate time their vaccination series should be completed.

The treatment of tetanus may require sodium pentothal to control the severe spasms that are associated with the disease. Constant nursing is re-quired along with monitoring of the fluid electrolyte status. Intubation may also be required.[2]

RABIES

Because of the risk of rabies, hunters should be instructed to see their primary care physician if attacked or bitten by animals. This disease, though described in literature for hundreds of years,[3] is still frightening and incurable. Postexposure vaccination remains the only hope for individuals who have been in contact with rabid animals. In a recent year every state with the exceptions of Hawaii, Rhode Island, and Vermont had confirmed cases of rabies. Over 3000 cases were documented in 1977 in the United States.[4] Approximately 30,000 people each year have to receive rabies prophylaxis because of contact with rabid animals. Rabies is not generally spread by domesticated dogs and cats; the skunk is its chief reservoir in the United States, although bats and foxes are also known to be infected frequently with the rabies virus.[5] Rabies prophylaxis should thus begin immediately for individuals bitten by abnormally behaving skunks, foxes, or bats. Rabies has not been generally found in rodents such as hamsters, gerbils, mice, rats, or squirrels in most parts of the country. Animals attacking people must be observed for 10 days, have proof of recent rabies immunizations, or their brain must be examined microscopically to determine if the victim should receive rabies prophylaxis.

Dogs are allowed for hunting in some states for both small and big game. Most allow the use of dogs at night to hunt for raccoons and in the daytime for hunting rabbits. Bird dogs are used by quail hunters to locate the birds, and duck hunters use retrievers to bring in the downed ducks. Dog bites among these hunters are infrequent.

The human diploid cell rabies virus vaccine (HDCV) is now available in many locations. Prophylaxis may be reduced to only a few injections as opposed to the previous series of 20 or more. Individuals who are likely to have contact with rabid animals (researchers, animal wardens, and cave explorers) usually require prophylactic vaccination.

Immune titers are available and a titer of greater than 1:16 is evidence of immunity to rabies.[6] The titer should be checked every 2 years. Prophylactic rabies vaccination has not been recommended for the general public and is reserved for only those individuals who have come in contact with a possibly rabid animal. Hunters bitten by wild or domesticated animals should see their primary care physician, who must be able to determine if rabies prophylaxis is necessary.

GUNSHOT WOUNDS

Most serious and/or fatal accidental injuries in hunting are related to the weapons used (see Fig. 26-3). For the nonhunter it may be difficult to understand how hunting gunshot wounds occur since hunted animals and hunters do not look alike. One trip to a deer camp can be quite revealing. Alcohol is taken to these camps almost as frequently as guns. Many hunters take two rifles to camp with them—"in case one fails." Perhaps as many as one-fourth of all deer hunters take a handgun or pistol to the camp to be carried in pockets or holsters. In 1979 these weapons accounted for over one-fourth of the hunting-related gunshot wounds in Colorado. The revolver, with its exposed hammer, is very likely to discharge if it is dropped or falls and the hammer strikes first. A case report from a wildlife commission in a Rocky Mountain state reads:

> Pistol laying in seat. Victim was moving the pistol to make room for others in party to sit in seat. Victim picked up gun by the barrel to put under the seat, bumped gun on gearshift and gun went off.[7]

The primary care physician should campaign for gun safety and urge state legislators to limit hunters to one gun apiece in the woods.

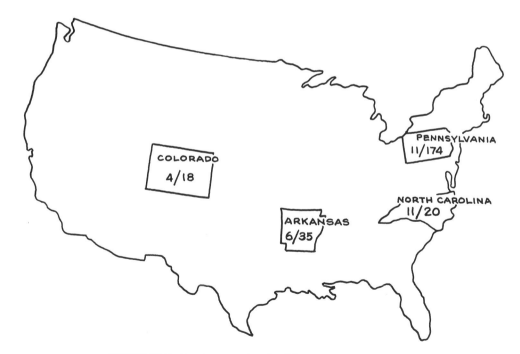

FIGURE 26-3. Hunting gunshot fatalities/injuries in four states.

The use of camouflage clothing without an orange vest should be illegal. A fatality case report from Arkansas reads:

> Victim was trying to trick his hunting partner. He snorted and scraped the leaves like a deer. Shooter thought he saw the tail end of a deer. He fired. Victim was wearing camouflage clothing.[8]

The use of a fluorescent orange piece of clothing is mandatory in some states. These legal statutes usually prescribe the number of square inches of this material that must be worn. This clothing works unquestionably well (Fig. 26-4): in the 9 years before Colorado enacted its statute, 91 hunters died from gunshot wounds; in the 10 years since, only 45 hunters died from gunshot wounds.[9]

Hunter safety education courses are now required in several states before the new hunter may purchase a license. Hunting gunshot fatalities can be markedly reduced. North Carolina had 19 fatalities during 1964 to 1965 but, after an education program was started, only seven in 1978 to 1979.[10]

The use of alcohol and other abused chemical substances in hunting poses a grave threat not only to the individual using the substance, but to other hunters in the area. This is illustrated by the following case report from a state wildlife commission:

> People in deer camp were intoxicated and playing with a .357 magnum pistol. It fell from a table, discharged, and struck victim in both legs.[11]

Adult supervision of underage hunters is not legally required in all states. Two case reports bear out the fatal consequences:

> A .410 shotgun discharged hitting a 13 year old in the stomach as a 12 year old handed him the gun, muzzle first.[12]

> After squirrel hunting two boys began shooting cans. Later they started pointing their guns at one another. Victim was fatally wounded when his companion's gun discharged.[11]

Adult supervision and instruction in gun and hunting safety might have prevented these two deaths.

A frequent cause of hunting gunshot wounds is the "brush shot." Some hunters take shots in dense brush at any noise they hear. Fluorescent orange hunting vests might somewhat reduce the chance of death. Visual acuity exams for hunters would be helpful, but hunter safety education has been shown to produce superior results.

Another common cause of gunshot wounds results from a combination of factors. Very often in "still" hunting the hunter quietly sips a beer while awaiting the prey, dozes off, and either discharges the gun directly by accident or falls from the nest, discharging the gun in the process. Climbing up or down from the nest with a loaded gun has resulted in genital and extremity gunshot wounds. Simple education can prevent many of these injuries.

OTHER HUNTING INJURIES

Target and competition skeet shooting are now popular sports in the United States. Contestants may use handguns, rifles, or shotguns for tournament competition and may fire 300 shells or more in each competition. Because of the noise volume protection must be offered for the ears since hearing damage occurs with long exposure to repeated weapon fire.[13] Shooter's earmuffs or ear plugs prevent hearing loss.

Injuries associated with bow and arrow hunting are often orthopedic in nature: fractures, dislocations, sprains, and strains. Accidental injuries in hunting related to neither guns nor bows include lacerations, fractures, sprains, dislocations, back strains, frostbite, exposure hypothermia, drowning, carbon monoxide asphyxiation, and burns. Hypothermia can be a killer for those caught unprepared in rapidly changing winter weather. The temperature does not have to be sub-Arctic, as the chill factor at 14° is −27° in a 30-mph wind. Clothing and any form of shelter may be life saving. Hands and feet must be kept warm and dry. Numbness or skin color change (gray or yellow–white) may be the first signs. These areas must be gently and progressively warmed. Placing the hands next to the abdomen may accomplish this (see Chapter 10).

Big game or small game hunters face all the hazards of any outdoorsperson when camping. *Fires*

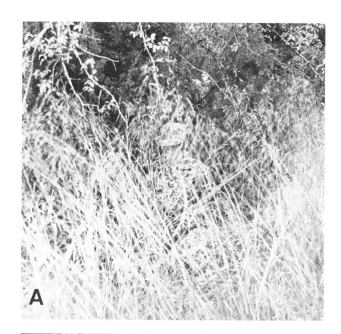

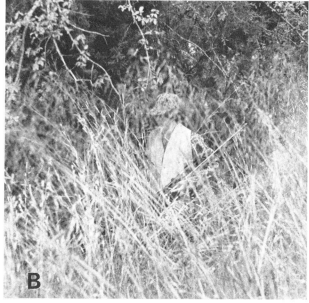

FIGURE 26-4. A. Hunter crouched in front of tree wearing camouflage clothing. **B.** Same hunter, same location with fluorescent orange (600 square inches). Note: Big game, such as deer, are color blind.

remain the cause of serious injuries and deaths. The use of gasoline to start a fire may produce a bomb-like explosion that can result in flash burns even at a distance from the fire. The Boy Scout method of setting up a campfire area can prevent these problems (Fig. 26-5).

Campers in recreational vehicles often use unvented heaters which may result in carbon monoxide asphyxiation deaths. This may also occur in tents that are closed. The use of only vented heaters or of down-filled clothing or sleeping bags may be an acceptable substitute in more moderate climates.

For the hunter poison ivy can be a source of much discomfort. It may have variable appearance making it difficult to avoid. Individuals coming in contact with poison ivy should wash the area affected to remove the oleoresin from their skin; this may require a degreaser. Those individuals developing the rash of poison ivy may be treated conservatively with calamine lotion as needed every 4 hours. Those developing more significant problems with ruptured vesicles may require moist com-

presses and/or an astringent wet dressing. Those who develop oozing lesions which become secondarily infected with bacteria may require antibiotic treatment, such as erythromycin 250 mg q.i.d., and antihistamines may be necessary to help reduce the itching. For those with larger involved areas, corticosteroids may be required.[14] The usual choice is prednisone, 60 mg initially on day 1, tapering to 5 to 10 mg 10 days after therapy was started.

HUNTING-RELATED ACCIDENTS AT HOME

Hunters' families have a greater risk of accidental injuries with some of these being catastrophic. The storage of camping equipment at home should be evaluated. All sharp equipment such as knives, hatchets, axes, and tent stakes should be kept in an area that is not easily accessible to young children. All combustible materials such as fuel for gasoline lanterns and cook stoves should *not* be kept in an

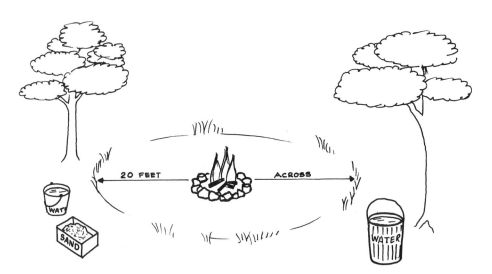

FIGURE 26-5. Appropriate method starting and extinguishing a fire: (1) Select a site that is clear of grass, leaves and twigs, etc. for a diameter of 15 to 20 feet and without overhanging limbs; (2) Build the fire on dirt, sand, or rocks; (3) Keep containers of water and sand nearby to extinguish blaze. The containers should be clearly marked. Lantern fuels should be stored separately at least 20 feet from the fire; (4) To extinguish the fire, cover with water, turn embers, water again, and then cover with dirt or sand.

unventilated closed space. The garage, often used for storage of this fuel, is a very poor choice as it often houses water heaters. Gas water heaters may supply a spark that can trigger an explosion from the gaseous vapors of lantern fuel.

Many hunting-related gunshot wounds occur at home with guns that are "unloaded." All guns should truly be unloaded and *verified* as unloaded. These guns should be kept under lock and key in a gun cabinet or an area that is not accessible to children. Trigger locks are available; these prevent the trigger from being engaged when the lock is in place and may be purchased at hunting supply stores. Ammunition should be stored in child-resistant containers in separate locations *away* from the guns.

PHYSICIANS AND ACCIDENT PREVENTION

The *Survival Manual* is printed for free distribution by the Colorado Department of Natural Resources, Division of Wildlife, and is particularly recommended for outdoor activities. Six rules for survival are given and should be reviewed by the physician along with the patient[15]:

1. Tell someone where you are going and when you plan to return.
2. Never go alone.
3. Take enough food for possible emergency use.
4. Take a compass and a map.
5. Wear proper clothing and equipment.
6. Plan your outing so you may return before dark.

First-aid courses should be recommended by the primary care physician for those planning to make hunting trips for extended periods of time or to remote areas. These courses provide the knowledge that may be life saving or may prevent disabling wounds. The control of hemorrhage by compression and/or tourniquet and the simple splinting of fractures may significantly reduce morbidity and mortality for hunters. It is imperative that the counseling physician discuss the hazards of hunting when prescribing it. The approach must be one of education through prevention. It is not enough

to advise patients to "go hunting" or to leave instructional materials like survival manuals or hunter safety books in the reading room. A brief but careful, thorough review of the salient aspects of hunting should be made by the practitioner. These features are summarized below:

1. Hunter education courses
2. Fluorescent orange vests for the hunter
3. Not mixing alcohol and guns
4. Visual acuity exams for the hunter
5. Annual physical endurance assessment before going on extended trips to rugged areas
6. Survival training
7. Acclimation to altitude for those planning to hunt at altitudes of 3500 feet or more above sea level
8. Proper clothing
9. Adult supervision of children who hunt
10. Use of vented heaters
11. Starting and extinguishing fires by the method recommended by the Boy Scouts
12. Use of appropriately loaded shells
13. Use of only those guns in good working order and those rated to handle the shells used
14. Unloading of guns before entering vehicles, houses, shelters, or nests, and before crossing fences, climbing trees, or when walking up steep hillsides or on slippery surfaces

REFERENCES

1. Robinson C: Normal and Therapeutic Nutrition. New York, Macmillan, 1972, p 76.
2. Schwartz SI, Shirer GT, Spencer FC, Storer EH: Principles of Surgery. New York, McGraw-Hill, 1979, pp 204–207.
3. Kaplan MM, Koprowski H: Rabies. Sci Am 242 (1): 120–134, 1980.
4. U.S. Public Health Service: Morbidity and Mortality Weekly Report 27: 499–501, 1978.
5. U.S. Public Health Service: Morbidity and Mortality Weekly Report 30: 363–354, 1981.
6. Wilcox K: Rabies, in Conn HF (ed): Current Therapy. Philadelphia, WB Saunders, 1981, pp 58–62.

7. Hunter accident case reports, personal communication, Colorado Department of Natural Resources, Division of Wildlife, 1979.

8. Hunter accident case reports, personal communication, Arkansas Game and Fish Commission, 1979.

9. Caskey RB: Personal communication, Colorado Department of Natural Resources, Division of Wildlife, August 28, 1980.

10. Hunter accident case reports, personal communication, North Carolina Wildlife Resources, 1979.

11. Hunter accident case reports, personal communication, Arkansas Game and Fish Commission, 1978.

12. Hunter accident case reports, personal communication, Arkansas Game and Fish Commission, 1980.

13. Baxter D: A study of noise induced sensorineural hearing loss in adult male hunters native in Greenland and to the Baffin zone in Eastern Canadian arctic. J Otolaryngol 8(4): 315–325, 1979.

14. Selpan A: Poison ivy dermatitis, in Conn HF (ed): Current Therapy. Philadelphia, WB Saunders, 1981, pp 672–673.

15. Survival Manual, Colorado Department of Natural Resources, Division of Wildlife, 1979.

BIBLIOGRAPHY

Ormon C: Complete Book of Hunting. New York, Harper, 1962.

Morris D, Strung N: Family Fun On and Around the Water. New York, Cowles, 1970.

27
The Role of the Primary Care Physician in Cardiac Rehabilitation

Franklin E. Payne, Jr.

Two major questions are appropriate in a discussion of the primary care physician and cardiac renabilitation:

1. Should the primary care physician be relegated to a secondary role in the reconditioning and restructuring process after the discovery of coronary heart disease?
2. Is cardiac rehabilitation a worthwhile endeavor for any physician when morbidity and mortality are considered?

The answer to the first question must be soundly in the negative. The patient remains a whole person, not a diseased heart, with many related needs and problems which necessitate the primary physician's care and management. The second question must be answered in the affirmative. In fact, the development of cardiac rehabilitation programs prior to the experimental evidence to support the implementation of such programs points out the validity of the logical application of epidemiologic data. A balanced summary recently presented by the AMA Council on Scientific Affairs[1] reflects a widespread acceptance among physicians. In addition, experimental evidence is now accumulating to substantiate the benefits of such rehabilitative programs. In Canada sustained physical activity has shown a fivefold decrease in the probability of both fatal and nonfatal recurrences of the infarction.[2] This cannot be fully explained by other changes in health habits or disease severity. In the United States an early report of the National Exercise and Heart Disease Project after a 3-year follow-up reveals data "consistent with an assumption of substantial benefit from exercise."[3] An earlier study had shown a decreased progression of atherosclerotic lesions documented by cardiac catheterization.[4] Additional evidence is expected to continue to accumulate in the establishment of the effectiveness and safety of cardiac and other multiple risk factor programs (e.g., MRFIT).[5]

COMPREHENSIVE PATIENT MANAGEMENT

The primary care physician should consult with the cardiologist for expertise in the areas of technical evaluations and medical management of coronary heart disease on both an acute and chronic basis. Other dimensions of the patient's heart disease (job, family life, hobbies) are best managed by the patient's personal physician. Additional risk factors must be discussed and treated: smoking, high serum cholesterol and triglycerides, weight loss, diabetes mellitus, hypertension, stress, and lack of exercise. Patient compliance is more probable if only one or two changes at a time are implemented because of the difficulty in making any change in the established lifestyle of a middle-aged or older individual. Once a goal is reached, another change may be initiated. Such an approach reduces patient non-compliance and physician frustration.

Complicating diseases of the patient require the physician's continuing management. Poorly controlled diabetes makes the rehabilitative program difficult at best. The interactions of cardiac and ancillary medications must be considered to prevent detrimental synergistic or antagonistic effects. Another disease may preclude the use of certain cardiac drugs, e.g., β-blockers in a patient with recurrent asthma or diabetes. The primary care physician knows the patient from longitudinal experience and is able to make appropriate decisions.

The above emphasis upon limited changes and comprehensive management requires a carefully designed, simple, but progressive plan for the patient with an acute infarction. The plan outlined in Table 27-1 is an example of such a plan. It begins with the patient in the cardiac care unit (CCU) and progresses toward maximal rehabilitation. The phases are helpful to remind the physician and the patient that the plan is progressive. The patient should be able to visualize his or her progress, and the physician should be careful not to expect too much from

---

TABLE 27-1. PHASES OF CARDIAC REHABILITATION

Phase 0:   Patient with acute infarct is in cardiac care unit.

Phase 1:   Two to four days after myocardial infarction, the patient begins exercise, progressive mobilization, counseling, and psychologic conditioning. Modified treadmill test is done on (or soon after) day 10. If pain, a fall in blood pressure, ECG changes, or arrhythmias occur, the patient is at high risk of sudden death during the first four to six weeks and should be managed accordingly.

Phase 2:   Patient returns to hospital twice weekly to attain target heart rate of 90 to 115 while on telemetry. This phase lasts four to six weeks. Patient and spouse receive counseling. The high-risk patient is identified and managed.

Phase 3:   Patient begins active, long-term, outpatient rehabilitation program. Management includes determination of target heart rate and periodic evaluation with special treadmill test. Other aspects involve emphasizing progressive exercise, teaching self-responsibility and providing job training. The patient should be given advice about sexual activity, exercise, work, diet, and coping methods. Resources are provided to patients who are not able to participate in the program on a long-term basis.

Phase 4:   Patient leaves program to enter community (employment, retirement, new loction, etc.) and adapts his or her lifestyle to patterns learned in the rehabilitation process.

(From Payne FE, Boineau JP: Cardiac rehabilitation. Am Fam Physician published by the American Academy of Family Physicians; 22(4): 152–156, 1980, with permission.)

the patient too soon. The plan also allows for checkpoints that determine whether more attention is needed to particular areas or whether alternative plans are necessary. Upon completion of phase 4, the physician should continue to have frequent contact with the patient to follow each area and intercede if the patient regresses from accomplished lifestyle changes. Other specifics of these phases are in the following text.

Psychological and emotional considerations may be the most important areas in which management is needed. Patients frequently become cardiac cripples when they become aware of covert or overt heart disease. In one study 80 percent of patients who were employed at the time of coronary bypass surgery continued to be unemployed 4 years later.[6] Cardiologists are emphasizing the role of the primary care physician in the movement of heart disease patients toward normal living.[7] Most patients who survive a myocardial infarction have little or no decrease in myocardial function. Although the extent of disease in the individual patient must be considered, most patients can achieve a level of conditioning higher than that maintained prior to the onset of their cardiac disease. Marathon running is the ultimate example.[8] If such goals are achieved, the discovery of heart disease in a patient can actually be a positive event! The physician's continuing surveillance of total patient needs, combined with a clear focus on the realities of cardiac rehabilitation, can engender a positive attitude and improved compliance on the part of patients.

PSYCHOLOGICAL MANAGEMENT AND COMPLIANCE

Psychological testing and interview assessment define the patient's attitude toward his or her illness and the rehabilitative process. Obviously, serious cognitive conflicts with the accompaniment of strong emotional states exist in a cardiac patient who feels confronted with the possibility of sudden death and other manifestations of the disease. As individual attitudes and emotions are identified, the staff can appropriately and accurately interact with patients.

Denial may prevent a patient's acknowledging

illness to him- or herself, even though thoroughly understanding the disease process. Thus, personal identity with the disease itself accurately determines the patient's motivation.[9] The subtlety of this patient process can easily be overlooked if not investigated specifically and routinely. An understanding of the patient's own anatomical and functional capacity best overcomes denial. Those patients with little or no limitations, particularly, must be convinced of the normal lifestyle, and even increased activity, of which they are capable.

The spouse is essential to the rehabilitative process. Any disease affects the marital relationship (or a relationship with similar commitment) in its complexity of interaction. Pre-existent areas of conflict retard or even prevent rehabilitation. A severe psychological problem can develop from the synergistic effect of an overprotective spouse and an increasingly passive, dependent patient. Only detailed identification and discussion of these complex attitudes and feelings prevent their negative impact on cardiac rehabilitation. Marriage-role redefinition may need to occur because of changes in employability and other factors.

Sexual activity must be discussed, as neither patient nor spouse often initiates such a discussion.[10] An inaccurate perception of the energy level required for the performance of sexual foreplay and intercourse exists among patients and physicians. Initially, the distinction should be made between sexual activity within marriage and outside of marriage. (This discussion centers on physiology, not morality.) Extramarital sex is more stressful with higher pulse rates and, according to several studies, is related to increased risk of cardiovascular morbidity and mortality.[11] In sexual activity with one's spouse, pulse rates usually do not exceed 120 per-minute. The energy level of the latter compares with the stress of many daily activities: climbing stairs, walking at 3 miles per hour, and emotional states produced by family disagreements, problems in the work environment, and situations encountered in simply driving a car in congested traffic. Thus, post-infarction patients can tolerate the mild-to-moderate stress on the myocardium produced by sexual activity with one's spouse. If patients' sex lives are discussed in an open atmosphere, considerable quality can be added to their life on a two-fold basis: lack of fear related to a sexual encounter and an enhanced marital relationship.

Patients must be involved early in the rehabilitative process. Exercise stress testing and other physical activities have repeatedly been shown to be safe within 1 or 2 weeks of an infarction.[12,13] This approach prevents the 20 to 25 percent decrease in work capacity that occurs after 3 weeks of bed rest[14] and a psychological adaptation to inactivity. The patient's early experience of rehabilitation produces a mindset for later increased activity. In addition the exercise relieves depression and anxiety by its direct effects. A detailed description of a hospital and outpatient program has recently appeared in a primary care publication.[15]

Immense benefits in positive reinforcement occur by periodic retesting to allow the patient to see objective evidence of an increase in exercise performance. Such retesting does not necesssarily need to be the full performance of a treadmill protocol, but may be abbreviated; e.g., a three-lead system. Additional support is gained if the patient is also informed of dropping blood pressure, cholesterol, weight, and other objectively improving parameters. Patient education and psychological assessment can also be carried out during the hospitalized period.

ACTIVITIES

Treadmill stress testing determines the energy level at which the patient may begin (Chapter 7). Common and inexpensive charts describe exercises and daily activities at these energy levels that must be monitored by the patient, physician, and staff.[16] From the patient's treadmill performance the appropriate level of physical activity can be determined from Table 27-2 according to mets (metabolic equivalents). (One met is the required energy at rest and is approximately equivalent to 3.5 milliliters O_2/kilogram body weight/minute.) Caution is required to prevent the patient's becoming overly zealous in personal or group competition. Occasionally the staff must be reminded of the necessity for restriction of activities within the patient's functional level.

A balanced program does not overemphasize personal exercise to the neglect of other activities. Recreational activities should consist of games and social activities that motivate patients through mutual support and encouragement. These positive group dynamics result from the association of patients with similar underlying disease processes. Other interactions include support of dependency needs interpersonal education, peer pressure, and other covert means of behavioral and attitudinal reinforcement. These interactions should be encouraged and even designed into the overall program.

Group exercise (e.g., aerobic dancing), as well as individual programs, can be staged according to treadmill performances of those patients in the group. Groups may even be identified on this basis and, as each member improves his or her exercise capacity, the energy level of the group exercises may be proportionately increased.

Nutritional education should be designed for group support. The dimension of the program should be practical and include the actual preparation of meals designed to be "heart healthy." Obviously, kitchen equipment must be available. The patient's spouse should participate since dietary modifications impact heavily on the entire family. The spouse also needs to understand how and why meals need to be prepared in a specific manner.

The primary care physician, whether involved in the cardiac rehabilitation program or not, will probably be managing the cardiac patient once phase 3 has been completed. Both patient and physician may wonder what activities are appropriate for the patient returning to the community. A sound basis for these activities is the patient's performance during cardiac rehabilitation and the pathophysiology of the patient's heart. Decisions at this point are highly individualized. Many infarcts are small, ejection fractions are normal, and the patient has no other symptoms of heart disease. This person may pursue any activities fitting anyone of a similar age. On the other hand, patients may be limited to class III or IV because of their pathophysiology and may continue to have symptoms. In either case, however, the monitoring that occurred during rehabilitation warns of possible arrythmias associated with exertion. The same level of exercise that was

TABLE 27-2. RELATIVE MERITS OF VARIOUS EXERCISES IN INDUCING CARDIOVASCULAR FITNESS

Energy Range[a]	Activity	Comment
1.5–2.0 Mets[b] or 2.0–2.5 Cals/min. or 120–150 Cals/hr.	Light housework such as polishing furniture or washing small clothes	Too low in energy level and too intermittent to promote endurance.
	Strolling 1.0 mile/hr.	Not sufficiently strenuous to promote endurance unless capacity is very low.
2.0–3.0 Mets or 2.5–4.0 Cals/min. or 150–240 Cals/hr.	Level walking at 2.0 miles/hr.	See "strolling."
	Golf, using power cart	Promotes skill and minimal strength in arm muscles but not sufficiently taxing to promote endurance. Also too intermittent.
3.0–4.0 Mets or 4–5 Cals/min. or 240–300 Cals/hr.	Cleaning windows, mopping floors, or vacuuming	Adequate conditioning exercise if carried out continuously for 20–30 minutes.
	Bowling	Too intermittent and not sufficiently taxing to promote endurance.
	Walking at 3.0 miles/hr.	Adequate dynamic exercise if low capacity.
	Cycling at 6 miles/hr.	As above.
	Golf—pulling cart	Useful for conditioning if reach target rate. May include isometrics depending on cart weight.
4.0–5.0 Mets or 5–6 Cals/min. or 300–360 Cals/hr.	Scrubbing floors	Adequate endurance exercise if carried out in at least 2 minute stints.
	Walking 3.5 miles/hr.	Usually good dynamic aerobic exercise.
	Cycling 8 miles/hr.	As above.
	Table tennis, badminton and volleyball	Vigorous continuous play can have endurance benefits but intermittent, easy play only promotes skill.
	Golf—carrying clubs	Promotes endurance if reach and maintain target heart rate, otherwise merely aids strength and skill.
	Tennis, doubles	Not very beneficial unless there is continuous play maintaining target rate—which is unlikely. Will aid skill.
	Many calisthenics and ballet exercises	Will promote endurance if continuous, rhythmic, and repetitive. Those requiring isometric effort such as push-ups and sit-ups are probably not beneficial for cardiovascular fitness.
5.0–6.0 Met or 6–7 Cals/min. or 360–420 Cals/hr.	Walking 4 miles/hr.	Dynamic, aerobic and of benefit.
	Cycling 10 miles/hr.	As above.
	Ice or roller skating	As above if done continuously.
6.0–7.0 Mets or 7–8 Cals/min. or 420–480 Cals/hr.	Walking 5 miles/hr.	Dynamic, aerobic, and beneficial.
	Cycling 11 miles/hr.	Same.
	Singles tennis	Can provide benefit if played 30 minutes or more by skilled player with an attempt to keep moving.
	Water skiing	Total isometrics; very risky for cardiacs, pre-cardiacs (high risk) or deconditioned normals.

(continued)

TABLE 27-2. (Continued)

Energy Range[a]	Activity	Comment
7.0–8.0 Mets or 8–10 Cals/min. or 480–600 Cals/hr.	Jogging 5 miles/hr.	Dynamic, aerobic, endurance building exercise.
	Cycling 12 miles/hr.	As above.
	Downhill skiing	Usually ski runs are too short to significantly promote endurance. Lift may be isometric. Benefits skill predominantly. Combined stress of altitude, cold and exercise may be too great for some cardiacs.
	Paddleball	Not sufficiently continuous but promotes skill; competition and hot playing areas may be dangerous to cardiacs.
8.0–9.0 Mets or 10–11 Cals/min. or 600–660 Cals/hr.	Running 5.5 miles/hr.	Excellent conditioner.
	Cycling 13 miles/hr.	As above.
	Squash or handball (practice session or warmup)	Usually too intermittent to provide endurance building effect. Promotes skill.
Above 10 Mets or 11 Cals/min. or 660 Cals/hr.	Running 6 miles/hr. = 10 Mets 7 miles/hr. = 11.5 Mets 8 miles/hr. = 13.5 Mets	Excellent conditioner.
	Competitive handball or squash	Competitive environment in a hot room is dangerous to anyone not in excellent physical condition. Same as singles tennis.

[a]Energy range will vary depending on skill of exerciser, pattern of rest pauses, environmental temperature, etc. Caloric values depend on body size (more for larger person). Table provides reasonable "relative strenuousness values," however.

[b]Met = multiple of the resting energy requirement; e.g., 2 Mets require twice the resting energy cost, 3 Mets triple, etc.
(From Beyond Diet: Exercise Your Way to Fitness and Heart Health, by L Zohman, MD, CPC International, Englewood Cliffs, New Jersey. Reprinted with permission.)

safe during rehabilitation should be safe for 1 or 2 years after an infarction, bypass, or other cardiac event. An increase in exercise level beyond this baseline is a real possibility, but should be gradual. The more severe the disease, the less should be the incremental increase. Based upon exercise tolerance and other symptoms, repeat exercise testing continues to advise the patient and physician on the appropriate level of exercise. Probably, the most critical management by the primary care physician is the prevention of a decline in the level of a patient's exercise once the program is left. Such decline is a real and common occurrence and detrimental to the cardiac status of the patient.

STAFFING REQUIREMENTS

The ideal staff in a cardiac rehabilitative program is presented in Table 27-3.[17] Many programs, however, may be designed with fewer people, and most positions require only a part-time commitment with main duties elsewhere. As in any organization, one person must assume administrative responsibility to develop, maintain, and coordinate all dimensions of the program. That person can be any health professional with experience or training in such a program. A physician must play the overseer to maximize the medical care of patients and minimize possible complications. His or her time may be

TABLE 27-3. STAFF FOR A CARDIAC REHABILITATION PROGRAM[a]

Medical director	A family physician, cardiologist or other physician trained in cardiovascular disease and rehabilitative medicine to direct patient care.
Administrator	The medical director may assume this function. If he or she does not, however, another health professional with experience in such programs may serve in this capacity.
Cardiology consultant (if available)	
Psychologist	
Exercise physiologist	
Therapist (physical, corrective, occupational, or recreational)	
Nutritionist	
Social and vocational counselor	
Psychiatric consultant (if available)	

[a]This is an optimal staff and not all of these disciplines are necessary. *(From Payne FE, Boineau JP: Cardiac rehabilitation. Am Fam Physician, published by the American Academy of Family Physicians; 22(4): 152–156, 1980, with permission.)*

minimal on an ongoing basis but should be committed and consistent.

Community size should not restrict the possibility of a well designed program. With creativity and volunteer efforts it is possible to minimize costs. On the other extreme, a large program might finance several full-time salaries and have elaborate physical facilities. Financial support may be obtained from private or governmental organizations within the community. Essential components are the administrator, the physician, and space. Third-party payments are available in some areas of the country and may be designed into local payment programs.

Every staff member should be initially and repeatedly trained in cardiopulmonary resuscitation (CPR). Regular meetings of all personnel should be held in order to discuss patients and allow the communication necessary to develop common goals and objectives. Considerable overlap of functions exists and requires flexibility and openness by the entire staff. In fact, the most essential component is the enthusiasm and mutual cooperation of the staff.

Many primary care physicians are graduating from programs with exposure to a cardiac rehabilitative program and can be called upon for their assistance. In addition, continuing education and on-site training programs are becoming available. With the prevalence of ischemic heart disease, every community should have at least one physician who is involved in cardiac rehabilitation. This is necessary to ensure the best medical advice in this complex disease process which consists of both physical and psychological components. It is a tragic gap in modern medical care to allow patients who have been extensively evaluated and hospital treated for heart disease essentially to vegetate in their inactivity because of the fear and lack of availability of a supervised rehabilitation program; such patients later become unfortunate victims of progressive disease or sudden death.

REFERENCES

1. Council on Scientific Affairs: Physician-supervised exercise programs in rehabilitation of patients with coronary heart disease. J Am Med Assoc 245:1463–1466, 1981.
2. Shephard RJ, Corey P, Kavanagh T: Exercise compliance and the prevention of a recurrence of myocardial infarction. Med Sci Sports Exercise 13(1):1–5, 1981.
3. Shaw LW: Effects of a prescribed supervised exercise program on mortality and cardiovascular morbidity in patients after a myocardial infarction. Am J Cardiol 48:39–46, 1981.

4. Selvester R, Camp J, Sanmarcos M: Effects of exercise training on progression of documented coronary arteriosclerosis in men. Ann NY Acad Sci 301:495–508, 1977.

5. Neaton JD, Broste S, Cohen L, Fishman EL, et al: The multiple risk factor intervention trial (MRFIT). VII. A comparison of risk factor changes between the two study groups. Prev Med 10(4):519–543, 1981.

6. Anderson AJ, Barboriak JJ, Hoffman RG, et al: Retention or resumption of employment after aortocoronary bypass operations. J Am Med Assoc 243:543–545, 1980.

7. Wenger NJ: Rehabilitation after myocardial infarction. J Am Med Assoc 242:2879–2881, 1979.

8. Kavanagh T, Shephard RJ, Pandit V: Marathon running after myocardial infarction. J Am Med Assoc 229:1602–1605, 1974.

9. Oldridge NJ: Compliance in exercise rehabilitation. Phys Sports Med 7(5):94–103, 1979.

10. Masur FT: Resumption of sexual activity following myocardial infarction. Sexuality and Disability 2(2):98–114, 1979.

11. Veno M: The so-called coition death. Jpn Legal Med 17:535, 1963.

12. Sivarajan ES, Bruce RA, Almes MJ, et al: In-hospital exercise after myocardial infarction does not improve treadmill performance. N Engl J Med 305:357–362, 1981.

13. Fein SA, Flein NA, Frishman WH: Exercise testing soon after uncomplicated myocardial infarction. J Am Med Assoc 245:1863–1868, 1981.

14. Saltin B, Blemquist G, Mitchell JH, et al: Response to exercise after bed rest and training. Circulation 37–38 (Suppl 7):1–55, 1981.

15. Rucker TW: Cardiac rehabilitation in a family practice setting. J Fam Pract 10(3):407–414, 1980.

16. Zohman LR: Beyond Diet . . . Exercise Your Way to Fitness and Heart Health. Englewood Cliffs, NJ, CPC International, 1974.

17. Payne FE, Boineau JP: Cardiac rehabilitation. Am Fam Physician 22(4):152–156, 1980.

BIBLIOGRAPHY

Cardiac rehabilitation, in Milvy P (ed): The marathon: Physiological, medical, epidemiological, and psychological studies. Ann NY Aca Sci 301:455–515, 1977.

Symposium on exercise in the post coronary patient. Med Sci Sports 11(4):365–385, 1979.

Wenger NJ (ed): Exercise and the heart. Philadelphia, FA Davis & Company, 1978.

28
The Child and Adolescent in Sports: A Psychosocial Profile

Bruce C. Ogilvie

The primary care physician is most often the professional in the best position to provide information as to health maintenance of the child's physical and psychosocial development. It has been estimated that more than 20 million male children are now actively participating in competitive youth sports. It has not been possible to estimate the number of female participants, but certainly half that number would be a reasonable guess. We must therefore assume that the greatest proportion of these children will have their first professional contact with their family physician. It is hoped that a review of some of the central issues with regard to the psychological and social implications of sports participation may serve as a guide in the physician's role as an effective counselor. The emphasis here is on the relationship of such activities to the child's psychological readiness for competitive programs and how they might best serve the sociological needs of the child. The issue of the role that parents play in the determination of whether or not the sport experience enhances the child's development should not be underemphasized.

Few are better equipped than those in the primary care specialties to have a grasp of family dynamics that can provide the basis for sensitive and intelligent counseling. The President's Counsel on Fitness and Sport and the American College of Sports Medicine have each been advocates for the primary care physician to take an even greater role in terms of an active concern for the physical and mental health of children in sports. A stated goal of these and other professional organizations is the education of the general public in order that every child may experience an increase in self-esteem and remain an active participant in lifetime sports.

INTERNAL VERSUS EXTERNAL SPORTS MOTIVATION

There is no single psychological insight that has equivalent value for the clinician as that of determining the degree to which the sports activity is fulfilling the child's internal needs. The study of both the long- and short-term effects of sports participation always leads to seeking answers to the following questions: Is this particular child involved in an activity that has intrinsic value? Will it eventually contribute to increased feelings of self-worth?

At some point during the physical examination gentle inquiry should be directed toward making a discrimination as to the degree of internal compared with external motivation.

Once this has been established, one is in a strong position to direct the sports experience toward emotional growth and increased self-acceptance. Such an insight has particular significance in relation to the child's desire to master the whole range of motor skills essential for feeling good about him- or herself as a performer. It is during the advances from the unstructured, low-pressure level of recreational games to the highly structured, high-pressure level of competitive sports that the emotional and physical dangers intensify. It is during this transitional phase that the counseling physician must determine if the most fundamental needs of the child are being sacrificed for values that contribute least to the long-term health and happiness of the child.

Study of the child's early participation in sports and games at the loosely organized neighborhood level finds that the child's need fulfillment is almost exclusively intrinsic in nature. Investigators have found that freedom of expression, joy, and emotional release interact with important social rewards in terms of peer acceptance and form the basis for their continued interest. The significance of peer relationships is so fundamental that it becomes the environment for establishing a positive identity which is supported by the integration of important human values. The physician must be particularly on guard in the role of counselor with respect to those children who are more gifted in motor skills or mature earlier and are enticed into the next level of organized sports. It is at this point that one is able to gather data as to the anticipated role the parents will play in the athletic life of the child. Independent of how insightful the physician becomes in determining the child's needs, the ability to filter out the parents' motivations is absolutely essential when counseling the family with respect to wholesome sports motivation.

It is vital at this transitional point in the child's athletic life that he or she be provided with an opportunity to explore the significance and meaning of the activity in the most personal terms. This can only be approached in private where the physician can offer a nonjudgmental setting where the child feels totally free of any form of parental coercion. An open inquiry may be framed by posing such questions as:

- What are you seeking from sports competition?
- Can you tell me why you have such a compelling interest in competing?
- What do you find so attractive in competitive sports?

Any of a number of good questions that start the process of reflection on the part of the child is suitable. The open nondefensive response to such questions provides the directional cues for exploration of the child's personal motivation. The responses are more valid when he or she is guaranteed privileged communication.

DANGERS WITHIN HIGHLY COMPETITIVE PROGRAMS

Lest some take these warnings as a blanket condemnation of competitive sports, it should be stated that many sports psychologists heartily support the philosophy that there must be provisions for those who are more gifted, independent of the areas of performance that are examined. This should not blind us to the inherent dangers that Pop Warner football, Little League baseball, age group swimming, league soccer, figure skating, and many other highly competitive programs may contain.

A particularly insidious danger is the disproportionate increase in external rewards that are typically utilized to motivate participation. Many children are all too readily seduced by material rewards and special privileges, such as being selected to a special "in" group. The socially naïve young athlete is even more vulnerable. Each child also experiences in varying degrees an inner struggle as the demands of the competitive program begin to clash with his or her recreational needs. Far too many become involved in a values struggle with which they have insufficient life-experience to cope. The social pressure that is inherent in the competitive situation forces the majority to acquiesce, relinquishing values that would be better retained as the basis for making important life decisions.

Physicians who may choose to use this conflict as a means for the exploration of values, whereby the young athlete examines his or her life priorities and then makes the most rational choice of action will be impacting upon one of the sports worlds most cherished values. When the child commits to the motivational influences of being evaluated, graded, selected, and all other forms of external judgments, he or she begins to lose total control of the worth of the activity and, in a sense, submits to the evaluation of others. The physician who takes the responsibility for helping the young athlete not to succumb to such external manipulations is accused of attempting to get the athlete to avoid the reality of natural selection as it operates in sports. This Darwinian imperative has provided the basis for the rationalizations for "survival of the fittest" that so characterizes competitive sports programs. After making a commitment to the competitive program, the youngster quickly introjects the American value with respect to winning. Though there are signs that some educators are coming to question this value, there is little evidence that a values reorientation is occurring.

It should be the physician's responsibility to try to counter the loss of touch with innermost feelings as the pressures from external rewards take their toll. The physician must act as the purveyor of the often lost truth—that there are human activities that contribute more to a child's growth as a person when devoid of the harsh selective processes that typify most youth programs.

SUBJUGATION OF THE CHILD TO THE POWER OF OTHERS

This aspect of the child's world is the natural consequence of moving into competitive youth programs and requires a special form of vigilance on the physician's part—particularly regarding the powerful role the coach plays in the life of the child. Such persons play many roles in the lives of their charges and, for some children, the quality of their relationship with a coach can form the basis for personal feelings that are lifelong in nature.

Depending on the lack of fulfillment at home, some children place the coach in the role of mother or father, and for so many others this may be the only close personal relationship they ever share with a meaningful adult. It was not surprising, therefore, to have found in one study of the world class and Olympic female swimmers that 12 years later they still rated their coaches as the most significant persons in their lives.[1] In many youth programs it has been observed that a significant number of children place the coach in the role of a divinity. The general public tends to remain oblivious to the abuse of power that can occur by those coaches who are either insensitive or untrained with respect to the needs of children. Inherent in this role is the power to complement the psychological and social growth of the child or to create emotional scars that haunt the child for the remainder of his or her life.

Children who attempt to use sports participation as the primary means of establishing self-worth are in greatest danger of experiencing emotional trauma, particularly those who suffer most from low self-esteem and have serious doubts as to their personal worth. The physician must communicate to those responsible for the development of the child that every program must provide protection for such children. When such children transfer the determination of their worth as human beings, the authority role of the teacher becomes very complex. The complex nature of such relationships are compounded by the fact that the authorities donating their time to youth sports programs are rarely trained or certified with respect to child growth and development. The overwhelming majority are generous adults who have been participants in the sport but have no formal training in coaching. The primary care physician would be rendering a great service by offering a short course to the neighborhood coaches immediately before the start of each season.

VULNERABILITY TO TRAUMA

It is unfortunately true that there is too little research to use as the basis of identifying the vulnerable child; but what has appeared in the literature supports what is known about failure-prone children in any other learning situation. Based upon three separate studies of highly competitive youth programs in northern California, three trends were found to be consistent within sports and for both boys and girls. The children who were in the attrition samples were measurably more anxious and tense with an elevated fear of criticism for failure. They were more sensitive to criticism and experienced higher levels of guilt feelings. They measured slightly lower in their ability to deal with abstract learning material.[2]

Parents, coaches, and others should be taught to take warning from some of the most recent research which indicates the potential for trauma for a given number of children. An important study published in 1978 indicated that the self-esteem of the child must be considered if it is presumed that the best should be provided to all children. These authors reported that the sports experience may contribute to the child's self-esteem only when other important psychological factors are taken into consideration. First is the child's attitude with respect to the attraction of the activity for the child; second, the degree to which the child believes him- or herself capable of achieving success. Personal worth or value is integrally bound to these two factors. These studies reinforce previous findings in that those children with favorable self-perceptions of their physical ability were those who were well adjusted and without neurotic problems or personality disorders.[3]

It is unfortunate that most of what has been learned about the potential negative effects of the stresses found in competitive youth programs has been from the clinical study of those who have been referred for some form of emotional crisis. There are no longitudinal studies in the literature that would provide a factual basis for categorizing the emotional traumata that one sees in daily practice. Although it must be generalized from research experience with extreme examples, such as those who become emotional casualties, there is one fact that cannot be overlooked; the ego commitment any given child makes—which forms the basis for the motivation to turn out five times a week for 2 or 3 hours and remain in a highly structured program—is bound to influence positive or negative self-regard. There is almost a universal belief by the professionals in the mental health field that a positive sense of identity is far more essential for confronting reality from a substantial positive base than any other human emotional set.[4] The motivation to compete should not be used against the child in ways that lead to exploitation and a lessening of positive self-regard.

DANGER OF EXPLOITATION

The danger for the more dependent child, or the child who is forced to relinquish all control over his or her life in order to remain in a competitive program, acts as a weeding process: for the most part, only the survivors are visible. Children who remain after the intense selective process may experience a more subtle danger: the potential for becoming an extension of the coach, team, organization, and sometimes even the fans. Within this select group are those children who are exploited by media exposure. It is so easy for the child's needs to become lost in this maze of engaging in an activity in order to satisfy questionable needs of the adults around them. It is at this point where the physician must question whose needs are being met.

In counseling the youthful athlete it is extremely important to provide assistance in defining his or her responsibilities to the adults involved and where they must end. Particularly, the child must come to recognize that his or her participation in sports may be compensating for the unfulfilled needs of these adults, and be taught ways to ward off the exploitation of any guilt feelings. Parents of the competitive child seem to be masters at provoking guilt whenever their child's performance does not enhance their selfish egos. There is sufficient stress for any child when not living up to his or her own image of an idealized self; adding responsibility for the neurotic needs of others is unwarranted. The child should be prepared to accept an important reality about human performance: the quest for excellence in any area of life is a selfish pursuit. This does not necessarily imply a lack of appreciation for the needs of others; but since the quest is ego centered, pleasing others is a secondary concern.

WHAT IS THE IDEAL ENVIRONMENT FOR THE CHILD ATHLETE?

It has been documented in northern California that it is difficult to distinguish between the gestalt of youth programs and what is experienced in National Basketball Association (NBA), National Football League (NFL), and National League baseball camps. The coaching model employed with children was essentially identical to that in any professional sport. It appeared that both coaches and parents had designed their programs from their observations of training programs shown on television. The teaching aid that has been most effective in terms of modifying coach and parent behavior has been to expose them to their own behavior via the use of video playback. It has been found that they are not unwilling to change; however, they had been unconscious of the role they were playing and no one had taken the time to teach them alternative role models. They must be aided in recreating a child-centered environment that attends to the needs of the whole child, not just the child as an athlete.

CONCERN FOR THE WHOLE CHILD

If our concern is for the whole child, then it is essential that the theoretical and practical lessons of child development be understood and applied. Specific to the discussion is the process by which the child establishes a unique sense of identity. The noted child authority Eric Erickson wrote of the fundamental nature of the period between 7 and 12 years of age in terms of solidifying one's identity.

This period is of particular importance because each child must be provided with an opportunity for mastering feelings of inferiority. This is the same span of years in which children have the highest probability of participating in some sport activity. There is no better setting for testing their identities than that provided during their social and physical interactions with their peers. Recreation, group games, and play provide objective feedback as they test their role by acting out in relation to their playmates. These early experiences form the foundation for their consciences and become the stable basis for deep values which serve as a guide for future judgments and actions. It is through these interactions with other children that they learn the boundaries of their own existence and integrate a highly individualized self-concept.

If a positive environment for social learning is provided, it has been found that the child exhibits the following strengths: recognition of the importance of personal sacrifice, the capacity to identify with the needs of others, the ability to honor consensus rules or agreements, and a wholesome dependency relationship with others.[5]

RECOGNITION OF THE CHILD'S POTENTIAL

Certainly there is no other area of concern where the primary care physician is better equipped by training to be an effective educator than that of establishing the physical, social, and psychological readiness of the child. In treating the child athlete, one of the most prevalent emotional crises has been caused by the adult's inability or unwillingness to honor the child's biologic or psychological time clock.[6] Adults must constantly be reminded that motor skills acquisition is dependent on constitutional factors and that physical maturation is under the control of the individual's unique inner time clock. The upper limits such as bone length, motor efficiency, and muscular strength have been predetermined. In relation to the psychological time clock and the issue of physical size in relation to the child's social behavior, it is clear that adult expectations are frequently out of focus. There is a general tendency to project adult norms of conduct simply because a youngster has an early maturing body. Adults fail to understand that psychologic readiness may be proceeding at quite a different pace. Adults directing youth programs should continually be reminded that chronologic age can only be used as a rough measure of a child's psychologic and physical readiness for competitive sports. It has been observed in consulting with the U.S. Figure Skating Team that referring these young elite athletes for bone age analysis was necessary in order to alter parental or coaching perceptions of the child. These children were referred because they were experiencing decrements in performance or were not demonstrating expected levels of excellence during actual competition. Discrepancies of between $1\frac{1}{2}$ and 2 years were found between bone age and chronologic age. Though the referral sources were acting upon the assumption that there was some psychologic basis for performance problems, these were children who were experiencing the normal plateau in their curve of motor skills acquisition. The adults seemed to have lost sight of one of the basic laws of human development: every aspect of human development proceeds on a unique schedule and it is essential to honor this inner biologic time clock.

This fact is certainly one of the most frequent causes of the crisis with which the physician may be confronted when attempting to serve the needs of children in elite athletic programs. So many parents and adults involved in such programs have lost sight of the reality that they are dealing with children in a child's world. Too many behave as if they have to stamp out the childhood years and force the child to meet the imposition of adult standards. These highly motivated children rarely are able to discriminate between reasonable goals that are appropriate physically and psychologically from those that are imposed by neurotic adults. They generally are found to be experiencing deep feelings of guilt because somehow they have not measured up to someone's unreasonable standards. The physician, in the role of authority, can contribute greatly by educating adults to the fact that chronologic age is not a reliable measure of any given child's psychologic, emotional, or even mental age.

IDENTIFYING THE CHILD'S NEEDS

In order to intervene and guide each child as to the best course to take, it is helpful to attempt to gain a more objective measure of his or her feelings.[7] The use of a standard set of questions touching upon the various aspects of the sport experience affords the child an opportunity to reflect his or her innermost needs while at the same time providing the physician with counseling insights. Questions should be asked as to the level of emotional commitment to sports, the degree of physical confidence brought to the activity, how the child feels about possible failure or criticism during participation, and what he or she expects the role of the coach to be. Questions touching upon these areas can become the basis for exposing deeper or subconscious motives that can be used to give intelligent direction to a child's athletic life.

As a guide for the development of an objective list of questions, here is a sample from the Los Angeles Children's Hospital Inventory, designed to seek evidence that could help act as a guide in counseling the child athlete. It was not the intent of this standardized inventory to classify children with respect to specific athletic traits, but rather gain directional cues for exploring their basic motivation. The first series of questions are selected from the 25 used to identify ego commitment to sports, or athletic motivation:

I set high goals for myself in sports.
a. never b. sometimes c. frequently
To be successful in sports is of great importance to me.
a. never b. sometimes c. frequently
I respond to athletic challenges.
a. never b. sometimes c. frequently
I think about myself as succeeding in sports.
a. never b. sometimes c. frequently
I set high goals for my teammates.
a. never b. sometimes c. frequently[6]

An important area of inquiry is the degree of self confidence the child brings to the sport activity.

I feel that I have what it takes to be a successful competitor.
a. rarely **b.** sometimes **c.** frequently

It is easy for me to concentrate and learn a new skill.
a. sometimes **b.** most often **c.** frequently

When the coach demands it I can give more.
a. rarely **b.** sometimes **c.** frequently

I like to match my skill off against others.
a. rarely **b.** sometimes **c.** frequently

I can talk back to my opponents.
a. rarely **b.** sometimes **c.** frequently[6]

The values and philosophy that have been expressed are entirely consistent with those of the American College of Sports Medicine and the President's Counsel on Fitness and Sport. In the light of the very special role that the physician is called upon to play he or she is asked to become an agent for the following goals:

1. Ensure that the sports program is designed to permit every child with an opportunity to develop strong positive feelings about his or her body.
2. Insist that the end effect of every program results in a "positive body image" which can become the integrating core for the whole personality.
3. Ensure that the sports experience contributes positively to the child's ability to identify more sensitively with others.
4. Provide the opportunity for the child to build positive bridges of feelings for others.
5. Ensure that the natural process of failure and success provides a growth experience that will lead to the development of the empathic human quality.
6. Provide a sport experience that conditions attitudes that health maintenance through physical expression increases one's joy of living.
7. Educate the child to anticipate that there are few areas of life that can afford as much opportunity for self-actualization and even, for some individuals, peak experiences.[6]

The other areas of inquiry that have proven to be of most value have been insights into a child's emotional control, attitude toward aggression, ex-

perience in relation to pre-event tension, ability to handle criticism and failure, and capacity to place faith in others. This last dimension has proven to be the most valuable insight into the youthful competitor because it forms the basis for everything we offer as counselors. It is important to warn anyone using such a method of inquiry that responses to such questionnaires must not form the basis for making judgments, but simply deepen the nature of inquiry.

Should a young patient answer a question that indicates an inability to bounce back after making an error, or that he or she never sets high goals in sports, the physician is in a better position to determine just what this response means to the child. If an athlete reveals an inability to express aggressive feelings without eventually feeling guilty, or to place faith again in anyone, the physician has some valuable profound insights available.

Redefining the physician's goals as counselor to the athletic child, they fall into these priorities:

- Help the child to gain insight into his or her primary needs.
- Enable the child to comprehend the dangers of succumbing to extrinsic motivational factors.
- Guide the child away from making the sports activity the measure of self-worth.
- Enable him or her to comprehend that the pursuit of excellence can only be measured in very personal, individually determined terms.
- Above all propound that no matter how remarkable the physical gift, it can never be used as the proof of one's worth as a person.

REFERENCES

1. Ogilvie BC, Gustovson J: How competition affects elite female swimmers. Phys Sports Med 8:113–116, 1980.
2. Rohde L: The relationship of personality factors to participation in age-group tackle football. MA Thesis, San Jose State University, 1969.
3. Sonstroem RJ: Med Sci Sports 97–102, 1978.
4. Gergen KJ: The Concept of Self. New York, Holt, 1971.

5. Erikson E: Childhood and Society. New York, Norton, 1963.
6. Ogilvie BC: The child athlete: Psychological implications of participation in sport, Ann Am Acad Polit Soc Sci 445:47–58, 1979.
7. Ogilvie BC: Meeting children's needs in sport. School Nurse Natl Assoc Schools 12:13–20, 1980.

BIBLIOGRAPHY

The Cooperative Sport and Games Book. New York, Pantheon Books, 1978.
Cratty BJ: Learning About Human Behavior Through Active Games. Englewood Cliffs, N.J., Prentice-Hall, 1975.
Cratty BJ: Movement Behavior and Motor Learning. Philadelphia, Lea & Febiger, 1962.
Fisher AC: Psychology of Sport. Palo Alto, Calif, Mayfield Publishing, 1976.
Kane JE: Psychological Aspects of Physical Education and Sport. Boston, Routledge & Kegan Paul, 1972.
Klavora P, Wipper AW: Psychological and Sociological Factors in Sport. University of Toronto, School of Physical and Health Education, 1978.
Martens R: Social Psychology and Physical Activity, New York, Harper & Row, 1970.
McGlynn GH: Issues in Physical Education and Sports. Palo Alto, Calif, National Press Books, 1974.
Ogilvie BC, Tutko TA: Problem Athletes. London, Pelham Books, 1966.
Orlick T: Winning Through Cooperation. Washington, D.C., Acropolis Books, 1978.
Rushall EBS: The sports environment: "A capacity to enhance—A capacity to destroy," in Status of Psychomotor Learning and Sports Psychological Research. Dartmouth, Nova Scotia, Sports Sciences Associates, 1975.
Sabo DF, Runfola R: Sports and Male Identity. Englewood Cliffs, N.J.: Prentice-Hall, 1980.

29

The Physician as Fitness Motivator

Maynard A. Howe and Bruce C. Ogilvie

Few physicians understand the impact they have on their patients' lives. This impact extends far beyond the immediate office setting and influences the patient's well-being. Society attributes a position of power and influence to physicians, and they are therefore imbued with a tremendous responsibility.

Physicians fulfill a variety of roles within their practices. The primary role is that of diagnostician and healer. People usually seek out physicians when they are ill or notice changes in health that concern them. They want to understand the cause of the discomfort and want the symptoms to go away. Physicians are well aware that people seek psychological comfort and aid from them. For example, psychological needs are often masked when the patient repeatedly complains of vague, ever-shifting symptoms that persist even after extensive testing indicates no organic basis. Physicians who are comforting and reassuring can speed up the curative process in patients who are genuinely ill. Another important role of the physician is that of educator and director of preventive health care programs for patients and their families. It is in this role that the physician can become the critical element in aiding patients in adopting a fitness program and supportive lifestyle changes.

The primary care physician, more than other medical specialists, has the opportunity to have many more insights into family members' physical condition and problems as well as their overall lifestyles. The physician's unique position allows the promotion of general health care, especially those programs aimed at self-care and physical exercise.

IMPORTANCE OF PHYSICAL EXERCISE

It has now been clearly established that physical exercise yields both physiologic and psychological benefits. Both medical and psychological literature strongly support this fact which has resulted in increased advocacy of physical exercise by health professionals.

Every professional body concerned with human health, such as the American College of Sports Medicine, the AMA Council on Fitness and Health, and the International Council of Sports and Physical Education, holds personal health maintenance as its primary goal. Their advocacy is based as much upon cost efficiency of health care as on ameliorating the quality of life for the general public. It is almost impossible to attend any regional or national meeting in the medical field without being exposed to the data concerning the major stresses of our time—pollution, poor nutrition, and destructive lifestyles are some obvious ramifications of a fast-paced existence. Health professionals are increasingly being asked to encourage the general public to take more responsibility for their own health maintenance which would aid in controlling the costly epidemic of physical and emotional disorders.

There is overwhelming evidence for the value of maintaining cardiovascular fitness as the target and/or measure of overall systemic fitness. Since 1978, there has been a significant reduction in cardiovascular diseases, with the most important cause of this hopeful sign being attributed to the geometric increase in routinized running. This increase has been substantial, from approximately 40,000 runners in 1968 to over 40 million in 1978.[1] Recent data indicate that many other forms of physical exercise have also had measurable gains, and not only have a powerful positive impact on the cardiovascular system, but also can lead to significant improvements in emotional health and general well-being.[2]

Research on running during the past decade has provided a valuable insight into other activities. It has now been well documented that psychologic and physiological gains can be expected from a program that increases the heart rate to 60 percent of maximum for 30 minutes 3 days a week.[3] The evidence strongly supports that running and similar forms of aerobic exercise result in significant gains in emotional and mental attitude. These highly reliable changes have been reported in investigations involving a wide range of research subjects.[4,5]

Postcardiac and sedentary patients showed significant improvements in emotional health, according to several studies. The greatest change measured within these groups was the transition from severe depression and low self-esteem to high self-esteem and emotional integration. Weight, digestion, and sleep patterns were greatly improved, apparently in proportion to the level of cardiovascular endurance.[4]

Several recent studies have demonstrated that fitness training significantly affects cognitive performance. Exercise programs may be helpful as a means of reversing or arresting the physical degeneration involved in aging.[6,7] It has also been found that improvement in physical fitness increases oxygen transport capacity, thereby increasing recovery in mental performance following physical fatigue,[8] and that aerobic fitness training improves mental performance during physical exertion.[9]

One of the most important aspects of regular physical exercise is its effect on a variety of human behaviors. In studies involving work behavior, fitness training has been positively associated with reduced absenteeism and increased productivity. Exercise breaks on the job appear to improve output and reduce errors. Moreover, a general improvement in work performance and attitudes has been reported by employees who participate in exercise programs.[10] Regular physical exercise has also been found to improve sleep behavior. This improvement is most notable among females who had not previously engaged in physical activities.[5] Improvement in behaviors associated with interpersonal functioning, social adjustment, desirability, and popularity has also been positively related to fitness and sports activities.[7]

Studies investigating the effect of physical fitness upon emotional functioning have yielded consistently positive findings. Fitness training has been associated with improvements in mood, especially among subjects who are more distressed or physically unfit at the outset. Much of the research relating exercise to affect has focused on the reduction of anxiety and other stress conditions. In the vast majority of cases, anxiety, tension, and depression have been decreased, whereas positive feelings and moods have increased, resulting in a better sense of well-being.[4]

While there has been much research relating physical exercise to changes in personality variables, no evidence as of yet has supported the claim that major changes on personality tests can result from active physical exercise. Much of this research, however, has concentrated on short-term training and testing programs; longitudinal studies are only now being conducted.[11] The one personality variable which has consistently shown measured improvement in the research is self-concept. It has been hypothesized that improvements in self-concept have been caused by changes in body image resulting from physical exercise. With almost every population studied, positive changes in self-concept and body image have been found.[4]

Other interesting phenomena receiving current research support are the values reorientation, shift in perspectives, and improvements in imagination and creativity that occur in men and women who become positive health addicts.

What all these data ultimately mean is that there are valid reasons for the physician to devote a portion of patient contact time to fitness motivation. Focusing on this aspect of preventive medicine is likely to enhance patients' health maintenance and greatly reduce the incidence of adverse physical and mental conditions.

EXERCISE ETHIC

Recent research has shown that there is only a small portion of the general public that is already strongly committed to regular exercise. These people continue to move toward greater self-health maintenance and exercise consciousness aimed at prevention rather than treatment.[12]

While the number of participants in this movement continues to rise, they are still a minority of the population. Within this minority there are people who have engaged in physical activity since childhood and possess an "exercise ethic." They engage in sport and physical exercise because it is enjoyable. They are personally motivated and require little or no external prodding. In fact, regular physical exercise plays such an important role in their lives that it can be likened to an addiction. In many cases, the classic signs of addiction can be seen, especially when the "addictive" physical activity must be discontinued. Many times "withdrawal symptoms" may include restlessness, free-floating anxiety, irritability, sense of loss, feelings of guilt, and a pervasive depression.[13] The most exemplary cases of withdrawal are found when a professional or world class athlete must cease his or her athletic career. The depression that follows such termination can be so devastating that suicidal feelings and ideation can occur.[12]

Addiction to physical exercise can primarily be positive or negative. A positive addiction to exercise not only improves physical health but greatly enhances psychological functioning in almost every aspect of a person's life. A negative addiction, on the other hand, drains energy from other parts of a person's life in order to feed the addiction. It seems as though negatively addicted individuals use their involvement in physical exercise to escape or avoid other aspects in their lives such as interpersonal relationships, feelings of inadequacy, or anxiety-producing situations. In contrast, positively ad-

dicted individuals use involvement in physical exercise to enhance other areas of their lives, gaining psychological strength from their addiction.[14]

Regardless of the nature of the addiction, this segment of the population has deep abiding values which were developed and reinforced early as to the importance of physical exercise. Unfortunately, most people do not have an "exercise ethic." They lead rather sedentary lives and give little thought to participating in any physical activity.

The desire to participate actively in exercise is a direct result of social learning. Engaging in regular physical activity is a socially acquired behavior, and it is easy to see how these attitudes and behaviors have become relatively dormant in today's society. The continuous development of new and improved automation has virtually eliminated the need for any form of vigorous exercise on the job or in the home. Many adults passionately avoid activity. Our sedentary society has a love affair with labor-saving devices. Escalators and elevators have replaced stairs, and automation has decreased the need for physical labor on the job.

Physical inactivity is widespread in our society. The increasing coverage of athletic events by the media, especially television, has made avid spectators out of those who might have previously had some desire to participate. According to the President's Council on Physical Fitness and Sport children have shown a consistent decline on tests of strength and endurance over the past decade. In addition, recent cutbacks in physical education programs within the school system have either eliminated or greatly reduced the number of programs now offered. Statistics released by the Council have shown that over 50 percent of all the deaths in the United States result from medical problems that could be partially attributed to a lack of exercise. While this figure appears alarming, the same report stated that over 50 million adult Americans *never* engage in any form of physical activity.[3,15] The average American is inactive and is paying the consequences.

Generating and instilling an "exercise ethic" in adulthood is difficult but not impossible. With some knowledge of the psychological factors involved in motivation and resistance, it is possible for the family physician to include and reinforce a physical fitness regimen within a total preventive program. This is not to suggest that motivating and guiding patients toward effective self-care is an easy thing to do. All of the physician's medical and personal expertise is needed to motivate patients to exercise. Any medically sound fitness program the physician provides should pay special attention to the psychology of motivation. It is highly unlikely that the initiation and implementation of any physical fitness program will have lasting results unless the patient is personally motivated.

Many insights into the process of motivation have been developed through intensive research during the past 50 years. Pertinent to the physician's role as fitness motivator is the discovery that motivation may either be intrinsic or extrinsic in nature. Stated briefly, motivation is considered to be *extrinsic* when the behavior is performed as a means of reaching an end. For example, if a child participates in an activity because his or her father likes watching and offers approval and affection, then the child's motivation to perform is primarily extrinsic. However, if the child participates in an activity because there is nothing he or she would rather be doing at the time, then the primary motivation is *intrinsic*. The segment of the population referred to earlier as having an "exercise ethic" is most likely motivated intrinsically. The establishment of this ethic was probably rooted in a developmental growth of external and internal rewards and reinforcement from childhood. Such people require little or no extrinsic reward or reinforcement to continue their physical activity. They are well on their way to maintaining a lifelong program of self-care and preventive medicine.

Inactive people pose the greatest challenge to the physician. It is important to determine what approach is best for instilling an exercise ethic in a population of individuals who have an aversion to any form of exercise. The physician must first find the "ignition key" (the appropriate incentives) to get these patients started and keep them going on a fitness regimen.

Once the appropriate incentives are discovered, a system of reinforcement can be established and individualized for each patient. It is important to realize at this stage that extrinsic incentives and reinforcers alone do not have an enduring effect on the patient. If, however, the behavior schedule is properly introduced and implemented, the extrinsic rewards and incentives soon give way to intrinsic reinforcers as the patients experience benefits and rewards, which then become their motivation to continue. Therefore, the primary care physician's goal of promoting physical fitness can be accomplished by determining appropriate incentives and rewards, reinforcers that motivate their patients.

Examining motivational strategies can help the physician discover what rewards work best. One approach to motivation is to look at existing psychological and social needs within each person; they provide the motivating force necessary for prolonged participation in physical activity. The closer the activity can be tied to the already established needs of the patient, the greater the chance that the patient continues to exercise.

Every individual has psychological and sociologic needs. These needs express themselves in different behaviors associated with the satisfaction of the need. Pertinent to this discussion, the need or needs in every individual are social, achievement, and ego/esteem needs.[16,17]

People are basically social beings even though the concept of "rugged individualism" is valued highly. Human interaction and a feeling of belonging are important to almost everyone. The fear of social isolation or rejection can be one of the most powerful human motivators. Alienation and loneliness usually generate anxiety that causes a person to seek out interpersonal contact. Much of a person's daily activity is concerned with establishing, maintaining, or restoring positive emotional relationships.

People vary in the amounts and types of interpersonal contacts they prefer. Some enjoy being with small groups, perhaps just one or two close friends. Their needs for affection, communication, and personal validation are fulfilled by a small circle of friends. This type of individual tends to shy away from larger groups and organizations. Then there are people who seek both; they have intimate friends but also feel at ease in large groups and associations. Being in groups provides members with the opportunity to compare themselves with others and to see how valuable their abilities are.

Social interactions tend to confirm one's sense

of reality by a continual testing of views against societal norn.s. It is in this manner that identity is in part established and self-confidence maintained. Affiliative needs are easily satisfied by people perceived as similar to one's self. Therefore, to gain acceptance by others, it would be most effective to perform those activities that are attractive to other people who are like oneself. Physical activity can provide one means of interacting with others and is a way to gain acceptance and satisfy social needs. It allows for the establishment of close personal and social bonds as well as providing an avenue for receiving admiration and approval of others.

A person characterized by high social needs would not fare well in a solitary fitness program. This person might be encouraged to attend a running clinic, join a fitness club, or become active in an aerobic class.

Participation in physical activities and sports can lead to an increase in social status. One's estimation of a person wearing a "10 kilometer" race T-shirt differs from one's opinion of a person wearing a "marathon" T-shirt. Playing tennis at the local junior college does not carry the same social status as belonging to a prestigious tennis club. It is important to assess a patient's status needs while exploring various forms of fitness involvement.

In addition to affiliative needs, there are people who can be characterized as having high needs to achieve and excel. Achievement needs are filled not so much by the enjoyment of success as by the process of striving toward mastery and success. Research has demonstrated that individuals high in achievement needs prefer situations in which they have a moderate (50 percent) chance of success.[17] They measure their worth by their success and therefore activities which give the most feedback are preferred. Success at a very simple task gives little information about the individual's true capabilities, whereas failure is almost inevitable at tasks that are extremely difficult. Therefore, they prefer taking calculated risks and always take personal responsibility for their own success or failure. They like receiving immediate and concrete feedback on how they have performed.

Achievement needs can be met in two different but complementary ways. First, one can focus on competition with others, relying on external standards. Activities that include systems of scoring such as racquetball and tennis could be preferable for those patients whose needs require measurable outcomes in competition. Alternatively, one can focus on the mastery of a task relying on a more internal sense of satisfaction. Many skiers focus more on perfecting their form rather than racing with others. Similarly, some tennis players enjoy hours of rallying in order to perfect their strokes rather than keeping score as a means of measuring the outcome of their effort. Once an individual is able to measure his or her own capabilities with others or with some absolute external standard, it is generally easier to solidify internal standards of excellence.

While ego/esteem needs incorporate many of the characteristics of social and achievement needs, individuals successful in fulfilling high ego/esteem needs are generally described as being self-confident, self-assertive, highly motivated and successful in attaining realistic goals. These individuals tend to set high goals for themselves, function effectively in new situations, and experience comparatively low levels of anxiety. They perceive themselves as effective in governing their life and capable of achieving goals, even when initially they may meet with failure. Their ego needs involve a strong desire to be a prime mover and to be self-determined, and they believe they can control their lives. They are willing to assume responsibility for their actions, believing that what they do has a direct effect on the outcome of their endeavors. These individuals generally resist social influence; however, they are concerned with the image they have of themselves and, to some extent, the image others have of them. Their ego/esteem needs are satisfied and enhanced when their desires for strength, adequacy, competence, confidence, independence, and freedom are complemented with their desires for prestige, recognition, personal impact, and appreciation.[17]

While these individuals are generally involved in many activities, they may not be aware of the importance of maintaining physical fitness. These patients are easily motivated once provided with concrete and practical fitness prescriptions.

Although the psychologic and social needs just described are representative of pure types, most individuals have a combination of these needs, with at least one need being primary and the others secondary. Research from various governmental social surveys has shown that individual motives for participation in physical activities are based on the attractions and incentives involved in each activity and parallel the needs theory mentioned above. For example, when individuals were asked on a forced choice questionnaire why they participated in physical activity, the unanimous choice for women was "the chance to mix with other people," followed in order by "keeping fit," "takes your mind off other things," and "the pleasure of competition." The men in the study ranked the following, in order, as their motives for participation: "keeping fit," "the chance to be with other people," and "the pleasure of competition." In another study that analyzed the various factors which influenced participation in an exercise fitness program, social aspects/camaraderie ranked evenly with the desire for recreation and the need to keep fit. Although the need for affiliation ranked relatively low initially, it was considered by all the participants as the primary factor which influenced their program adherence.[18]

Another study of men found that 90 percent of the participants who responded indicated that they preferred to exercise with a group or with another person. These men felt that by participating with others they enjoyed the activity more, felt more of a personal commitment to continue, and experienced camaraderie while offering themselves a chance to compare their fitness levels with others.[19]

BEHAVIOR SCHEDULING

Although there appears to be no foolproof system of motivation, there are highly reliable generalizations that can contribute to and enhance the development of an exercise program for all individuals. Once the basic need or needs are identified and associated with a particular physical activity, it becomes necessary to incorporate a behavioral schedule of reinforcement.

When most individuals are confronted by their physicians with the issue of an exercise program, they generally agree to the need for such a program;

but they are often reticent when asked to investigate or generate goals relative to such a program. The patient wants to know the answers to questions such as these:

- "Why do I continue to behave in ways that are detrimental to me?"
- "What do I do to motivate myself to change these behaviors?"
- "How can I become what I want?"
- "How do I sustain myself long enough to achieve my goals?"

There is a subtle, underlying insecurity in these queries. They want to know what their chances are of obtaining a goal before they are willing to pursue it. They are, at some level of mental functioning, running a probability picture of success to failure through their mind's computer. While it is difficult to know what kind of mental tape is running, it is important to gain some insight into the success to failure ratio they have had with respect to other aspects of their lives. This is particularly significant when one seeks to help those who are just beginning in a physical activity.

The person who has been traumatized by participation in some physical activity, especially during their pubescent or adolescent years, may have a success/failure ratio that is detrimental to their initial participation. These individuals, many of whom have developed an aversion to exercise and have become overwhelmed with anxiety at the thought of physical activity, approach exercise needing much more external support. Whether the patient has had a high- or low-probability ratio of success to failure, he or she may need help in making an adjustment to the inevitable delayed rewards associated with initiating any fitness program. In order to make this adjustment a wholesome one, there must be a partial reward system built into the program, so that there are positive reinforcers along the way to nourish the incentive to continue to the goal. Personal attention and the achievement of short-term goals is a critical predecessor to total acceptance of long-term goals. That is, permanent behavioral and attitudinal changes are best achieved by small increments accompanied by confirmation that small efforts have been productive. The patient develops "ownership" of an attitude or behavior by doing this. Thus, when a new attitude or behavior has gained commitment through minor short-term successes, it becomes a part of the individual's value system and no longer requires as much external reinforcement.

For the primary care physician embarking on the role of fitness motivator, this psychologic truism suggests the need for an organized plan of steady reinforcement of small gains that can be gradually phased out as the person develops internal motivators necessary for continuation.

In addition to the reinforcement necessary to modify the patient's behavior, the following steps may be applied in developing a behavioral schedule once the patient has made a commitment to an exercise activity.

1. Initial Assessment. Have the patient bring to the first appointment an exercise journal in which he or she has recorded every physical activity engaged in during a 2-week period. In addition, the physician should select the medical history variables that provide the soundest evidence for structuring a fitness program. These may include blood pressure, body weight, heart rate, oxygen uptake, and the physician's opinion of the existence of psychologic factors. This overall assessment provides the patient and the physician with a physiologic and behavioral baseline from which to set realistic goals and expectations.

2. Selecting a Fitness Activity. Because motivation to begin an exercise program is heavily dependent upon the personal attraction of the activity, care should be taken in exploring with the patient as many fitness options as possible. This can be done prior to the initial appointment by means of a questionnaire or printed handout materials, or with the assistance of the physician or medical staff. Brainstorm many possible activities before narrowing down. It is important for the patient to be creative, to feel free to be completely unrealistic and to think of activities that would be fun. From the resultant list, the patient should select one or two activities that are most attractive and realistic. In selecting the activity, it is important to keep in mind the patient's *intrinsic needs* as well as build on

existing strengths and work with personal resources. Activities that enrich a person's life are usually more successful and are certainly more enjoyable than activities that would be experienced as a drudgery.

3. Setting Goals. Help the patient define personal short- and long-term goals in the chosen activity. The ability to explore and set reasonable goals requires great skill and invariably proves to be the most reliable motivational force when these goals are successfully accomplished. State the short- and long-term goal or goals precisely and program the specific steps required to reach them. It is important to realize at this stage that distant goals such as protection against heart disease, building muscle mass, longevity of life, or because "it is good for you" are elusive. These are not sufficient enough to continue motivation toward adherence to the activity.

4. Objectifying Improvement. Help the patient, if necessary, design some means of objectifying the course of improvement. A visual "signpost" that allows the patient and physician (or medical staff) to determine exactly where they are in relation to the goals set might be weight loss or body measurements, or resting and active pulse rates. If possible, have a member of the medical staff prepare a data-based graph or schedule such as those of Ken Cooper, where the patient can make a commitment based upon age, personal fitness, time, and energy expenditure.[20] Personal knowledge of the progress and results is unequivocally the most reliable motivational factor in the determination of human behavior. Therefore, if patients are provided with constant, objective data with regard to their progress, they are in the best position to produce change.

5. Monitoring Improvement. Once the patient has accepted the physician's counsel and has the means to observe his or her own progress, preparation should be made to monitor change and to maintain relatively frequent checks. A strong recommendation here is that the physician give someone in the office the responsibility for weekly and eventually monthly checkups to determine patient adherence to the prescribed program.

6. Build in Freedom. Allow the patient to be flexible enough to alter or change the program or activity as the "signpost" dictates. Because of the wide range of variability of patient response to health programs, some flexibility should be allowed so that a readjustment in goals is experienced instead of a "failure" to meet specific goals. For example, weight loss targets must be offered with consideration for a wide range of patient variability. Even the most rigid adherence to exercise programs by some patients does not result in the targeted goals, simply based upon physiologic differences.

7. Reinforcement. Help the patient build in short- and long-term rewards based on his or her improvement, even if only minor improvement is noticed or recorded. Improvement may be either physiologic or psychological.[21] The bottom line for changing any form of human behavior is that the change must result in some form of ego enhancement. Nothing strokes one's ego more effectively than the sight of (and the reward received for) an improvement, no matter how modest the gain is.

8. Engineer Environment. Investigate with the patient ways to engineer his or her life so that it continues to reinforce the new lifestyle. This may require restructuring with regard to time, place, habits, and positive support systems.

ATTENTION TO GOAL SETTING

The application of these steps or conditions can be helpful in almost any situation requiring the modification of a specific behavior. For example, suppose a patient who is following the physician's advice for an exercise prescription chooses to take up jogging. The long-term goal might be to achieve a heart rate of 60 percent maximum for 30 minutes 3 times per week. Together, the physician and patient must then specify a certain date by which to achieve this goal based on the patient's ability to adhere to a schedule, systematized training, and the tolerance for physical discomfort. Increments of gain should be based upon a realistic self-appraisal. Books on jogging or an experienced jogger may be consulted if the patient is uncertain about what to expect from this new endeavor. Once targets are defined, the patient must be encouraged to become some-

what compulsive about keeping records, graphs, or any visible measurement.

Continued follow-up and monitoring are highly reinforcing for some patients. This can take many forms. A phone call from the physician or a member of the medical staff, initially at 2- or 3-week intervals, can be scheduled. The next office appointment should be set at an advanced date according to the medical need for monitoring, and can be scheduled when the fitness program is introduced. Some physicians may find it useful to reserve specific hours, 1 day a week, when they or a medical staff member are available for routine monitoring. In some communities, public health nurses can be called upon for this kind of continuous monitoring access. Patients with questions can be encouraged to phone the physician's office and to write down less immediate questions for consideration during the monitoring session or the next office visit. Regular doses of praise, reassurance, and admiration from the physician and staff can also have a remarkable reinforcing effect.

PATIENT RESISTANCE MODES

Within any population the personal value of fitness ranges from those who are exercise addicts to those who have a total aversion to exercise in any form. Among the latter are the individuals so sedentary that they might declare, as George Bernard Shaw did, "Whenever I feel the need for exercise I lie down until the feeling goes away."

An exercise prescriptionist can expect to encounter the same treatment problems as those professionals treating any form of maladaptive behavior. These include physical lethargy, habitual avoidance, and a whole range of psychologic defense mechanisms. These resistant individuals can be divided into two groups: "The recalcitrant" and "the willing."

In any population there are a relatively small number of individuals, called *recalcitrant,* who will probably never embark on a fitness program. Their immediate reasons, although often a basic resistance to authority, are usually couched in much the same terms as voiced by the willing. The difference between the truly recalcitrant and the willing is primarily a matter of degree. Recalcitrants have deeply ingrained characteristic styles that are absolutely resistant to any normal reasoning or attempts to guide. These people may in fact need psychotherapeutic help before being able to make any commitment to a self-care program. Personal experience with people and their protective devices can enable the practitioner to recognize when the line is crossed, i.e., when an expression of resistance is so strong as to be adamant rather than simply an unwillingness restrained by easily overcome fears.

A majority of the uncommitted public fall into the category called "the willing," which includes young people whose family ethic has not provided role models that would instill an exercise ethic. Some are embarrassed by their bodies (as either too fat, too skinny, or too something) or their degree of strength or agility. They often believe that "exercise" can only be performed in groups or where they are exposed to public view or ridicule. Others are frightened by gossip about active people who have suffered heart attacks (not realizing that such disasters are apt to be the result of inappropriate or unsupervised physical activity). Then there are the numerous individuals who are dedicated bowlers, fishing enthusiasts, golfers, or the like who simply do not realize that some outdoor or sports activities do not provide the cardiovascular effort they need. There are also many who believe that they must give up smoking or drinking or some other entrenched social habit *before* entering a fitness program. This group may eventually give up such habits but, if they do, it is a result of, rather than a prerequisite for, a fitness regimen. The list of objections held by the willing is almost endless. The important thing about these people is that their resistance can be overcome in many ways.

The following are some brief summaries of classifications of the reactions most frequently displayed when a patient is forced to face the reality of a need to engage in some form of fitness regimen.

Rationalization Mode

When an exercise prescription is prescribed to patients who tend to rationalize, they embark on a long list of priority concerns each of which they feel must be taken care of before they can begin. In essence this form of rationalization helps the patient justify his or her behavior and buffers the patient from feeling the full impact of failure. When this resistance mode is encountered, it is easy to be seduced into using a counterrational approach. This may lead to a fun, competitive intellectual debate; however, little if any progress is to be made toward the patient actually embarking upon a fitness regimen. In fact, a counterargumentation approach only serves to further entrench the patient in his or her original rational objectives. If the patient's reasons are confronted or questioned persistently, he or she will become upset. Therefore, the physician should avoid arguing with the patient, acknowledge but not accept the rational excuses, and speak directly to the resistance. When a person really wants to do something, he or she finds a way. This message should be at the heart of the communication conveyed to the patient.

Denial Resistance Mode

These patients fail to identify with or relate to medical data presented as a basis for health concerns. They have a tendency to minimize their physical condition, which is a way of averting anxiety. A physician can detect if denial is being employed by the obvious disparity between the actual condition of the patient and the patient's personal perception of his or her condition. While many patients are unaware of the extent to which they are distorting the facts, some make a conscious effort at distorting reality as a means of preserving their self-image and the image they present to others. These patients do not acknowledge the reality of their condition in order to avoid the fear and shame that would accompany the awareness. Therefore, it is vital for the physician to present the patient's condition in a nonjudgmental and supportive manner designed to reduce the fear and anxiety that increase the tendency for denial. Threats and scare tactics rarely work. It is productive to raise anxiety levels moderately, provided that clear, practical, and personally relevant steps toward eliminating the problems are conscientiously prescribed.

Since self-image and societal image are of importance to patients employing denial, it is possible to appeal to those factors in helping to motivate patients toward fitness. Pointing out the patient's present physical appearance or condition interferes with the positive image he or she wishes to project.

Neurasthenia Resistance Mode

Neurasthenia is a neurotic condition characterized by complaints of chronic weakness, fatigue, and sometimes exhaustion. It is difficult for neurasthenic individuals to concentrate, and they often have feelings of inferiority, lack of enthusiasm, and dependency behaviors. The patient complains of an inner sense of exhaustion and finds his or her symptoms unpleasant and distasteful. This sense of exhaustion can often be selective; i.e., the patient may generate energy when engaging in activities or behaviors that are of interest and importance. These patients have an extremely low tolerance to stress and have learned to avoid stressful situations by exhibiting mental and physical fatigue and exhaustion.

The physician should be supportive in exploring with the patient an activity that is interesting and low in stress potential. The program should begin with a fairly minimal level of activity and progress slowly in small increments. A program of short walks through areas that would be of interest to the patient might be a starting point.

Hypochondriacal Mode

This character formation presents a difficult challenge because these patients have devised support systems that preclude exercise. Their reliance has been upon pharmacologic agents or other more esoteric health guarantees which help contain their anxiety about bodily functions. It takes great skill to substitute a reasonable exercise program enabling them gradually to relinquish their dependence on emotional crutches.

Constant reassurance is called for, particularly during the early phase of their exercising involvement when they may experience discomfort or minor strains. These individuals are almost bound to overreact to every physical adjustment that is a necessary part of any fitness program. The trusted physician may find that the patient's concern for his or her well-being has a powerful influence on the ultimate value of staying with a prescribed fitness program. The key word here is "prescribed." The patient must be regularly reminded that the fitness program can be as therapeutic as a pharmacologic prescription. Because bodily overconcern has been a lifelong means of channeling their anxiety, a dramatic turnabout must not be expected.

Type A Resistance Mode

This lifestyle presents some special problems in terms of inculcating and reinforcing the exercise ethic. These patients always seem to be running on an emotional high. With a hyperanxious approach they appear to be constantly vigilant and ready to defend themselves against a dangerous world. Type A personalities are time-obsessed and spend much of their time fighting to manage time while angrily dedicating their lives to proving that they are *not* time-obsessed. In actuality they are gradually wearing themselves out on a personal treadmill to oblivion.

The art of redirecting these workaholics is to include in their program some form of exercise that requires diligence and patience. Theirs is not a lifestyle that is relinquished unless they are forced to confront the distorted nature of their nebulous goals. Type A lifestyle has proven to be the most challenging to alter, even when the health professional documents the relationship with the stressors that abound in the lives of these patients. It is important to redirect these patients from their natural inclinations to see a fitness program as just another form of competition. The recreational aspects might be reinforced, concentrating on the quality use of their time. They should be encouraged to engineer a life space in which their ultimate achievement is to achieve a peaceful, relaxed state, thus relinquishing the need for winning or setting superhuman goals.

These brief sketches of patients' possible lifestyles necessarily leave out other significant, more pathologic aspects of an individual's attempts to allay fear or anxiety. Other extremely complex styles would require discussion more extensive than is appropriate in this review. However, these few examples should provide a brief overview sufficient to include a significant number of patients. The physician's role as healer, counselor, and teacher is a very special one indeed.

THE FITNESS DROPOUT

For all of the effort expended toward motivating, monitoring, and reinforcing, every fitness program or endeavor inevitably has its dropouts. Sometimes it helps the fitness motivator to know, in advance, the rationales behind the thinking of those who quit. Some research has extracted the following statements as reasons:

- "I get discouraged easily."
- "I don't work any harder than I have to."
- "I'm just not the goal-setting type."
- "I don't impose much structure on my activities."

On the other hand, research also gives some insights into what kinds of people stay with a program:

- "I seldom, if ever, let myself down."
- "I'm good at keeping promises, especially the ones I make to myself."
- "I have a hard-driving, aggressive personality."
- "I can persist in spite of pain or discomfort."

These statements raise several issues pertinent to the medical profession. The first and probably most difficult to contend with is the aversion to any form of physical discomfort. Those individuals who have spent the past 15 to 20 years escaping into sedentary pursuits become extremely apprehensive and frightened and may emotionally panic when they find themselves experiencing muscle twinges or the increased heart rate and respiration that occur.

As the patient adjusts to the new health regimen, some level of physical discomfort is inevitable. The old adage, "no pain, no gain," is a near universal experience. The physician is left with the responsibility of reinforcing the worth of some physical stress until the patient begins to experience psychological rewards, the first of which is usually

an elevation of self-esteem and a sense of accomplishment.

This stage of involvement necessitates a blending of the physician's medical knowledge and sensitivity about the patient in order to estimate the threshold of tolerance for any fitness program. The patient's tolerance is dependent on both physical and psychological thresholds. In order to be an artful motivator, the physician must always be cognizant as to what constitutes a personal threat to the patient. As an example, one would have to exhibit special concern for the obese patient who has lived a sedentary lifestyle for many years and who now becomes convinced that some fitness program is necessary. Even when the program is supervised by a qualified exercise physiologist, such patients have a body image conflict that blocks their initial wish to participate. Being able to place such persons in any program where there is little or no threat to their self-esteem is vital. Knowing that the obese subject experiences a slight gain in weight due to increased muscle mass before weight loss begins enables the physician to be supportive during the tough initial phase of weight loss. Those who are new to the experience need advanced warning and continued reassurance that their chosen exercise is not life threatening and that early discomforts are to be expected, are not serious, and will eventually disappear.

Another common deterrent occurs when an individual exceeds the prescribed medically sound regimen and develops some mild injury or new source of bodily pain. One of the best examples of this has been the medical findings associated with novice runners. The female novice has almost a 100-percent chance of experiencing some bodily injury within the first 6 months of training; the male has about a 50- to 80-percent chance. These are mostly mild strains of the lower leg; however, these overuse syndromes are sufficient enough to cause a reduction in motivation for the activity chosen.[22]

Both of these major deterrents can be greatly reduced by controlling the training schedules and devising realistic fitness goals. The basic fitness rule is that of setting goals that produce a fitness effect while avoiding overuse or physical threshold boundaries. The physician, as the exercise prescriptionist and authority, must assist patients in determining the fitness targets and the time schedules by which goals can be achieved. This requires a great deal of flexibility in program design and constant early monitoring of the exercise behavior. The skill and artistry the physician manifests in assisting patients in program selection, goal setting, and monitoring determines the success in changing patients' health habits. Within such a medically sound program, the physician is able to engage in preventive health medicine while protecting patients from possible excesses that frequently occur when individuals seek to institute a fitness program.

One of the many contributions that Ken Cooper has made to the fitness movement in the United States is based upon his research data. These enable the professional to prescribe methodically fitness routines that help reduce the major deterrents discussed above.[20] Using his normative data based upon sex, age, preferred activity, and time and distance goals, the physician can now systematically program a cardiovascular activity and goal for almost every interested patient.

PERSONAL SUPPORT OF THE EXERCISE ETHIC AS ROLE MODEL

In order to join the ranks of the health advocates, the physician must accept physical fitness as a personal value. This does not mean that the physician has to advocate any particular type of exercise, but it does require that he or she accept and act upon the medical evidence. While this requirement may seem the most demanding of all, the physician must recognize that his or her own physical fitness is the fundamental focus of attention in preparing to counsel others. Independent of one's status, the physician is at a serious disadvantage if he or she has neither maintained personal physical health nor shows some evidence of active participation in that which is being advocated to the patient. A physician who is 40 pounds overweight could have a negative motivational impact in attempting to counsel in the area of weight reduction. Addicted smokers and drinkers are rarely effective in changing these behaviors in others.

Here are the unfortunate realities about the medical profession. When a cross-section of physicians in southern California was given thorough medical examinations, it was found that most were in very poor condition. One out of five smoked, two out of three were overweight, one in four had high blood pressure, one in five had abnormal ECGs in a stress test, and more than half had high serum lipid levels.[3] The importance of such findings leaves those responsible for promoting exercise habits and quality health care in a challenging posture.

SUMMARY

Physicians have the power to affect their patients' mental and physical lives dramatically. Their advice can have an enormous impact on patients who are searching for direction. They can educate patients as to why regular exercise is one of the most powerful forms of preventive medicine for a healthy mind and body.

A fitness program should be carefully planned and individualized for each patient. This can be accomplished by researching the patient's interests, socialization patterns, psychological strengths and weaknesses, and environmental surroundings. Physicians can successfully alter a sedentary lifestyle only if the appropriate motivational cues are discovered.

Once the program is initiated, the physician or medical staff member can assist the patient in monitoring his or her progress. This is a crucial motivational phase. The patient must be able to observe some gain, however small, or else the desire to continue dissipates.

There is no foolproof method for trying to change an ingrained behavior pattern of inactivity. The physician may have to employ a trial and error method. The key word here is flexibility: Find what works for the patient. An exercise program that enhances one's lifestyle is more apt to be continued than is a program which disrupts a previously peaceful existence.

Empathy on the physician's part helps to allay the patient's fears about any new fitness routine that is about to be undertaken. Positive reinforcement builds confidence and self-esteem, and an awareness of the patient's avoidance techniques makes it easier to discern the proper course of action. Finally, and most important, it is essential that the counseling physician have a deep, abiding personal value in physical fitness. Physicians must become living examples of the values they seek to instill in their patients.

REFERENCES

1. Cooper K: Runner's World exclusive. Runner's World (Dec), 1979.
2. Heinzelmann AF, Bagley R: Response to physical activity programs and their effects on health behavior. Public Health Rep 10: 85, 1970.
3. National Center for Health Statistics, United States Bureau of the Census: Washington, DC, US Government Printing Office, 1980.
4. Folkins CH, Amsterdam EA: Control and modification of stress emotions through chronic exercise, in Amsterdam EA, Wilmore JH, DeMaria AN (eds): Exercise and Cardiovascular Health and Disease. New York, Yorke, 1977.
5. Folkins CH, Lynch S, Gardner MM: Psychological fitness as a function of physical fitness. Arch Phys Med Rehab 53:503–508, 1972.
6. Powell RR: Effects of exercise on mental functioning. J Sports Med Phys Fitness 15:125–131, 1975.
7. Stamford BA, Hambacher, Falica A: Effects of daily physical exercise on the psychiatric state of institutional geriatric mental patients. Res Q 45:34–41, 1974.
8. Gutin B: Effect of increase in physical fitness on mental ability following physical and mental stress. Res Q 37:211–220, 1966.
9. Weingarten G: Mental performance during physical exertion: The benefit of being physically fit. Int J Sports Psychol 4:16–26, 1973.
10. Donoghue S: The correlation between physical fitness, absenteeism and work performance. Can J Public Health 68:201–203, 1977.
11. Ismail AH, Young RJ: Effect of chronic exercise on the personality of middle-aged men by univariate and multivariate approaches. J Hum Ergol 2:47–57, 1973.
12. Ogilvie BC, Howe MA: Career crisis in sport. Paper presented to the World Congress on Sport Psychology, Ottawa, Canada, 1981.
13. Ogilvie BC: A running psychologist speaks of running. Paper presented to the American Academy of Orthopedic Surgeons, September 1980.
14. Glasser W: Positive Addiction. New York, Harper & Row, 1976.
15. President's Council on Physical Fitness and Sports: Editorial. Washington, DC, March 1980.
16. Deci E: Intrinsic Motivation. New York, Plenum Press, 1975.
17. Maslow AH: Motivation and personality, ed 2. New York, Harper & Row, 1970.
18. Stevenson CL: Socialization effects of participation in sport: A critical review of the literature. Res Q 46:287–301, 1975.
19. Teraslinn R, Pantanch T, Koskela A, Oja P: Characteristics affecting willingness of executives to participate in an activity program aimed at coronary heart disease prevention. J Sports Med 224–229, 1969.
20. Cooper K: Aerobics. New York, M Evans, 1968.
21. Layman EM: Psychological effects of physical activity, in Wilmore JH (ed): Exercise and Sports Science Reviews. New York, Academic Press, 1974.
22. Bittker T: Running gluttony. Runner's World 12:10–12, 1977.

30
Legal Aspects of Sports Medicine

Elmer J. Walker, Emidio A. Bianco, and
Peter M. Hartmann

The purpose of this chapter is to familiarize physicians with basic legal principles applicable to sports medicine. The authors intend that the readers not be intimidated by either the law or lawyers, but rather view medical negligence as a reasonable concern for society and physicians. A basic understanding of medical malpractice law should not only diminish the fear of being sued, but should also encourage physicians to practice medicine according to acceptable medical standards, which is the best defense against being sued successfully.

No physician is totally immune from being sued. When a suit is brought by a person who sustains an injury during a sports event, the plaintiff's attorney may include any person or institution that is vulnerable for money damages arising from the alleged injury. Although the attorney may name anyone connected with the injury, such action does not necessarily imply that all the defendants are to be found liable. This chapter discusses physician liability where the physician treats or evaluates an injury sustained during a sports event sponsored by an educational institution, or an injury sustained during an amateur athletic contest.

A physician attending an amateur athletic contest may be doing so in one of the following capacities:

1. As a spectator who may render gratuitous medical services in an emergency to an injured athlete

2. As a volunteer who provides medical services gratuitously to one of the institutions or teams involved in that specific athletic event
3. As a physician employed by the institution or team to provide necessary medical services during a specific athletic contest
4. As an independent contractor with the local school board or educational institution to be a team physician

Irrespective of which category is accurate, the physician may be liable. The potential for legal action arising from sports injuries is emphasized by the fact that from 1975 to 1978 over 22.5 million men and women participated in sports events and over 1 million injuries occurred.[1,2]

While it may be that a physician *implicitly contracts* with patients that he or she possesses and will exercise a reasonable degree of care, skill, and learning, malpractice is predicated upon the *failure to exercise requisite medical skill*. The duty owed by the physician to the patient to exercise ordinary care and skill is imposed by law, and arises irrespective of whether the services are rendered gratuitously or for a fee.[3]

Until recently a team physician or a Good Samaritan was almost totally immune from litigation; few court cases arose from injuries sustained in the amateur sports arena. However, there are recognizable trends indicating that the physician who evaluates or treats an amateur athlete may be named among the possible defendants in a medical malpractice suit.[2]

BREACH OF CONTRACT

Almost all malpractice cases are based in medical negligence rather than in breach of contract. Unless there are specific contract terms between the physician and the patient or legal guardian, or the physician has made specific guarantees, the court bases the suit in medical malpractice law, i.e., negligent performance by the physician. (The elements of medical negligence are discussed later in this chapter.) Specific contract terms include such things as guaranteeing a cure, promising to restore health within a definite time period, or specifying that a given prescription will unequivocally relieve the patient's symptoms.

A breach of contract requires the plaintiff to demonstrate: (1) words or conduct illustrating a promise to provide a cure or special treatment, (2) a failure to abide by the agreement's terms, and (3) damages resulting from the breach.[4,5] Breach of contract does not require showing negligent performance by the physician who renders medical services, but only proof of a failure to achieve the promised results. Any physician willing to guarantee a specific result is liable for damages where the guarantee is not fulfilled.

GOOD SAMARITAN

Every physician irrespective of the type of relationship with a patient is personally liable for any negligent performance. A doctor who becomes a Good Samaritan, or volunteers to provide professional services, must understand that altruism does not shield him or her from a lawsuit. Hoping to encourage medical and health care personnel to render aid in emergency situations, many states have passed laws commonly known as Good Samaritan Statutes.

The general rule of law in the United States is that no person is legally required to come to the aid of another person in distress unless there is a previously existing *legal* relationship, e.g., parent/child, physician/patient, or public servant (police, firefighter, or lifeguard on duty). However, once aid or rescue is attempted, the rescuer has a duty not to abandon the rescue and to use whatever reasonable means are immediately available to continue the rescue attempt.

Vermont, under certain conditions and exceptions, *requires* any person to give reasonable assistance to a person in grave physical harm. Exceptions to the rule are as follow:

1. One is not expected to give assistance that causes "danger or peril to himself."
2. The rescue attempt cannot remove the rescuer from "important duties owed to others."
3. One is not expected to render assistance where "assistance or care is being provided by others."[6]

At the time of this publication, no Vermont appellate decision has been rendered concerning the requirement to be a Good Samaritan. The exceptions make the law appear very difficult to enforce. Perhaps the intent of the law is to jog the conscience of society and to encourage reasonable attempts to rescue a person in peril. The Vermont Statute like most Good Samaritan Statutes immunizes the rescuer from ordinary negligence, but not gross negligence.

The Maryland legislature recently enacted a typical Good Samaritan Statute. A person, licensed by the State of Maryland to provide medical care, who renders medical aid, care, or assistance for which no fee or compensation is charged (1) at the scene of an emergency, (2) in transit to medical facilities, or (3) through communications with personnel rendering emergency assistance is *not* liable for any civil damages as the result of any professional act or omission by him or her not amounting to gross negligence.[7]

Unless otherwise stated, Good Samaritan Statutes do not immunize a physician from *gross* negligence; i.e., where a person sustains an injury because the physician's act or failure to act caused an injury and the physician was aware (or should have been aware) of a *clear and present danger*.

For example, a physician is aware that an injured athlete in no distress is sprawled on the playing field and has sustained a head injury, but nevertheless moves the head before understanding the mechanism of injury or before examining the athlete's head, neck, and extremities. Immediately thereafter the person becomes quadriplegic. The physician may be liable for gross negligence because every physician is aware, or should be aware, that head injury may be associated with cervical spine injury, and that movement of the cervical spine in such cases may worsen a spinal cord injury (a clear and present danger). On the other hand, assume the same patient to be in acute respiratory distress and all reasonable attempts to clear the airway by chin lift or jaw thrust fail. Cardiopulmonary resuscitation must be administered, and unfortunately quadriplegia follows *after all reasonable attempts* were made to clear the airway, including a modified head tilt. The maximum legal action possible, if any, in this desperate situation is ordinary negligence, because only the reasonable physician standard may be applied. Therefore, the physician *is not* liable because the Good Samaritan Statute immunizes the physician from ordinary negligence.

We recommend that physicians not trained or experienced in trauma refrain from acting where an injured person is not in acute distress or imminent danger of death. Where lifesaving procedures are the only course of action, then lifesaving takes precedence over inherent physical injury that may result from applying certain techniques. A plaintiff will have difficulty proving gross negligence against a physician in such cases because the dividing line between ordinary and gross negligence during a medical emergency is seldom exact, and reasonable physicians can respectably disagree as to where ordinary negligence ends and gross negligence begins during a lifesaving attempt.[8]

While medical providers are not legally required to render emergency assistance, most medical personnel feel morally obligated to help those in distress, but are reluctant to do so for fear of being sued. Good Samaritan Statutes are intended to encourage medical or health personnel to render aid to persons during a medical emergency.

MEDICAL MALPRACTICE

The *legal standard of care* (the legal test of whether or not a physician is negligent) is the requirement that a physician or surgeon possess and exercise that degree of skill and learning ordinarily possessed and exercised by physicians of good standing practicing in the community under similar circumstances. The *medical standard of care* refers to the medical propriety of certain procedures.[9,10] This standard is applicable to physicians who practice sports medicine irrespective of whether the services rendered are gratuitous or for a fee.

By undertaking (to render) professional service to a patient, a physician or surgeon represents that he or she possesses, and has as a *duty to possess,* only that degree of learning and skill ordinarily possessed by physicians and surgeons of good standing practicing in the same community under similar circumstances. It is his or her further *duty to use the care ordinarily exercised in like cases* by reputable members of the profession practicing in the same or a similar locality and under similar circumstances and *to use reasonable diligence and best judgment* in the exercise of that skill and application of that learning, in an effort to accomplish the purpose for which he or she is employed. A defendant physician must violate one of those duties before being guilty of malpractice.[11]

The key legal concept in medical malpractice liability is "negligence." A medical practitioner should know the elements of a legal cause of action for negligence. According to Prosser et al., a plaintiff patient must establish *each* and *every* one of the following elements in order to win a case of legal negligence against a defendant physician:

1. There must be *a duty,* which is an obligation recognized by law, requiring that a physician conform to a certain standard of conduct, for the protection of others against unreasonable risks.
2. There must be a *breach* of that duty, or a failure to conform to the standard required.
3. There must be a *proximate or legal cause,* i.e., a reasonably close causal connection between the physician's conduct and the resulting injury.

4. There must be *damages,* that is, actual injury, either temporary or permanent, which can be compensated in a dollar amount.[12]

A medical malpractice action has a more rigorous proof requirement than the breach of contract suit. The basis of medical malpractice is the allegation that *the physician failed to provide his (or her) services in accordance with the current level of medical knowledge and skill.*[13,14]

Medical malpractice theory is based upon three component duties that a physician owes a patient: (1) a duty to possess the *requisite knowledge and skill* such as possessed by the average member of the medical profession; (2) a duty to exercise ordinary and reasonable care in the application of such professional knowledge and skill; and (3) the duty to use his (or her) best judgment in the application of this knowledge and skill.[15,16] The physician should be aware of the prevailing sports medicine standards of practice. (Later in this chapter, the authors offer recommendations that provide the basic requirements for physicians contemplating the practice of sports medicine.)

Physicians may be called upon to perform physical examinations to certify that a person is capable of undertaking a particular role. For example:

- A student is physically able to participate in football or basketball.
- A student is physically capable of actively participating in a day-to-day physical education program.
- An employee is physically able to perform a demanding job.
- A person may participate in a community athletic program.
- A person is an acceptable insurance risk.

Such examinations must be thorough and appropriate so that the physician's recommendations are made in the best interest of the examinee, the examinee's family, and the organization requesting the examination. The physician who fails to perform an adequate physical examination may be person-ally liable even though employed by either a school district or a private firm.

Most schools appear to require physical examination of athletes, and many schools specify that physicians perform the examinations. These examinations are likely to be cursory. Although physicians unanimously agree that physical examinations should be detailed and complete, some examinees are nevertheless certified as physically capable when they are not. Under such circumstances, a plaintiff may argue that the examining physician is an agent of the school district and that if he or she is negligent, both he or she and the school district are responsible.[17]

CONSENT AND ASSUMPTION OF RISK

There is a legal maxim that *no legal damage is done to him who consents.* This maxim may create a misconception that the athlete who consents to participate in a sport assumes the risk of injury and therefore removes liability from the team physician or any physician who might have made the qualifying medical examination. Appenzeller, in his book *Sports and the Courts,*[2] makes the following observations:

> While the athlete may assume the risk of a sport, he or she is not responsible for the negligence of the physician. For example, the athlete would not be held responsible if he were examined by a doctor, and the doctor through negligence, erroneously found no medical condition making it inadvisable for him to participate in the sport.[2]

Weistart and Lowell, in *The Law of Sports,*[18] foresee athletes suing their physicians when they believe that an improper medical examination caused their injury:

> For example, if a football player died as a result of a heart attack it might be alleged that a doctor who gave the player a physical exam before the season began was negligent since death was the result of a

defect or injury that should have been discovered in the examination.[18]

While an athlete may assume the risk of injury inherent in sports events the physician remains liable for the examination. If the doctor claims to be a sports medicine specialist, he or she will be held to a higher standard and may be liable in a situation where the general medical practitioner would not be.[2]

Although an athlete does not assume the risk of injury resulting from physician negligence, he or she may be precluded from recovering money damages when he or she *is* guilty of assuming the risk. An example of *assumption of the risk* medicine is where an athlete insists on actively engaging and participating in contact sports such as football, wrestling, and boxing despite advice and warnings from the physician.

The following is taken from 57 American Jurisprudence 2d[19]:

> The cases arising out of injuries suffered by participants in games, sports, and contests which involve bodily contact or other hazards, furnish apt illustrations of the application of the principles underlying the doctrine of assumption of risk in its primary sense.* A person who voluntarily participates in a legal sport, game, or contest assumes the ordinary risks of such activity, and if he suffers injury or death as a result, there can be no recovery therefore, as against either a promoter or operator of the sport, game or contest,† or from his opponent or other participant.[20] In other words, a participant in almost any game or sport assumes all risks incidental to the particular game or sport which are obvious and foreseeable.[21]

The timeworn illustration of one willingly submitting to personal injury, whereby there can be no legal injury, is that of a prizefighter engaged in a legal bout. **Daniel v. Tower Trucking Co.,** *205 SC 333, 32 SE 2d 5.*

†*Annotation: 7 ALR 2d 704, 707 Section 3. The promoter of a "mere boxing exhibition or match" which was not an illegal prizefight, or a fight where each contestant sought an advantage by injuring the other, was not civilly liable for the death of a minor participant.* **Parmentier v. McGinnis,** *157 Wis 597, 147 NW; 007.*

EXPRESS AGREEMENT TO WAIVE LIABILITY

Promoters of certain sports events, particularly the martial arts, may require each contestant to sign a "waiver" that purports to immunize the promoting agent or the sports physician from liability. In essence, by express agreement the contestant assumes the risk of injury that may arise from substandard promotional activities or medical malpractice.

Courts may recognize agreements that exculpate a person from liability; however, certain requirements must be met by the person seeking exculpation or the exculpatory agreement will be ruled invalid. It must appear that the terms of the agreement were known and clear to the contestant; if not known, the promoter or physician must show that a reasonable contestant in the same position would have known. The expressed terms of the agreement must be applicable to the particular misconduct that gave rise to the alleged injury.[22]

The contestant must have actual knowledge of the risks to be assumed and must voluntarily incur the risks. In other words, a contestant does not assume the risk for failure of the promoter to correct dangerous defects known only to the promoter, or where the promoter fails to adhere to the building code, for example, which in turn causes a light fixture to crash on the contestant. One would not expect a reasonable athlete to voluntarily incur the risk of head injury by a crashing fixture. Generally courts do not recognize a contract that allows one party to escape the intent of protective legislation; in other words, if an act is prohibited by law, such an act cannot be the subject of a valid contract.[23] Therefore, the promoter cannot contract to avoid any duties imposed by the State Athletic Commission's Regulations or by the Building Code. Similar reasoning would apply to exculpatory agreements concerning medical malpractice, i.e., actual knowledge and voluntary acceptance of known potential medical malpractice by the physician. The physician cannot escape protective legislation such as athletic commission rules, commission on medical discipline requirements, or medical licensure laws. In the case of exculpatory agreements concerning physicians, the authors do not believe courts view such contracts favorably, particularly because of the gross disparity of knowledge between physicians and laymen and because of public policy concerns; i.e., a duly licensed physician who accepts an appointment to perform a specific task is expected to adhere to an acceptable standard of care. Courts do not favor contracts that place one party at the mercy of the other party's negligent act.[22]

RECOMMENDATIONS

Any physician contemplating the responsibility to be a "team physician" or "sports candidate examiner" should consider the following questions irrespective of whether the services to be rendered are either gratuitous or compensated:

1. Am I trained in cardiopulmonary resuscitation?

A physician lacking the basic skills of cardiopulmonary resuscitation but who nevertheless assumes the responsibility for "team physician" assumes a higher risk for liability than the physician trained in CPR. The American Medical Association, local Heart Association, the Joint Commission on Accreditation of Hospitals, and most hospital medical staffs encourage and in some cases require that physicians become trained in CPR and undergo periodic retraining. In the event that an athlete sustains a cardiopulmonary arrest in the presence of a team physician who is not trained in cardiopulmonary resuscitation, the liability is obvious because a physician lacking the skills to resuscitate an athlete breaches a standard of care. It is reasonable to expect that any physician taking on the responsibility of trauma care has the ability to perform basic life support procedures taught in readily available courses.

2. Do I know how to manage an acutely traumatized athlete with special concern for head injury and vertebral body injuries?

Any physician approaching an acutely traumatized athlete must not only know what to do, but more importantly what *not* to do in order to prevent serious debilitating injuries. The ABCs of trauma care have been specifically developed by the American College of Surgeons (Committee on Trauma) and are now available in a course on advanced trauma life support, which includes a detailed manual on how to manage a traumatized person during the first hour postinjury. Although many of the discussions in the advanced trauma life support course may not apply to athletics, the principles do apply. There is particular emphasis on head, extremity, and vertebral body trauma. The American College of Surgeons points out that the first principle in the care of any traumatized patient is *primum non nocere*— first, do no harm. Improper movement of the skull and spine may produce irreversible spinal cord trauma. Improper manipulation of an extremity may result in nerve and vascular injuries of a permanent nature (Chapters 12, 13).

The "team physician," therefore, must be skilled in basic life support and know the principles of trauma life support. If a course is not available or if the physician is unable to attend an advanced trauma life support course, the physician should at least become familiar with the principles of trauma life support. The local Fire Department has emergency medical technicians skilled in the management and movement of an acutely traumatized patient; we recommend that team physicians learn these principles. Fire Department EMT Instructors are usually quite competent and happy to accommodate physicians in this area.

3. Will my malpractice insurance extend to sports medicine?

No physician should endeavor to become a team physician without first inquiring about his or her malpractice coverage. During these days of increased liability and varying activities assumed by some physicians, one should expect that malpractice carriers place limitations on physician activities by denying coverage in specific areas. Call your insurance broker or agent. Make no assumptions concerning the scope of your insurance coverage.

4. Does the team or institution sponsoring the team have liability insurance to cover a team physician?

This question is of special importance where the physician's personal liability insurance does not cover team physician activities.

5. Has the athlete in question made available a consent form for the treatment of nonemergency injuries?

Consent forms are of extreme importance where the athlete requiring treatment has not reached the age of majority, which is usually defined by statute within any given state. In the United States, the general rule is that a minor may not consent to medical treatment in the absence of the legal guardian, which in most cases would be his or her parents. There are certain exceptions, however, to the general rule. These vary from state to state, but generally include the following situations where the minor may consent without parental or legal guardian consent:

1. The minor is a parent or married.
2. The minor is seeking treatment or advice concerning venereal disease, pregnancy, or contraception not amounting to sterilization.
3. Where the physician makes a judgment that a delay in treatment would adversely affect the life or health of the minor, the minor may consent or the physician may go ahead *without* such consent if the emergency is a life-or-death situation.
4. The minor may consent for treatment concerning drug abuse or mental illness.

The physician must distinguish between elective and emergency treatment. In an elective situation where treatment can reasonably be delayed, the physician should be certain that the consent forms had been previously obtained by the team or that a parent standing by gives oral or written per-

mission. In the event of an emergency where the athlete is unconscious or in cardiopulmonary arrest, the physician may move ahead without anyone's consent.

6. When does a sports physician become most vulnerable to negligence claim?

Vulnerability to a negligence claim increases where the team physician makes a judgment to permit an athlete to re-enter a sports event after being sidelined for an apparent injury. The physician should be able to distinguish muscle strain from ligament strain. Concussions should be sidelined and observed. Abdominal trauma must be evaluated carefully to rule out visceral injuries. A decision to permit re-entry after an apparent injury requires a medical judgment after a proper examination, and any doubt in the physician's mind should be resolved in favor of *no re-entry* irrespective of team pressures.

7. When I elect to be a Good Samaritan, how do I avoid liability?

Primum non nocere (first, do no harm)! Assess the medical problem. Learn the mechanism of injury. Start CPR where indicated and do not be concerned about injuries that may result from a properly administered lifesaving treatment: a dead patient has no opportunity to recover from injuries.

Do not attempt treatment you are not trained to administer. Remember that gross negligence is not sharply defined during a medical emergency and a plaintiff who survives death will have difficulty proving where ordinary negligence ends and gross negligence begins—particularly where the physician saved the plaintiff's life by providing an adequate airway, administering air or oxygen, or maintaining circulation.

EPILOGUE

Again, this chapter is not intended to frighten or deter physicians from assuming the responsibility of "team physician." For many physicians, particularly those who are former athletes, being a team physician may be rewarding and can be fun. There is no need to be overly concerned about liability for the care and treatment of athletes where the physician is trained in cardiopulmonary resuscitation and understands the basic principles of trauma life support. CPR requires "hands-on" skills which can be learned by taking appropriate courses. The management of a trauma patient can be learned from texts and attending 1- or 2-day seminars, or from local fire companies who have trained emergency medical technicians or instructors.

REFERENCES

1. Ryan A: The Prevention of Injuries in Sports and Physical Education, Sports Safety II. Chicago, Oct. 1976.
2. Appenzeller H: Sports and the Courts. pp. 223–240.
3. *Benson v. Mays,* 227 A.2d 220 at 223 (1967).
4. *Salem Orthopedic Surgeons v. Quinn,* 79 Mass. Adv. Sh. 661, 386 N.E. 2d 1268 (1979).
5. *Robbins v. Flintstone,* 308 N.Y. 543, 127 N.E. 2d 330 (1955).
6. Vermont Code, T.12, Sec. 519.
7. Annotated Code of Maryland, Article 43, Section 132.
8. *Am. Jur. P.O.P.,* 7:355, Proof 1.
9. *Am Jur* Physicians and Surgeons (1st ed, sections 78–90).
10. Physicians and surgeons: Standard of care and skill required of specialists. 21 ALR 3d 953.
11. 16 *Am Jur Trials:* Defense of Medical Malpractice Cases, Section 137 Standard of Care; Definition of Malpractice. p. 603.
12. Prosser WL, Wade JW, Schwartz VE: Torts, Cases and Materials, ed 6. Foundation Press, 1976.
13. *Hale v. State,* 53 A.D. 2d 1025, 386 N.Y.S. 151 (1970).
14. *Hirschberg v. State,* 91 Misc. 2d 590, 398 N.Y.S. 2d 470 (1970).
15. 53 A.D. 2d at 1025, 386 N.Y.S. 2d at 152.
16. Contractual liability of physicians, Buffalo Law Rev 28: 628–629, 1979 (ftn 16).
17. See *Beadling v. Sirotta* (1961) 71 N.J. Super 182, 176 A.2d 546. cited in 7 Am Jur Trials, Contact Sports Injury Cases, Section 2, p. 218. [Both the doctor and the employer were held responsible for the doctor's negligence.]
18. Weistart JC, Lowell CH: The Law of Sports. Indianapolis, Bobbs-Merrill Co., 1979.
19. 57 Am Jur 2d, Negligence, Sec. 285, p. 678.
20. *Gaspard v. Grain Dealers Mut Ins. Co.* (La App) 131 So. 2d 831 [injury by flying bat which slipped out of baseball player's sweaty hands]; *Rogers v. Allis-Chalmers Mfg Co.,* 153 Ohio St 513 92 NE 2d 677, 18 ALR 2d 1363 [golfer assumes ordinary risk of being hit by a golf ball while playing]. Annotation: 7 ALR 2d 704, 714, Section 7.
21. *Hawayek v. Simmons* (La App) 91 So.2d 49, 61 ALR 2d 1254.
22. Prosser WL: Law of Torts, ed 4. 1971, pp 442–445.
23. *New Jersey v. Brown* 143 N.J. Super 571, 364 A.2d 29 (1976).

Glossary

Daniel Garfinkel

With the marked growth of the field of sports medicine over the past 10 years, a new vocabulary has emerged. Therefore, physicians interested in this subject may be inundated with many new terms with which they have no previous familiarity. It is well known that medical schools are trying to teach students not to use proper names or slang terms, but as the field of sports medicine grows, so does the use of this strange vocabulary. Along with the new terms, sports medicine has also incorporated many of the long-term standards of orthopedics (indicated by an asterisk). This Glossary may clear up some of the communication problems primary care physicians may have to face.

Athlete's foot*: Tinea pedis (ringworm of the foot); produces itching, fissure formation, and inflammation.

Athlete's neurosis: Usually in men, with three components: (1) excessive and exclusive preoccupation with physical fitness; (2) sudden breakdown around age 40, when physical powers are beginning to wane; (3) breakdown almost immediately following some threat to physical well-being.

Athletic sickness: Weakness, nausea, lightheadedness; appears sometimes after vigorous exercise.

Back-pack palsy: Unexpected weakness, numbness, and wasting of arm and shoulder girdle, previously seen in military personnel but now seen in civilians. Due to compression by backpack straps of brachial plexus or peripheral nerve supply.

Baker's cyst*: Bursitis of the semimembranous and the medial gastrocnemius bursa, presenting as a large soft tumor mass in the poelteal space.

Barked shin: Contusion of shin.

Barton's fracture*: Marginal fracture of distal radius with volar or dorsal fragment plus subluxation of carpus.

Baseball finger: Avulsion of the extensor tendon from its attachment to the dorsal surface of the base of the terminal phalanx.

Bennet fracture*: Fracture dislocation of carpal metacarpal of thumb with fracture of some portion of the medial proximal margin of the base of the metacarpal.

Biker's knee: Occurs when saddle too high, causing excessive leg extension on the patella by the infrapatellar tendon, just before contraction of the quadriceps muscle group.

Black eye: Periorbital hematoma.

Black heel: Calcaneal petechiae secondary to repeated microtrauma, as in sudden stops and starts in the racket sports.

Blocker's exostosis: *see* Blocker's node.

Blocker's node: Myositis ossificans located in the middle third of the arm just over the deltoid insertion attachment on the lateral aspect of the humerus. Secondary to blocker throwing arm up to check impetus of opposing player.

Blowout fracture: Traumatic injury to the orbit of the eye, manifesting limited eye motion or double vision.

*Standard orthopedic term.

335

Bonking: Seen in endurance athletes when they run out of liver glycogen. The blood sugar drops, the patient gets dizzy, shaky, confused, cold sweats, and experiences lack of coordination.

Boot-top fracture: Comminuted fracture of tibia and fibula secondary to high-speed forward fall, angling leg over high rigid ski boot.

Bowler's thumb: Digital neuroma of distal interphalangeal joint (DIP) associated sometimes with osteoarthritis.

Boxer's fracture*: Fracture of the neck of the fourth and fifth metacarpal.

Boxer's knuckle: Traumatic bursa, chronically inflamed, over the metacarpal.

Buddy system: Alignment of a sprained finger to adjacent finger in order to immobilize it. (Also, pairing off of partners for safety, as in swimming.)

Burner: *see* Stinger.

Cauliflower ear: Hemorrhage between the perichrondrium and cartilage of the ear.

Charley horse: Contusion of elements of the quadricep muscles.

Clicking hip*: *see* Snapping hip.

Clothesline injury: Direct blow to the larynx with pain and difficulty in swallowing and inspiration. There may be acute laryngospasm.

Clutched thumb*: *see* Trigger finger.

Coaches' finger: Dislocation of the proximal interphalangeal (PIP) joint of the fingers—usually middle phalanx dislocated dorsal to the proximal phalanx. Generally result of hyperextension.

Colles' fracture*: Impaction of distal fragment of radius into proximal fragment dorsal with radial shortening and loss of volar angulation.

Crabs: Pediculosis pubis.

Crazy bone: Contusion of ulnar nerve in the ulna groove.

Cyclist's palsy: *see* Handle bar neuropathy.

Ding: also known as "Getting your bell rung"—a first-degree head concussion. There is no loss of

consciousness but the athlete may be slightly confused and have dizziness and ringing in the ears.

Foot drop*: Contusion of the peroneal nerve by direct blow. If significant swelling or hemorrhage, can cause loss of motor function.

Footballer's (English) ankle: Tenderness over the talar bone of the ankle and small osteophytes seen on x ray.

Frozen shoulder*: Adhesive capsulitis secondary to generalized inflammation within the glenohumeral joint. Causes pain and loss of motion.

Gamekeeper's thumb*: Rupture or chronic laxity of the ulnar collateral ligament of the first metacarpal–phalangeal joint.

Golfer's elbow: Inflammation of the flexor pronator group of muscles at their origin in the medial epicondyle or the humerus.

Golden period: First 20 minutes after an injury, when it is easy to identify an injury before swelling sets in.

Groin pull: Strain of hip flexors, adductors in the upper thigh.

Hammer toe*: Combination of contraction of flexors and extensor tendons so that one or more joints is in flexion and another is in extension.

Hamstring pull/tear: Usually appears in overdeveloped athletes, can be acute or gradual onset. Pain appears in the lateral or medial posterior thigh, usually a tear of the biceps femoris.

Handle bar neuropathy: Overuse syndrome associated with bicycling, manifested by an ulna neuropathy, appearing as weakness and loss of coordination in one or both hands after several days of bicycling.

Head case: *see* Space cadet.

Heat cramps: Painful spasms of muscles, usually those used most. Thought to be caused by falling serum sodium level.

Heat exhaustion: Weakness, sweating, or dizziness without a temperature rise; may be associated with dehydration and tachycardia.

*Standard orthopedic term.

Heat fatigue: Inefficient muscle function.

Heat stroke: When the internal or external heat load exceeds the body's cooling ability so much that the body temperature actually rises drastically and temperature control is lost.

Heel spur*: Plantar fasciitis. Inflammation reaction at insertion of the plantar fascia into the calcaneus.

Herpes gladiatorium: Herpes simplex infection; occurs in wrestlers.

Hip pointer: A contusion of the bone of the iliac crest.

Hitting the wall: Usually seen in hot weather among runners when their muscles run out of glycogen and they get severe muscle pain.

Hooker's elbow: Lateral epicondylitis secondary to ice fishing "hooking"—repeated jerking on a fishing line attached to a wooden stick.

Hot spots: Trigger points.

Hurdler's injury: Avulsion of ischial tuberosity at the attachment of the long end of the biceps and the semitendonosis, due to forcible flexion of hip with knee extended.

Jammed finger*: Variety of conditions, usually collateral ligament and volar plate injury. Could be an articular fracture or dislocation.

Jersey finger: Rupture of the flexor profundus, usually of the second or third finger.

Jock itch: Tinea cruris (ringworm of groin); may also be caused by monillia.

Jogger's foot: Trauma to the medial plantar nerve producing entrapment and inflammation, manifesting as burning heel pain.

Jogger's itch: *see* Judo itch.

Jogger's penis: *see* Penile frostbite.

Joint mice*: Usually visualized loose bodies, small and opaque, unattached to bone, and interspersed between joint surfaces.

Judo itch: Intense itching around ankles and wrists working up extremities to hips and shoulders. Appears after judo workouts and sweating.

Jumper's knee: Inflammation of the patellae tendon at its attachment to the inferior pole of the patella.

*Standard orthopedic term.

Little League elbow: Traction problem of the attachment of the flexor muscle mass over the medial epicondyle at the elbow, secondary to excessive throwing. X ray may show widening of epiphyseal plate.

Little League shoulder: Undisplaced fracture of the proximal humeral epiphysis with widening of the proximal humeral epiphyseal line.

Locked knee: *see* Trick knee.

Maisonneuve fracture*: Presents with tenderness on the medial side of the ankle joint. A fracture of the proximal fibula with sprain of the medial ligaments.

Malicious malalignment syndrome: Combines the elements of a broad pelvis, femoral anteversion, valgus knee, external rotation of the tibia, and pronation—a combination of minor imperfections that may cause sharp knee pain, such as condromalacia.

Mallet finger: *see* Baseball finger.

March fracture*: Fatigue fracture of the metatarsal shaft.

Medial epicondylitis: *see* Golfer's elbow.

Morton's foot*: Second metatarsal longer than the first, which causes weight and distribution problems and pain.

Morton's neuroma*: Interdigital mechanical neuritis that eventually leads to a fibrous reaction producing a neuroma usually into the third and fourth toes.

Musher's knee*: Iliotibial band irritation causing lateral knee pain while "mushing" dog team secondary to sharp backward kicking of the leg.

Overuse syndrome: Pain of an insidious onset, related to specific athletic activities, which disappears when one stops the activity. May lead to significant medical problems.

Pac-Man wrist: *see* Space Invaders wrist.

Penile frostbite: Burning sensation on penile tip, progressing to early frostbite, with tenderness and anesthesia. Secondary to tissue response at high velocity at below-freezing temperature through polyester fabric.

Pitcher's elbow: Repeated unrecognized injury to the medial aspect of the elbow causing loose bodies and osteophytes especially on inner aspect of the trochlea and in the medial ligament.

Positive addiction: Seen in regular exercisers who are mostly addicted to same and derive beneficial results.

Pudendal neuritis: Bilateral compression of dorsal branches of pudendal nerves between bicycle seat and pubic symphysis; may cause impaired sexual response.

Pump bump: Tender red nodule (bursa) lateral to calcaneal attachment of Achilles tendons.

Punch drunk: Permanent sequella secondary to multiple concussive blows to the head, with changes in the pyramidal, extrapyramidal, and cerebellar pathways. Results in slurred speech, dull facies, slowness of mentality, and tremor.

Reverse Colle's: *see* Smith fracture.

Rider's strain: Strain of adductor longus muscle of the thigh seen in horseback riders.

Runner's ache: Stitch or catch in the side, thought to be from stretching of the large intestine by a gas pocket.

Runner's fracture: Stress fracture of the lower end of the fibula.

Runner's knee: Usually refers to chrondromalacia patella, now called patella femoral dysfunction. However, used in conjunction with other ill-defined knee problems.

Runner's toe: *see* Tennis toe.

Second wind: Subjective feeling of getting breath. No definite physiological explanation—may be due to slipping back under anaerobic threshold.

Shin splints*: Pain along the anterior medial or lateral surface of the tibia. Thought to be periostitis of the attachment of the anterior tibia or posterior tibial muscles along the border of the tibia.

Ski fracture: Fracture of lateral malleolus.

---

*Standard orthopedic term.

Smith fracture*: Fracture of distal radius with increase in volar angulation, possibly associated fracture of the ulnar styloid.

Snapping hip: Due to a chronic bursitis with thickening of bursal walls and spasm of the tensor fascia lata so that on each step, as the tensor slides back and forth over the trochanter, an audible pop and snap occurs.

Snapping neck*: Snapping or popping neck, audible, or palpable. May be due to either irregularity at articulation or forced snapping of a tendon over bony prominences.

Snapping shoulder*: Subluxation of the biceps tendon produced when covering of the bicipital groove is torn.

Solar plexus: Blow to coeliac ganglia (the great sympathetic plexus and principal ganglia, so-called because of radiating fibers).

Space cadet: Athlete with persistent somatic complaints for which no physiologic cause can be found.

Space Invaders wrist: Probably minor ligamentous strain of the wrist secondary to repeated movement of wrist, secondary to playing the popular video game.

Sports anemia: Mild anemia occasionally seen in athletes. Thought to be due to subclinical hemolysis of red blood cells circulating through feet.

Stinger: Stretch or impingement of C5-6 of the brachial plexus.

Stone bruise: Bone bruise, traumatic periostitis.

Strawberry: Severe abrasion of skin usually with weeping secondary to sliding or rubbing on a floor.

Student elbow: Synonomous with olecranon bursitis.

Swimmer's ear: Acute otitis externa.

Swimmer's shoulder: Impingement of a swollen tendon of the rotator cuff under the coracoacromial ligament and the acromion (the coracoacromial arch).

Tennis elbow: Lateral epicondylitis with tenderness in same area, at the site of the attachment of the common extensor tendon and lateral collateral ligaments. May also be a radial humeral bursitis, or annular ligament sprain.

Tennis leg: Probably a tear of the plantaris muscle or possibly partial tear of gastrocnemius or soleus muscle. Usually appears as a snap or pop in the posterior calf region.

Tennis thumb: Tendonitis with calcification in the flexor pollicis longus secondary to repeated friction.

Tennis toe: Subungual hematoma produced by pressure; usually of the second toe, but also the first and third.

Tennis wrist: Occurs when butt of racquet hits the palm of the hand, causing fracture of the hamate bone. Patients may present with evidence of neuritis, tendonitis, and pain on top of hand.

Trick knee*: Due to cartilage injury, medial or lateral, that pops, clicks, or locks.

Trigger finger: Thickening of fibrous sheath over flexor tendon at metacarpal–phalangeal joint which narrows canal beneath them; underlying segments of tendon enlarge as nodule. Passage of nodule through restricting canal produces a snap.

Turf toe: Traumatic lesion of first metatarsal–phalangeal joint secondary to hyperextension caused by traction between toe and playing surface.

Unhappy triad: Tears of the anterior cruciate, medial collateral ligaments, and medial meniscus simultaneously when athlete is hit from the side.

Urban cowboy rhabdomyolysis: Myoglobinuria. Cramps and tenderness in muscle, may be accompanied by a reddish urine secondary to myoglobin urea. All secondary to strenuous activity—in this particular case, riding a mechanical bull—but also seen with prolonged exertion and in karate and marathoners.

---

*Standard orthopedic term.

Water skiing douche: During a fall, water under high pressure may enter a body orifice, resulting at times in significant trauma, e.g., to the large bowel, rectum (water skiing enema), tympanic membrane.

Water wart: Molluscum contagiosum.

BIBIOGRAPHY

Apple C: Medicine for Sports. Yearbook Medical Publishers, 1979.

Brady D, Kineche S: A study of 4000 running injuries. Running Times (54):22–29, 1981.

Burke K: Ulnar neuropathy in bicyclists. Phys Sports Med, 9(4):52–56.

Corkill G: Backpack palsy. West J Med 132(6):569–572, 1980.

Darl W, Matthews K: "Mushers" knee and "hookers" elbow in the athlete. N Engl J Med 304(12):737, 1981.

Galton L: Your Child in Sports. Frane-Watts Publishers.

Garnch J: Sports medicine—Symposia on common orthopedic problems. Pediatr Clin N Am 24 (November):11–77.

Glick I: Tennis wrist. Tennis Week. (Jan.) 1980.

Hershkowitz M: Penile frostbite—An unforeseen hazard of jogging. N Engl J Med:296, 1977.

Howland WP: Practical management of upper extremity dislocations. Consultant (February), 183–193, 1981.

Kizer KW: Medical hazards of the water skiing douche. Ann Emerg Med 9:268–269, 1980.

McCowan TC: Space Invaders wrist. N Engl J Med 304 (22):1368, 1981.

Mirkin H: The Sports Medicine Book. Boston, Little, Brown, 1978.

Nirschi G: Sports Favoring Arthritic Changes. Upjohn Co brochure, 1980.

O'Donoghue: Treatment of Injuries to Athletes, ed 3. Philadelphia, WB Saunders, 1976.

Powers RD: Urban-Cowboy rhabdomyolysis. N Engl J Med:304–427, 1981.

Rask MP: Medical plantar neuropraxia—Report of three cases. Clin Orthop (July/Aug.):134–193, 1978.

Romanurti T: Orthopedics in Primary Care. Baltimore, Williams & Wilkins, 1979.

Sullivan SN: Judo–jogger's itch. N Engl J Med:300–866, 1979.

Index